Monographs of the Physiological Society No. 39

Atrial receptors

ATRIAL RECEPTORS

R. J. LINDEN
and
C. T. KAPPAGODA
*Department of Cardiovascular Studies,
University of Leeds*

CAMBRIDGE UNIVERSITY PRESS
Cambridge
London · New York · New Rochelle
Melbourne · Sydney

Published by the Press Syndicate of the University of Cambridge
The Pitt Building, Trumpington Street, Cambridge CB2 1RP
32 East 57th Street, New York, NY 10022, USA
296 Beaconsfield Parade, Middle Park, Melbourne 3206, Australia.

© Cambridge University Press 1982

First published 1982

Printed in Great Britain at the University Press, Cambridge

Library of Congress catalogue card number: 81 10209

British Library cataloguing in publication data
Linden, R. J.
Atrial receptors. – (Monographs of the Physiological Society; no. 39)
1. Cardiovascular system
I. Title II. Kappagoda, C. T.
III. Series
611'.12 QM178
ISBN 0 521 24188 X

Monographs of the Physiological Society

Members of Editorial Board: *M. de B. Daly, (Chairman); R. A. Gregory, C. R. House, P. B. C. Matthews, S. Thomas*

PUBLISHED BY EDWARD ARNOLD

1. *H. Barcroft and H. J. C. Swan* Sympathetic Control of Human Blood Vessels, 1953*
2. *A. C. Burton and O. G. Edholm* Man in a Cold Environment, 1955*
3. *G. W. Harris* Neural Control of the Pituitary Gland, 1955*
4. *A. H. James* Physiology of Gastric Digestion, 1957*
5. *B. Delisle Burns* The Mammalian Cerebral Cortex, 1958*
6. *G. S. Brindley* Physiology of the Retina and Visual Pathway, 1960 (2nd edition, 1970)
7. *D. A. McDonald* Blood Flow in Arteries, 1960*
8. *A. S. V. Burgen and N. G. Emmelin* Physiology of the Salivary Glands, 1961
9. *Audrey U. Smith* Biological Effects of Freezing and Supercooling, 1961*
10. *W. J. O'Connor* Renal Function, 1962*
11. *R. A. Gregory* Secretory Mechanisms of the Gastro-Intestinal Tract, 1962*
12. *C. A. Keele and Desiree Armstrong* Substances Producing Pain and Itch, 1964*
13. *R. Whittam* Transport and Diffusion in Red Blood Cells, 1964
14. *J. Grayson and D. Mendel* Physiology of the Splanchnic Circulation, 1965*
15. *B. T. Donovan and J. J. van der Werff ten Bosch* Physiology of Puberty, 1965
16. *I. de Burgh Daly and Catherine Hebb* Pulmonary and Bronchial Vascular Systems, 1966*
17. *I. C. Whitfield* The Auditory Pathway, 1967*
18. *L. E. Mount* The Climatic Physiology of the Pig, 1968*
19. *J. I. Hubbard, R. Llinás and D. Quastel* Electrophysiological Analysis of Synaptic Transmission, 1969*
20. *S. E. Dicker* Mechanisms of Urine Concentration and Dilution in Mammals, 1970
21. *G. Kahlson and Elsa Rosengren* Biogenesis and Physiology of Histamine, 1971*
22. *A. T. Cowie and J. S. Tindal* The Physiology of Lactation, 1971*
23. *Peter B. C. Matthews* Mammalian Muscle Receptors and their Central Actions, 1972
24. *C. R. House* Water Transport in Cells and Tissues, 1974
25. *P. P. Newman* Visceral Afferent Functions of the Nervous System, 1974

v

PUBLISHED BY CAMBRIDGE UNIVERSITY PRESS

28 *M. J. Purves* The Physiology of the Cerebral Circulation, 1972
29 *D. McK. Kerslake* The Stress of Hot Environments, 1972
30 *M. R. Bennett* Autonomic Neuromuscular Transmission, 1972
31 *A. G. Macdonald* Physiological Aspects of Deep Sea Biology, 1975
32 *M. Peaker and J. L. Linzell* Salt Glands in Birds and Reptiles, 1975
33 *J. A. Barrowman* Physiology of the Gastro-intestinal Lymphatic System, 1978
35 *J. T. Fitzsimons* The Physiology of Thirst and Sodium Appetite, 1979
39 *R. J. Linden and C. T. Kappagoda* Atrial Receptors, 1982

PUBLISHED BY ACADEMIC PRESS

34 *C. G. Phillips and R. Porter* Corticospinal Neurones, Their Role in Movements, 1977
36 *O. H. Petersen* The Electrophysiology of Gland Cells, 1980
37 *W. R. Keatings and M. Clare Harman* Local Mechanisms Controlling Blood Vessels, 1980
38 *H. Hensel* Thermoreception and Temperature Regulation, 1981

Volumes marked with an asterisk are now out of print.

CONTENTS

		page
	Preface	xiii
1	**Introduction to the reflex responses from the atria**	1
	The consideration of a reflex	1
	Receptor	1
	Afferent nerve	2
	Efferent limbs of a reflex	3
	Effector organ	3
	Central nervous connections	3
	The reflexes from atrial receptors	4
2	**Histology of sensory nerve endings in the heart**	6
	Light microscopy	7
	General review	7
	Some particular investigations	9
	Complex unencapsulated endings	13
	End-net	21
	Electron microscopy	23
	Conclusion	29
3	**Electrophysiology of atrial receptors**	31
	Receptors which discharge into myelinated fibres in the vagi	31
	Histological studies	36
	Conduction velocities	37
	Isolated tissues	37
	Spontaneous patterns of discharge	38
	Invoked changes in pattern of discharge	41
	Natural stimulus to atrial receptors	44
	Type B receptors	45
	Type A receptors	48
	An alternative hypothesis	50
	Conclusions	56

Contents

		page
	Receptors which discharge into non-myelinated fibres in the vagi	57
	Spontaneous discharge	57
	Natural stimulus	63
	Receptors which discharge into the sympathetic nerves (so-called 'sympathetic afferents')	65

4 Method of establishing reflexes from atrial receptors — 74

The stimulus – the manner of its application — 74
Left atrial receptors, small balloons — 76
Right atrial receptors, balloon and bypass — 77
Left atrial pouch — 79
Monitoring atrial pressure — 80
The stimulus – its nature — 81
  Attempts to grade the stimulus — 82
  Electrophysiology — 83
Specificity of the stimulus — 90
Reflex pathway — 91
  Afferent pathway — 92
  Efferent pathway — 93
Care of experimental animals — 94
Anaesthesia — 95
  Blood gases and the acid–base state — 97

5 Reflex effects on the heart, I: review of previous work — 101

Infusion experiments — 102
  Vagal pathways — 105
  Non-vagal pathways — 108
  Haemorrhage — 109
  Direct action on the sinu-atrial node — 110
  Conclusions — 111
Perfusion experiments — 112
Discrete distension of parts of the heart — 117
  Right atrium — 117
  Left atrium — 120
Stimulation by methods not involving distension — 124

6 Reflex effects on the heart, II: discrete stimulation of atrial receptors — 128

Evidence for an increase in heart rate — 128
Afferent pathway of reflex — 137
  Vagal section or cooling — 138

		page
	Electrophysiological evidence	139
	Grading the stimulus	141
	Differential cooling of the vagi	144
	Non-vagal pathway	155
	Efferent pathway of the reflex	156
	Blockade of sympathetic nerves	156
	Electrophysiological evidence	158
	The vagal efferent component	161
	No bradycardia	167
	No positive inotropic response	171
	Summary	171

7 Atrial receptors: the systemic and pulmonary circulations — 173

Receptors within the chest — 173
Cardiac receptors — 174
'Cardiopulmonary' receptors — 176
Pulmonary artery receptors — 177
Aortic baroreceptors and chemoreceptors — 178
Receptors in the lungs — 179
Summary — 180
Atrial receptors and the systemic circulation — 180
Atrial receptors discharging into myelinated vagal fibres — 180
 Left atrial receptors — 180
 Right atrial receptors — 183
Receptors discharging into non-myelinated vagal fibres — 187
 Discrete stimulation of atrial receptors — 192
Afferent fibres in sympathetic rami — 195
Summary — 200
Atrial receptors and the pulmonary circulation — 200

8 Central connections of atrial receptors — 203

General background — 203
Spontaneous activity in the brain stem — 205
Supramedullary influences — 207
Termination of afferent fibres from atrial receptors — 208
Convergence of afferent fibres — 212
'Interaction' of reflex effects in man — 217
Summary — 217

9 Various interventions and the kidney — 219

Changes in urine flow — 219

Contents

	page
Negative pressure breathing	220
Nature of the responses	223
Altered gravitational forces: centrifugation	225
Immersion	227
Changes in the cardiovascular system	227
Changes in the concentration of ADH	229
Alterations of vascular and extracellular fluid volume	230
Infusion experiments	231
Dialysis experiments	234
Injection of drugs	234
Atrial receptors and renal blood flow	235
Atrial receptors and the renin–angiotensin system	240
Effect of cooling the vagi	241
Effect of changing volumes of various parts of the circulation	243
Atrial receptors and steroid hormones	245
Atrial receptors and prostaglandins	249
Conclusion	249

10 Atrial receptors and urine flow — 251

	page
Distension of the left atrium: obstruction of mitral orifice	251
Time course of response	255
Nature of the response	257
Effect on the cardiovascular system	261
Evidence for the reflex nature of the diuresis	261
Conclusion	261
Distension of the right atrium: obstruction to flow	262
Distension of localised regions of the atria: no obstruction to flow	263
Stimulation of left atrial receptors using small balloons	263
Features of the increase in urine flow	267
Stimulation of right atrial receptors using small balloons	268
Reflex nature of the responses	268
The afferent path	268
The efferent path	273
The blood-borne agent: is it ADH?	274
An alternative hypothesis	285
Efferent renal nerves: background	287
Atrial receptors and efferent renal nerves	291

Contents

		page
	'*Sympathetic*' *afferent fibres and renal nerves*	297
	Conclusion	301
	Atrial receptors, renal nerves and the urine response	301
	Conclusions	307
	Note on 'volume receptors'	307
11	**Atrial receptors in disease**	**310**
	Atrial receptors in heart failure	312
	Atrial receptors and cardiac arrhythmias	317
	Tachycardia and diuresis in animal models	317
	Effect of arrhythmias on the discharge from atrial receptors	319
	Atrial receptors and renal circulation in 'shock'	320
	References	**323**
	Index	**358**

PREFACE

The interest in cardiovascular reflexes took an immense leap forward with the publication of the monograph *Reflexogenic Areas of the Cardiovascular System* by Heymans & Neil in 1958. The main topics of that monograph rightly concerned the functions of systemic arterial baroreceptors and chemoreceptors. Any reflexes thought to be emanating from the heart, such as the Bainbridge reflex, were confined under a heading 'Cardiovascular Reflexes of Uncertain Origin'; and others, complex in nature, were said to be evoked by the injection of large quantities of drugs.

However, as pointed out, it had been known since the turn of the century that nervous end-organs, the histological description of which led the investigators to believe they were physiological receptors, had been discovered in most tissues in the heart. Thus interest in the function of cardiac receptors was re-awakened. Following this review and the experiments in which various drugs were injected into vessels near or in the heart in attempts to stimulate receptors, numerous investigators examined the functions of cardiac receptors with varying degrees of success. Obviously a suitable division of approach was to examine, separately if possible, the functions of receptors in the ventricles and the atria. Brief comment is made in this monograph on the functions of ventricular receptors as they have been investigated extensively physiologically, though not histologically, and the information is necessary background for a consideration of the function of atrial receptors. However, the main topic of this monograph, atrial receptors, has only recently become of interest but, as shown in Chapter 2, they were well described histologically many years ago. Much of their function, as described in Chapters 6 and 10, has been shown by discrete stimulation of the receptors, but some, for the present, must be

Preface

a matter of conjecture and extrapolation based on the known functions of ventricular receptors as described in Chapter 7. However, a story of reflex mechanisms involving atrial receptors, heart rate and urine flow is unfolding and is presented in this monograph.

As the results of experiments in whole animal preparations depend so much on the 'state' of the anaesthetised preparation some space has been allocated (particularly in Chapter 4, but throughout) to brief descriptions of laboratory practice, usually based on evidence, but often on experience alone. Without this comment it would not be possible for the reader to make adequate judgements on the posed explanations of differences, sometimes qualitatively diametrically opposite, between the results obtained by different investigators.

Following the first chapter which simply indicates some of the means available to obtain evidence of the existence of reflexes from atrial receptors and also, in anticipation, states the main conclusions as to their function, the chapters sequentially present a view of atrial receptors from different aspects, each chapter building on the previous one. In order are presented comments on histology, electrophysiology, reflex effects on heart, circulation and kidney and finally speculation on possible clinical implications. Sufficient repetition and cross references have been provided to allow each chapter to have its own entity.

I am grateful for helpful discussion before, during and after experiments, to all my colleagues in the Department of Cardiovascular Studies, and particularly to Dr Kappagoda who not only was a close colleague during many of the investigations, but as co-author of this monograph also helped with the early drafts of some chapters of this monograph which was conceived during Dr Kappagoda's stay in Leeds and completed after his departure for Canada. It is with great pleasure I place on record my thanks to Drs Hainsworth, Kidd and Mary, each of whom helped during the later stages of the preparation of this monograph. I am also indebted to the many authors and publishers who allowed reproduction of material and to the secretarial help who patiently reproduced copy after copy of the manuscript, without complaint.

Leeds   R.J.L.

1 INTRODUCTION TO THE REFLEX RESPONSES FROM THE ATRIA

The main object of this monograph is to consider the evidence for and against the presence of different types of nervous end-organs, receptors, in the atria and, as will appear, to attribute reflex function to them. A first consideration must be what a reflex is and the criteria, anatomical and experimental, which warrant the conclusion that effective reflexes exist.

The consideration of a reflex

In physiological terms, the word *reflex* has a specific meaning. It involves the application of an adequate stimulus to a receptor, the activation of which results in the transmission of impulses in afferent nerves into the central nervous system (CNS). This 'information' is then 'processed' in the CNS with the subsequent transmission of impulses in efferent nerves to an effector organ resulting in the response. Thus the anatomical basis for a reflex is a reflex arc. In designing experiments to investigate reflex mechanisms, particular attention has to be paid to the component parts of the reflex arc.

Receptor

The receptor in any reflex arc is physiologically attached to an afferent nerve and it is specifically stimulated to discharge by some change in its environment. Thus its function is to lower the threshold of that fibre to one form of energy. No attempts have yet been made to study the precise mechanisms responsible for the initiation of the impulse at the endings in the atrial endocardium, a point emphasised by Paintal (1972) who, in his comments on this process in atrial receptors, extrapolated from investigations of the Pacinian corpuscle. However, it is important

Introduction to reflex responses

to realise that the fibro-elastic tissues in which the receptors lie probably determine the main individual characteristics of the 'receptor area'. The receptor is usually recognised histologically, e.g. the unencapsulated endings in the atrial sub-endocardial tissue (see Chapter 2), but often may be unknown histologically and be recognised physiologically by its discharge characteristics in terms of the pattern of trains of impulses in its afferent nerve, e.g. see the evidence for a second and third group of receptors in the atrial wall which are known to discharge into the vagal and sympathetic nerves (see Chapter 3).

Other characteristics of a receptor involve a description of the adequate stimulus to it which evokes the response. Such a description may be in simple terms usually used in physiological texts when describing reflex functions or it could be in engineering terms involved in control theory (e.g. Milhorn, 1966; Guyton, Coleman & Granger, 1972). The former would involve the relationship of numbers, frequency and patterns of impulses to pressure, stretch and chemical stimuli, whilst the latter would demand these relationships be computed as transfer functions. However, as the atrial receptors and their function have not yet been investigated from the standpoint of control theory there will be no further consideration of this topic in this monograph.

Afferent nerve

The afferent nerve fibres involved in the reflexes from the atria may be large or small, myelinated or non-myelinated and are usually recognised by their conduction velocities, which characterise one group of myelinated fibres in the vagi (conduction velocities 9–35 $m \cdot s^{-1}$) as emanating from unencapsulated endings in the sub-endocardial tissue. Of the other two groups, both without known histological end-organs, one discharges into non-myelinated fibres (conduction velocities $< 2\ m \cdot s^{-1}$) in the vagi, and the other into both myelinated (conduction velocities 5–25 $m \cdot s^{-1}$) and non-myelinated fibres (conduction velocities $< 2\ m \cdot s^{-1}$) which pass into the spinal cord through the rami communicantes, the so-called 'sympathetic' afferent fibres. These three groups of fibres and some of the functions

The consideration of a reflex

attributed to them will be referred to again in subsequent chapters – particularly Chapters 3, 6, 7 and 10.

Techniques, dependent on the above properties, of cooling (e.g. Kappagoda, Linden & Sivananthan, 1979) and anodal block (e.g. Coleridge, Coleridge, Rosenthal & Dangel, 1973) are also used for the recognition of specific afferent fibres involved in particular reflex responses and the value of these techniques will also be discussed in Chapters 4, 6, 7 and 10.

Efferent limbs of a reflex

Where the efferent limb of the reflex is in peripheral nerves, the efferent fibres are recognised by techniques similar to those by which afferent fibres are observed. In addition, there is a possibility of obtaining the response and blocking the effect on the effector organ. For instance, when the response of the reflex is a change in heart rate caused by a change in the activity in the efferent sympathetic nerves, then as well as being able to section the nerves to abolish the response after first demonstrating its presence, it is always possible to use a β-adrenoreceptor antagonist to block the effect of the liberated noradrenaline at the receptor sites on the effector organ. This technique and other similar ones will be described in Chapters 4, 6 and 7.

Effector organ

In general this is the most obvious functional part of any reflex as changes in it are observed when measuring the response. For instance changes in the heart rate are easy to observe on a record of systemic arterial blood pressure or electrocardiogram and heart rate can be shown to change on applying the stimulus; such a response in the heart to stimulation of atrial receptors, and other responses in the kidney, will be described in Chapters 6 and 10.

Central nervous connections

This portion of a reflex arc is the hardest to define and research in this area usually awaits a fairly complete description of the

Introduction to reflex responses

parts of the reflex arc enumerated above. Little is known of the central connections of the reflexes attributable to atrial receptors because research in this area is only just beginning, but the evidence available will be described and criticised in Chapters 8 and 10.

The reflexes from atrial receptors

The evidence from some of the results of investigations into the function of atrial receptors has been anticipated in that it has been stated above that there are three distinct groups of receptors.

To anticipate further the contents of this monograph evidence will be provided to substantiate the above grouping of receptors and to support the following functions.

Much the most investigated of the groups of receptors are the unencapsulated end-organs within the sub-endocardial tissues which discharge into myelinated fibres in the vagi. Stimulation of these receptors results in a reflex increase in heart rate, with afferent fibres solely in myelinated fibres in the vagi, central connections in the medulla, an efferent pathway solely in sympathetic nerves to the heart and there is no concomitant positive inotropic effect. In addition, they cause a reflex increase in urine flow with a small increase in sodium excretion; the efferent limb of this reflex is both nervous and hormonal. The hormonal limb consists of a substance which is not the antidiuretic hormone (ADH), and is possibly a diuretic substance; the possibility that there may be a small change in the concentration of ADH in the plasma is not yet completely decided. The blood-borne agent causes only an excretion of water and not sodium. The inhibition of the activity in efferent renal nerves caused by stimulating atrial receptors results in a small increase in water excretion and is the main cause of the increase in sodium excretion. Some increase in water and sodium excretion may be caused by haemodynamic changes secondary to the increase in heart rate. Evidence for these conclusions will be presented and discussed in Chapters 3, 4, 6 and 10.

There is much less evidence for the function of the other two groups of atrial receptors mainly because they have only recently

Reflexes from atrial receptors

been recognised and because of the difficulty of studying them by discrete stimulation. There is a little evidence to show that stimulating atrial receptors discharging into non-myelinated fibres in the vagi causes a transient hypotension (and possibly bradycardia); but mostly, as with the receptors in the atria discharging into 'sympathetic' afferent fibres, their function is only to be derived by analogy from the function of similar ventricular and other cardiovascular receptors, which have been investigated in depth. The evidence appertaining to these areas of investigation is presented in Chapters 3, 4 and 7.

It is hoped the reader will keep these anticipatory conclusions in mind whilst weighing the evidence for and against them presented and referred to in the subsequent chapters.

2   HISTOLOGY OF SENSORY NERVE ENDINGS IN THE HEART

Surprisingly, relatively little is known of the exact termination of afferent and efferent nerve fibres within the heart. Of receptors attached to the two groups of afferent fibres, myelinated and non-myelinated, which course in the vagi and sympathetic rami, only receptor endings in the atrial endocardium discharging into myelinated fibres in the vagi have been described in any detail. Though, electrophysiologically (see Chapter 3), 'sympathetic' afferent nerve fibres, both myelinated and non-myelinated, have been shown to emanate from receptors in the heart, no histological structures have been accepted, unequivocally, as receptor end-organs. Some investigations have demonstrated fine nerve fibres coursing amongst the tissues of the heart, and on this basis and/or on the basis of degeneration studies, have alluded to these as being receptors (Woollard, 1926; Nettleship, 1936; Khabarova, 1963). No electron microscope studies are available to suggest that any structures other than the unencapsulated endings (see later) are receptor in function, and indeed such studies have suggested that some, at least, of the fine nerve fibres to these end-organs are sympathetic efferent fibres (Tranum-Jensen, 1979; see end of this chapter).

Of the two major means of histological investigation, light microscopy and electron microscopy, the latter has only just begun to be used even to look at these nerve endings. However, the available histological evidence of cardiac receptors, mainly atrial receptors, from light microscopy and electron microscopy studies, will be discussed in this chapter.

Light microscopy

General review

Sensory fibres from the heart were investigated first by Berkley (1895), Smirnow (1895) and Dogiel (1898); these fibres and their end-organs have recently received a good deal of attention. As well as the hearts of puppies, kittens and lambs, the hearts of the dog, cat, monkey and man have been examined thoroughly and a variety of end-organs described in the works of Michailow (1908), Woollard (1926), Nettleship (1936), Nonidez (1937, 1939, 1943), King (1939), Pannier (1940), Meyling (1953), Mitchell (1956), Coleridge, Hemingway, Holmes & Linden (1957), Holmes (1957a, b), Khabarova (1963), Semenov (1963), Abrahám (1964, 1969), Miller & Kasahara (1964), Volostchenko (1964), Williams (1964), Chervova (1965), Johnston (1968), Kumar (1971), Floyd (1979), Tranum-Jensen (1975, 1979) and Yamauchi (1979). Despite numerous studies of sensory nerve endings in the mammalian heart there still remains some disagreement concerning the types and distribution of these structures. In part, differences in histological technique probably account for much of the variation in observation and interpretation, but it is also unfortunate that few of the numerous published reports include photomicrographs of the described material. Since interpretation plays a considerable role in neurohistology, it is imperative that photographic evidence accompanies descriptive accounts and drawings. Accurate drawings are helpful particularly where three-dimensional structures are postulated, but always should be supported by photographic evidence.

In general in the earlier work, two different types of histological survey have been made. First, by the silver impregnation of the tissues followed by serial sections and secondly, by the supravital method of the infusion of methylene blue into the living animal or the soaking of tissue in methylene blue immediately after death. After the infusion of methylene blue the tissue is prepared so that whole thickness preparations can be viewed, for instance, from the endocardial surface, and it is this latter technique which has led to the better photographs and descriptions in the more recent work (e.g. see Fig. 2.1).

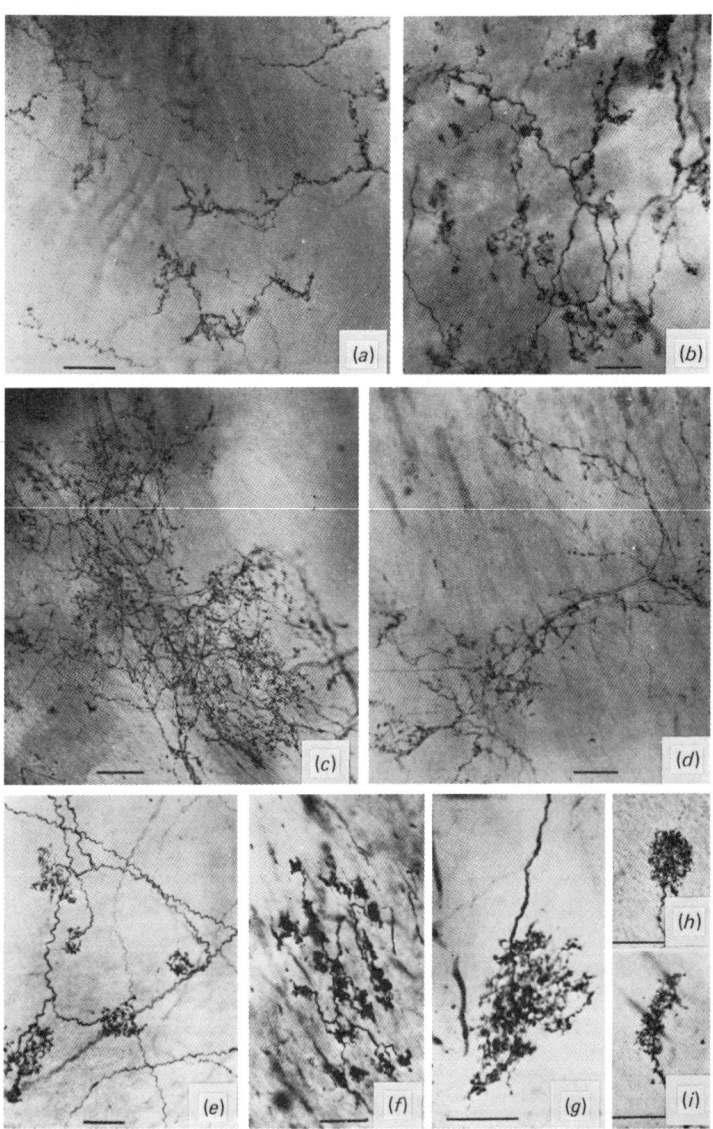

Fig. 2.1 End-organs observed in the atrial endocardium; stained with methylene blue by immersion or perfusion. The bar represents a distance of 100 μm. (a) Cat. Right atrial endocardium. Diffuse complex unencapsulated endings (CUE) with individual terminals tending towards compaction. (b) Cat. Right atrial endocardium. Diffuse CUE. (c) Lamb. Right

Light microscopy

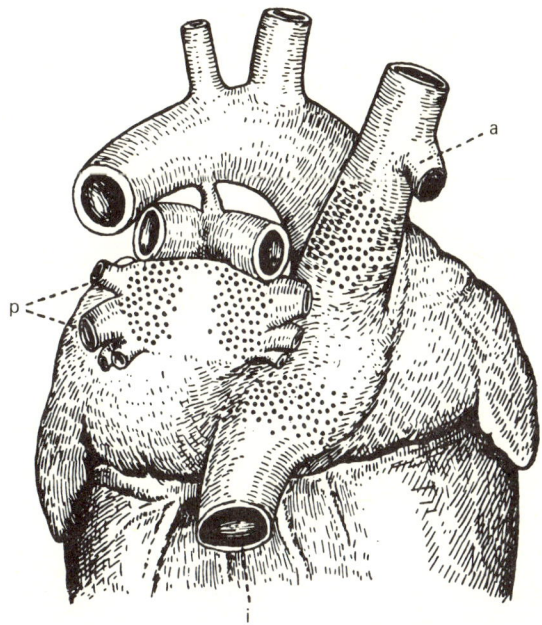

Fig. 2.2. Posterior view of the heart of a kitten showing the location of the receptor areas (dotted) at superior (a) and inferior (i) vena caval–right atrial junctions and pulmonary (p) vein–left atrial junctions. (From Nonidez, 1937.)

Some particular investigations

One of the most important contributions to the histology of atrial receptors was the investigation of Nonidez (1937), who, using the silver impregnation technique on the dorso-medial aspect of the junction of the superior vena cava with the right atrium, described a generous supply of sub-endothelial receptors which were vagal nerve endings. In addition to these

---

atrial endocardium. Diffuse CUE. (*d*) Monkey. Left atrial endocardium. Diffuse CUE. (*e*) Dog. Left atrial endocardium. Compact CUE. (*f*) Monkey. Left atrial endocardium. Compact CUE. (*g*) Lamb. Left atrial endocardium. Compact CUE. (*h*) Cat. Right atrial endocardium near inferior vena cava. Compact CUE. (*i*) Cat. Left atrial endocardium near entrance of pulmonary vein. Compact CUE. (From Miller & Kasahara, 1964.)

subendothelial endings in the new-born kitten which he found in the vena cava in its intrapericardial course, Nonidez also described similar nerve endings in the sub-endothelial tissue of the pulmonary veins encircling their circumference, again in the intrapericardial part of the veins (Fig. 2.2). Pannier (1940) repeated these observations using silver techniques in the adult cat and found sensory endings on the dorsal surface of the superior vena cava in the sub-endothelial part of the wall and endings in the sub-endothelium of the right pulmonary veins (Larsell, 1921; Nonidez, 1937; see also Lavrente, 1946).

Following investigations into many types of sensory endings found in somatic and vascular tissue, Miller & Kasahara (1964), using the methylene blue technique, examined the sensory nerve endings in the heart. Having previously arbitrarily and simply divided sensory nerve endings into three groups, (1) free fibre endings, (2) complex unencapsulated endings (e.g. Ruffini), and (3) encapsulated endings (e.g. Pacinian corpuscle), they concluded that similar types of endings occurred in the heart although only two types, the end-nets and the complex unencapsulated endings were consistently observed. The end-net was thought to be formed by the anastomosis (there is, as yet, no evidence from electron microscopy of axoplasmic continuity) of the branched dendrites of several apparently different myelinated fibres and is found throughout the entire endocardium; it is possible that the end-net represents the free fibre endings which otherwise seem to be totally absent from cardiac tissue. The end-net is not usually demonstrable with heavy metal techniques, therefore workers such as Nonidez (1939) and Khabarova (1963) did not describe these nerve endings but investigators working with methylene blue on the other hand have consistently described such structures (Michailow, 1908; Woollard, 1926; Meyling, 1953; Mitchell, 1956). The complex unencapsulated endings are usually described as two types, diffuse and compact type endings (e.g. Figs. 2.1 and 2.3), and arise from moderately sized myelinated fibres which are much branched and occupy considerable area. Encapsulated endings are rare in the hearts of mammals.

The atrial and ventricular epicardium show a variety of both diffuse and compact types of complex unencapsulated endings but the end-nets are generally absent from the epicardium.

Light microscopy

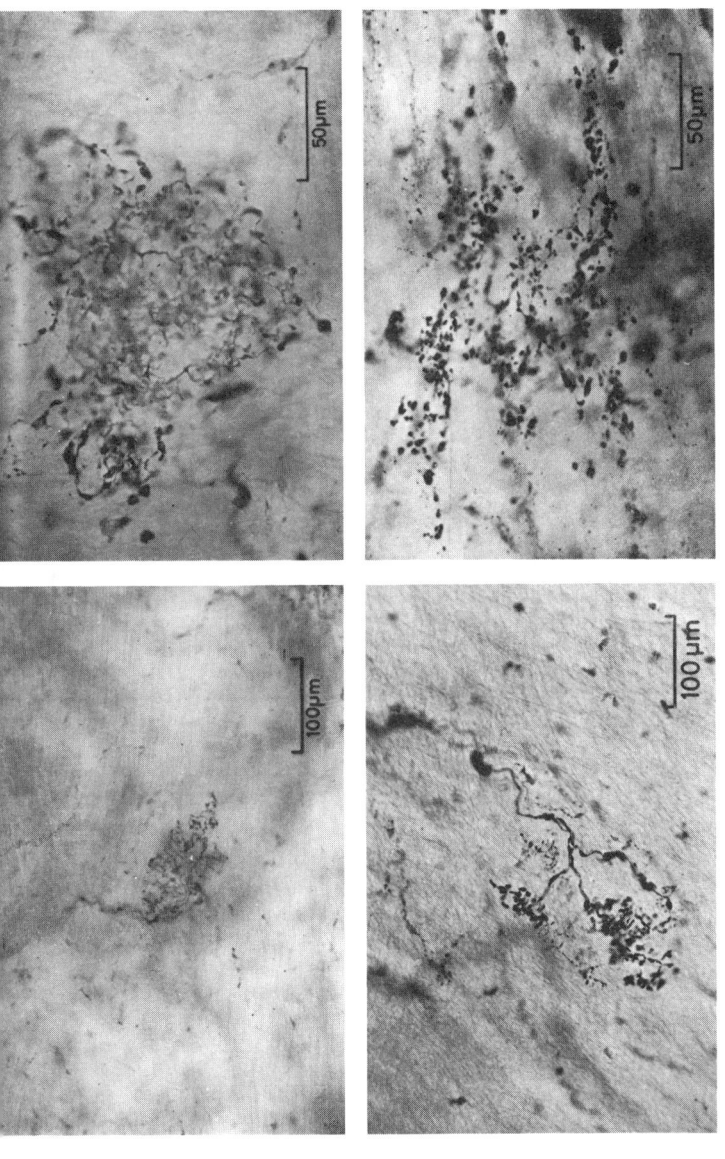

Fig. 2.3. Endocardium from pulmonary vein–atrial junctions of four dogs stained supravitally with methylene blue. Two different magnifications. Similarity of diffuse and compact endings is illustrated.

Histology of nerve endings in the heart

Miller & Kasahara (1964) in dogs, cats, lambs and monkeys did not find it possible to demonstrate nerve fibres terminating within the nodal tissue though such terminations were described by Torri (1962) using the electron microscope. Abrahám (1969) in the pig, calf and horse observed nerve plexuses within the sinu-atrial node and conducting systems. In the sinu-atrial node of the pig, but not the calf and the horse, Abrahám (1969) claims to have found not only efferent fibres but afferent fibres – some of which terminate in 'several small neurofibrillar end plates'.

King (1939) using methylene blue stain in the rat and examining only the myocardium has claimed to show two types of endings, (a) small encapsulated receptor endings frequently found between the muscle bundles, and (b) muscle spindles of varying degrees of complexity; only a few of these endings were observed and these only in the muscles of the ventricles. Only Plenchkova (1936) has also described muscle spindles in cardiac muscle, but Moravec-Mochet, Moravec & Hatt (1977) have suggested that there is an ultrastructural arrangement, resembling skeletal muscle spindles, in the atrioventricular junction of the rat heart. Miller & Kasahara (1964) did not comment on the work of King (1939) but stated they were unable to demonstrate sensory terminals ending along the myocardial muscle fibres although they could trace bundles of mixed myelinated and non-myelinated nerves through the connective tissue septa between muscle bundles. They considered these nerve fibres to extend ultimately to the endocardium. They concluded that there were no sensory endings in the myocardium. Abrahám (1969) agrees that, in general, there are few receptors in the myocardium. He found receptors only in the cat after also examining the dog, horse, pig, sheep and calf, and even these only in the right atrial wall and atrial septum; one type of ending consisted of a system of neurofibrillar end-plates and the other a spiral ending around the muscle resembling a muscle spindle.

Kumar (1971), using the silver impregnation technique, was unable to demonstrate unencapsulated endings or end-nets in the hearts of amphibia, in spite of showing, particularly in the endocardium, nerve fibres terminating 'in the form of free, end-ring, bulb-like, disc-shaped, oblong and club-shaped structures', in large numbers, which he claimed were receptors.

In *summary* it seems that, of all the histological studies so far

Light microscopy

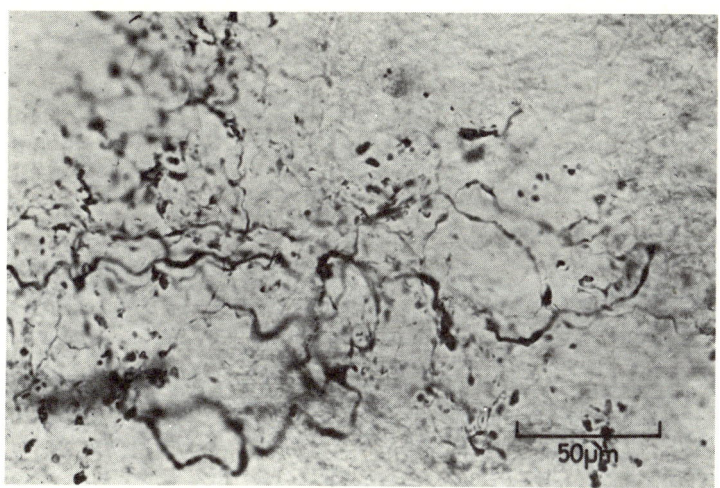

Fig. 2.4. Endocardium of pulmonary vein–atrial junction stained with methylene blue. High magnification of the receptor ending illustrates the three-dimensional (some parts out of focus) and diffuse nature of the ending allowing the conclusion that it may be a 'deformation' receptor.

described, the only structures worthy of further consideration as receptors are the complex unencapsulated endings and end-net described particularly by Miller & Kasahara (1964). The remainder of the chapter will consider these two endings, as observed in the atrial endocardium, in greater detail.

Complex unencapsulated endings

Most of the histological attention has rightly been paid to the atrial endocardium which is the most profusely innervated area of the heart and the most characteristic features of the atrial endocardium are the wealth and variety of complex unencapsulated sensory endings (e.g. Figs. 2.1, 2.3, 2.4 and 2.5) found only at the junctions of the superior and inferior vena cava and the right atrium and of the pulmonary veins and left atrium (as previously described (Fig. 2.2) by Nonidez, 1937) (also see Fig. 4.1), in the appendage and at the base of the inter-atrial septum. Nearly all the workers since Berkley (1895) and Smirnow (1895) have described many sensory endings in this location and all students of cardiac innervation have described and illustrated

Histology of nerve endings in the heart

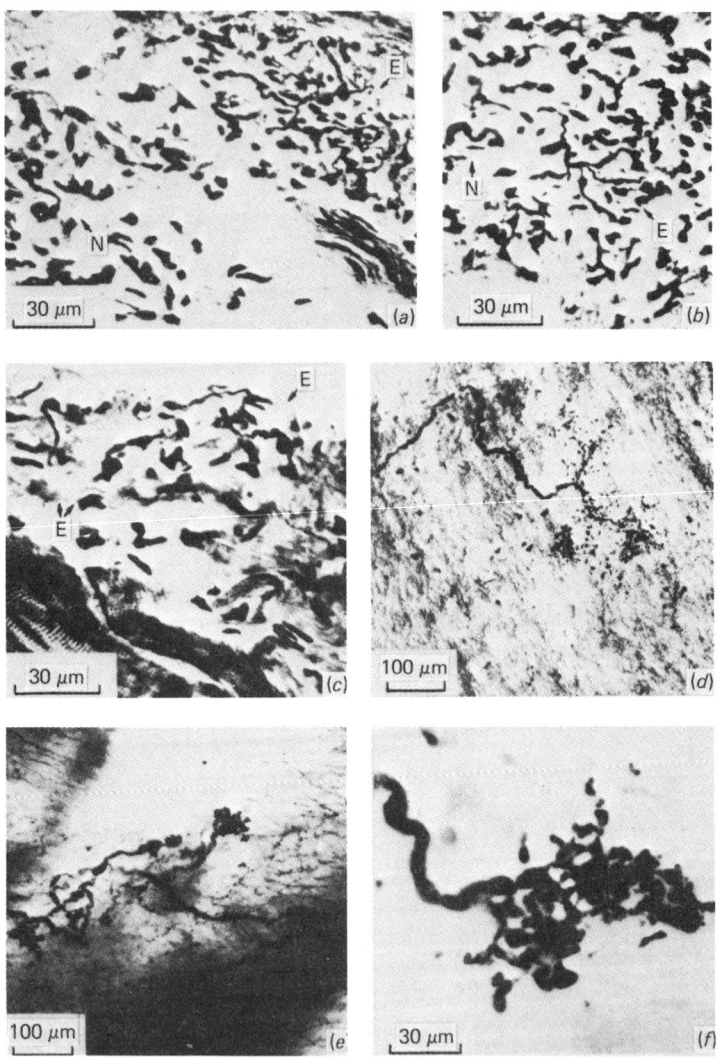

Fig. 2.5. (a)–(c) are sections taken from physiologically localised receptor areas of the atrio-venous wall of the dog. (d)–(f) are taken from whole thickness methylene blue preparations. All photomicrographs are untouched. (a) Tangential section through endocardium of pulmonary vein. To the left, a thick nerve fibre (N) is cut across several times; to the right, the fine branched nerve fibres and associated nuclei of a characteristic end formation (E). 12 μm section; silver impregnation. (b) Tangential section

Light microscopy

a large variety of complex unencapsulated terminals varying from diffuse to compact in general form (for references see above). Whilst numerous drawings of the endings are published (e.g. King, 1939), very few good photographs have appeared in print before the 1950s; as has already been pointed out it is imperative that photographic evidence accompanies the drawings and descriptive accounts. Only one study (Coleridge, Hemingway, Holmes & Linden, 1957) has defined the position of the receptors physiologically and then by using both the techniques (heavy silver metal and methylene blue) gone on to examine histologically the tissue beneath the surface of the small area (1 mm^2) of endocardium to which the stimulus was applied. The technique involved the recording of action potentials from a slip of cervical vagal nerve in the neck and by various snaring techniques and probing, first with the finger and then with a fine glass probe, a point of stimulation within the atria was obtained, the response to which was an increase in the trains of impulses recorded from the slip of the vagal nerve. The animal was killed, the atria opened and the small area located and marked and the tissues were examined histologically; in some animals the tissue was examined by the silver technique and in others prior to death methylene blue was infused in the animals and the tissue examined in endocardial surface preparations.

In the event complex unencapsulated endings were always

through endocardium of pulmonary vein. Again, a thick nerve fibre (N) and a typical end formation (E) are present. 12 μm section; silver impregnation. (c) Transverse section through right atrial endocardium. In the endocardial connective tissue, branched nerve fibres (E) and nuclei can be seen. 12 μm section; silver impregnation. (d) A thick nerve fibre in the atrial endocardium running to three end formations. Whole thickness methylene blue preparation, viewed from the endocardial surface. (e) Thick nerve fibres, ending as terminal expansions, in the posterior wall of the left atrium. In the background the fine plexiform fibres of the terminal nervous network can be seen. Whole thickness methylene blue preparation. (f) High-power photomicrography of a typical end formation. A thick nerve fibre terminates by branching into finer fibres which are partly obscured by deeply stained associated cellular elements. Note the essential similarity between this structure, seen in a whole thickness preparation, and the ending shown in the silver impregnated section in (b). (From Coleridge et al., 1957.)

Histology of nerve endings in the heart

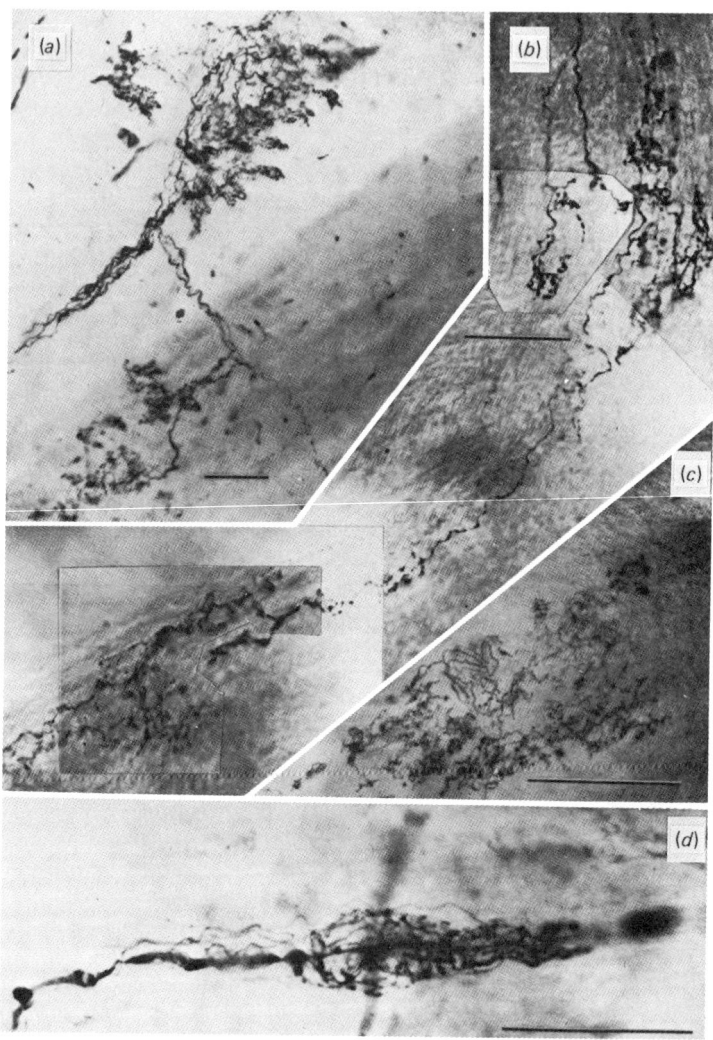

Fig. 2.6. The nerve endings demonstrated were stained by methylene blue immersion or perfusion. The straight black line in each photograph represents a distance of 100 μm. CUE: complex unencapsulated ending. (a) Large, diffuse CUE, on the inter-atrial septum, left atrium of a human heart. Endings similar to this are most often seen at atrio-venous junctions. (b) Diffuse CUE near the entrance of one of the right pulmonary veins into the left atrium of a human heart. This ending, like all other CUEs seen

Light microscopy

observed in these stimulated areas although the end-nets were also present in all preparations. Examples from this investigation are shown in Fig. 2.5 where it can be seen that silver staining shows end-organs similar to those observed after staining with methylene blue. Such an investigation also established the afferent nature of the unencapsulated organs.

Subsequently Holmes (1956, 1957a, b, 1958) examined many further preparations and included degeneration studies in his investigations. These degeneration studies allowed numbers of receptor end-organs in the right and left atria to be calculated. The total number of discrete endings in the whole atrial endocardium varies but may be of the order of 150 (Holmes, 1957a) to 300 (Miller & Kasahara, 1964). The distribution ratio between the right and left atria is variable but about two-thirds of the total number are to be found in the left atrium and one-third in the right atrium. The ratio of end-organs to nerve fibres is roughly two to one. The diffuse type of ending arises from fibres approximately 4–6 μm in diameter and branches of ramifications of one fibre may occupy an area of several square millimetres. Larger compact endings are usually the largest found in the heart and the fibres range from 8 to 14 μm in diameter. The terminal apparatus from these fibres varies in size from 50 to 350 μm. Saunders (1979) in a careful histological study has confirmed the results detailed above. In particular he found that though most of the axons which terminated in complex unencapsulated endings had only a single ending, some of the axons had many branches and had several endings; the mean number of endings per axon was 1.74 (S.D. ± 1.48; $n = 178$) which was within the range given by Holmes (1957a).

These findings in the atrial endocardium have been confirmed in man by Johnston (1968) who commented that more nerve endings were found in the atrial endocardium than in the endocardium of any other part of the heart, and observed that it was only in the atria that both complex unencapsulated

in this study, originated from myelinated fibres, seen entering at the top. (c) Compact type of CUE seen on the inter-atrial septum, left atrium of a human heart. (d) Compact type of CUE found at the entrance of the superior vena cava into the right atrium of a human heart. (From Johnston, 1968.)

Histology of nerve endings in the heart

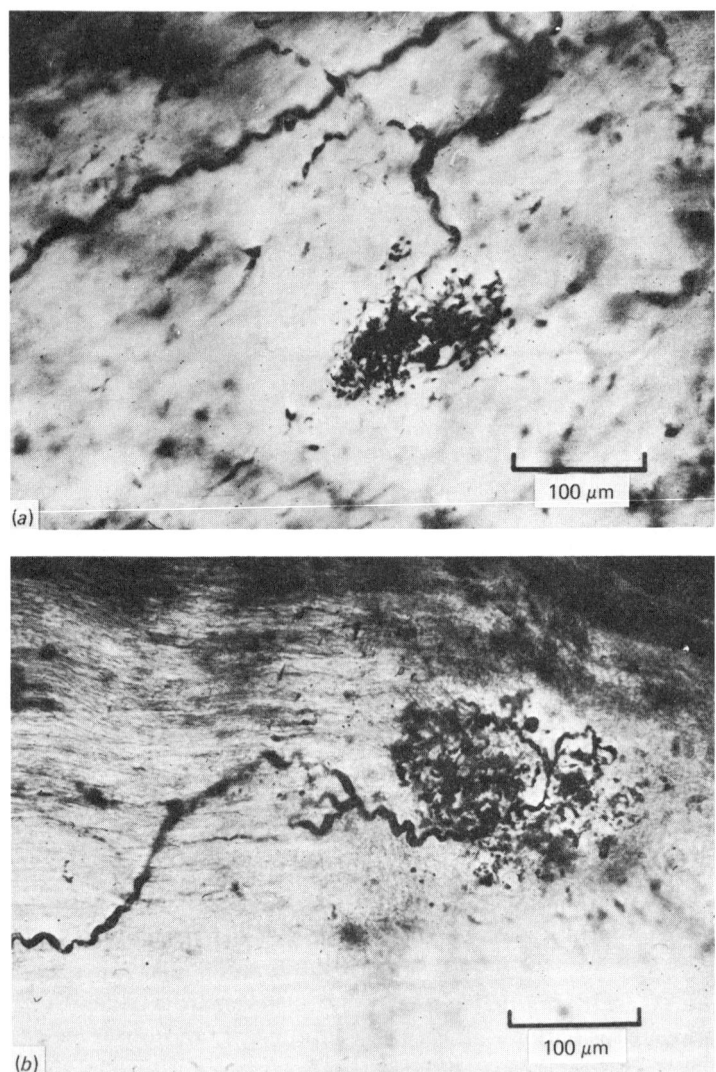

Fig. 2.7. Endocardium from left atrium of dog, stained supravitally with methylene blue and viewed from the surface in a whole thickness preparation: (a) one typical atrial receptor found at the upper pulmonary vein–left atrial junction, (b) another typical atrial receptor found in the endocardium of the appendage of the left atrium in the same dog.

Light microscopy

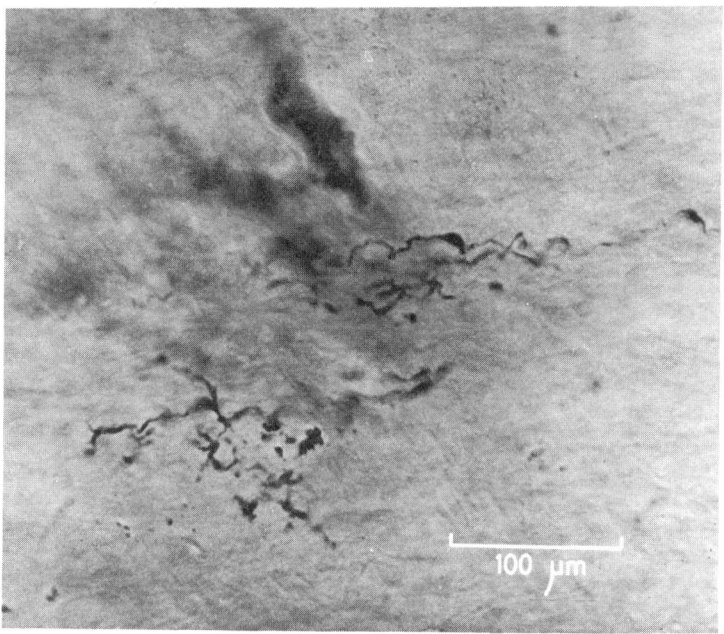

Fig. 2.8. Endocardium of left atrium of rabbit stained with methylene blue showing typical diffuse unencapsulated endings. (Linden & Mary, unpublished.)

endings and end-nets could be observed. He found also that, as in other mammals, complex unencapsulated endings are consistently found at the junctions of the superior vena cava and inferior vena cava with the right atrium and at the pulmonary vein–left atrial junctions (Fig. 2.6).

Although at least two investigations (Miller & Kasahara, 1964; Johnston, 1968) stated categorically that there were no receptor end-organs in the atrial appendages in dog and man, and that only an end-net was present, it was possible by distension of small balloons in the atrial appendages to elicit a reflex increase in heart rate (Kappagoda, Linden & Saunders, 1972*a*, *b*; see Chapter 5). Saunders (Floyd, Linden & Saunders, 1972) by careful staining using the methylene blue technique showed that there were about ten unencapsulated endings in the endocardium of each appendage (an example is shown in Fig. 2.7).

Histology of nerve endings in the heart

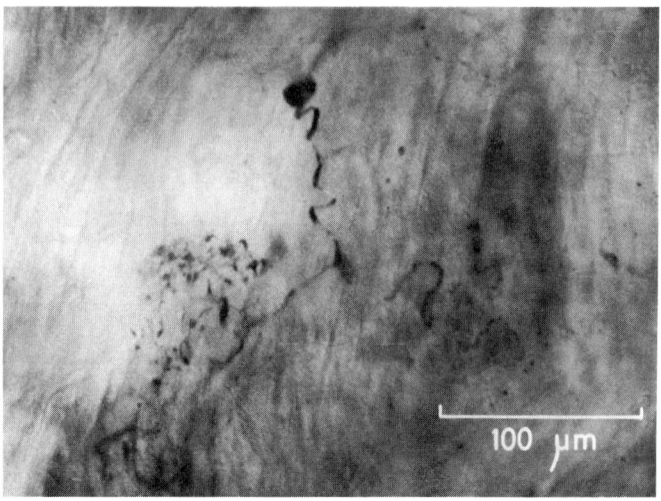

Fig. 2.9. Endocardium of left atrium of guinea-pig stained with methylene blue showing typical unencapsulated ending. (Linden & Mary, unpublished.)

Although the presence of unencapsulated endings in the rabbit had been commented on previously, no microscopic evidence was presented. Recently the presence of the same unencapsulated receptors has been shown in the atria of the rabbit both histologically (Fig. 2.8) and electrophysiologically (Kappagoda, Linden & Mary, 1977b). The presence on electrophysiological evidence, of the receptors in the rabbit had previously been denied though accepted on histological evidence (Rao, Fahim & Gupta, 1975). They are also present in the guinea-pig (Fig. 2.9).

That the unencapsulated endings were sensory nerve endings discharging into fibres in the vagi was confirmed using degenerative studies. Smirnow (1895) was unable to demonstrate complex endings following division of the vagi in the neck in the cat and the rabbit. Nettleship (1936) showed in the cat that the endings disappeared following bilateral vagotomy below the nodose ganglia, but not above, thus concluding that they were sensory in nature. Similarly, degeneration of the endings was observed by Holmes (1957a) following unilateral vagotomy in the dog. The unencapsulated endings remained intact following

Light microscopy

bilateral removal of the stellate ganglia (Woollard, 1926; Nettleship, 1936) and following removal of the sympathetic chains rostral to the eighth thoracic ganglia and the cervical sympathetic trunks (Nonidez, 1941).

End-net

In contrast to the findings in the atria, only end-nets are to be found in the ventricular endocardium and no other types of sensory ending have been observed (Miller & Kasahara, 1964). Johnston (1968), who included the heart of man in his studies of endocardium, also found that the ventricular endocardium showed end-nets similar to those found in the atrial endocardium but considered that fewer fibres made up this structure. He also observed that the ventricular end-net is best seen in the outflow tract of the right ventricle. Numerous end-nets and large complex unencapsulated endings were also observed in the adventitia of the base of the pulmonary artery and these structures have been thoroughly described and illustrated in the extensive studies of Abrahám (1955, 1956, 1961). Incidentally, no complex unencapsulated endings and no myelinated fibres were observed in the ventricular endocardium.

Examination of the endocardium of both surfaces of the leaflets of the mitral and tricuspid valves has shown both end-nets and occasional complex endings in the dog (Miller & Kasahara, 1964). However, these findings have not been confirmed in man (Johnston, 1968).

The end-net formation, so prominent in both the atrial (Fig. 2.10) and ventricular endocardium, was first recognised and described by Michailow (1908) but largely overlooked until the use of methylene blue by Meyling (1953), Mitchell (1956), Coleridge et al. (1957) and Holmes (1957a, b, 1958), which clearly depicted the network and emphasised that it was a structure separate from the diffuse and compact types of endings. It is surprising that the more recent Russian workers (e.g. Khabarova, 1963) failed to recognise this remarkable network and it is probable that their preoccupation with the heavy metal techniques explains this failure.

The reported results of the division of the vagal nerves on the end-net have been less consistent. Smirnow (1895) stated that

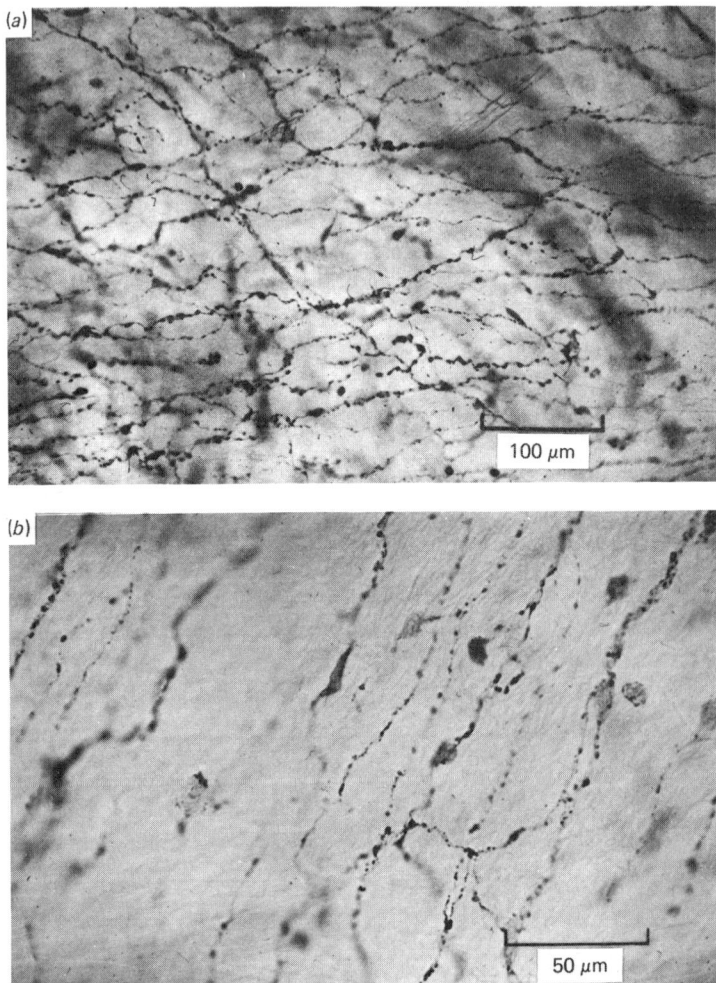

Fig. 2.10. Endocardium of left atrium of dog stained with methylene blue to show the end-net; illustration at different magnifications under light microscope.

he was able to visualise this structure following bilateral division of vagal nerves in the cat. Nettleship (1936) found that the network disappeared following bilateral vagotomy below the nodose ganglia in the cat. Bilateral removal of stellate ganglia in dogs and cats was shown to have no influence on the end-net

Electron microscopy

(Woollard, 1926; Nettleship, 1936). Holmes (1957a) found that the end-net was unaffected by vagal section and concluded that it was sympathetic in origin. Holmes (1957b) and Williams (1964) stained the endings to show non-specific cholinesterase activity and together with Miller & Kasahara (1964) concluded that the end-net was sensory.

Many of the above workers concluded, on the basis of light microscopy, that connections probably existed between the discrete unencapsulated endings and the end-net. However, it is not possible with light microscopy studies to demonstrate axoplasmic continuity which must await careful electron microscopy. Floyd (1979) on the basis of light microscopy and methylene blue staining observed discrete endings arising from fibres which were branching to form an end-net or arising directly from the meshes of an end-net. He thought the results, which presented evidence of interconnection and common innervation, indicated common features of morphology of the unencapsulated endings and end-nets, and postulated that any difference between the two were quantitative only, and that 'there seems to be no morphological basis to regard end-nets as anything other than extensive unencapsulated endings'. The methylene blue technique, however, does not distinguish between afferent and efferent nerves and Tranum-Jensen (1979) has pointed out that his studies showed that adrenergic fibres form a very considerable proportion of the plexus in the endocardium and in his opinion the end-net was, to a large extent, an efferent adrenergic plexus.

Recent techniques for selectively detecting the presence of neurotransmitters have made it possible to locate adrenergic and cholinergic fibres to the heart particularly to the coronary vessels (Denn & Stone, 1976). The evidence from this work suggests that the bead-like structures (which have often been described running through the ventricular epicardium) are probably parts of adrenergic efferent fibres.

Electron microscopy

Recently Tranum-Jensen (1975, 1979) examined atrial receptors using the electron microscope but pointed out that because the unencapsulated structures were so widely dispersed it was essential that the structures for study by the electron microscope should be localised, identified and selected for study by the light microscope and this limitation should be clearly recognised. In mini pigs of both sexes Tranum-Jensen (1979) also reported studies with fluorescence histochemical methods developed for examining catecholamines. Specimens for electron microscopy were obtained by a method previously reported (Tranum-Jensen, 1975) particularly in whole mounts stained for cholinesterase. In the whole mount preparations of pig atria stained for cholinesterase, accumulations of distinct circumscribed end-organs were found in the endocardium around the entrances of the pulmonary veins, endocardium of the superior vena cava and the adjacent atrial endocardium, on the right of the inter-atrial septum opposite the root of the aorta and in the anterior circumference of the mitral ostium a few millimetres above the valve. They were found less frequently around the inferior vena cava. The distribution was thus similar to that described above in other animals.

The position of the end-organ in the endocardium varied; some were located very close to the myocardium, occasionally bridged by a thin strand of myocardium, but others were located further away in the endocardial connective tissue. Collagenous fibrils but not elastic fibrils were observed in large amounts inside the end-organ. Strands of smooth muscle cells, frequently seen in the atrial endocardium, did not seem to have any special relation to the end-organ. Tranum-Jensen (1979) postulated that such differences in the location of the end-organs within the endocardium and their relations to connective tissue fibrils may influence their moment of activation during the cardiac cycle. This explanation of the difference between type A and type B discharges of atrial receptors is not thought to be an important one (see Chapter 3; Kappagoda, Linden & Mary, 1976, 1977a, b). However, Tranum-Jensen (1979) found that the cholinesterase activity in the pig was very likely to be of the so-called specific type in contrast to the largely non-specific cholinesterase activity he and others (Holmes, 1957b; Williams, 1964) had observed in the dog and the cat heart. There is no explanation for this difference.

Tranum-Jensen (1979) reported that the end-organ appeared as a disc-like aggregate of cells into which a thick nerve fibre entered, the thickness of the end-organ being usually about 20 μm and sometimes appearing as a single layer of cells. The thick stem fibre supplying a group of end-organs may lose its myelin sheath up to 100 μm before branching or it may retain its sheath on to the branches. Considering Paintal's (1972) model for receptor function such a branching would effect summation of stimuli first stated by Nonidez (1941). In sheep preparations of the endocardium, processed for the demonstration of adrenergic nerves, the course of thick myelinated fibres was followed using phase contrast optics. Microscopy of the same field in phase contrast and fluorescence clearly showed that the thick fibres were always accompanied by thin, fluorescent fibres (Figs. 2.11 and 2.12). Where an end-organ could be located a plexus of thin fluorescent fibres could be seen to surround the terminal portion of the thick portion. It was also frequently observed that fluorescent fibres, approaching from different directions, came into close relationship with the periphery of the end-organs.

Electron microscopic examination of the terminal portion of the thick fibre close to the end-organ frequently showed that a single Schwann cell enclosed both the thick fibre and its thin varicose fibres; the thin fibres contain accumulations of small vesicles which strongly suggest that they are efferent axons. In addition small separate nerves containing several similar thin axons were nearly always found in the immediate vicinity of the thick fibre. Synapses were not observed between the thick fibre and the thin fibres within the end-organ. Nevertheless, the findings are suggestive of a sympathetic efferent component to the end-organ. Adrenergic fibres have recently been identified entering the Pacinian corpuscle (Santini, 1969); previously in the study of end-organs of atrial nerves a relationship between the circumscribed end formations of thick fibres and the surrounding thin fibres had been noted (Lawrentjew, 1929; Holmes 1957a). Also, it has been demonstrated that catecholamines may influence the response of different mechanoreceptors, e.g. Pacinian corpuscles (Lowenstein & Altmirano-Orrego, 1956) and carotid sinus receptors (Zapata, 1975). However, physiological studies involving stimulation of sympathetic efferent nerves to the atria could not demonstrate a *direct* efferent effect on atrial mechanoreceptors (Zucker &

Gilmore, 1974b; Wahab, Zucker & Gilmore, 1975); only secondary effects were apparent.

The thick fibre splits into branches shortly after it has entered the end-organ, forming a dense arborisation of very irregular fibres with bulky varicosities containing numerous mitochondria and no specialised endings suggestive of receptor functions were observed. Morphologically all the cells of the end-organ were the same and they are considered to be modified Schwann cells, which ensheath the branches of the thick fibre except at the varicosities which are free of cellular covering. The exposed areas of the nerve membrane come into direct contact with the connective tissue fibrils, most of which are collagenous. The varicosities of the branches of the thick fibre were furnished with small protrusions which extend between the collagen fibrils. These protrusions contained small clear vesicles and occasionally a few larger vesicles with dense cores, but were devoid of larger organelles. Because these protrusions have the most intimate relation to the collagen fibrils, on a morphological basis they are considered an important part of the generator membrane of the

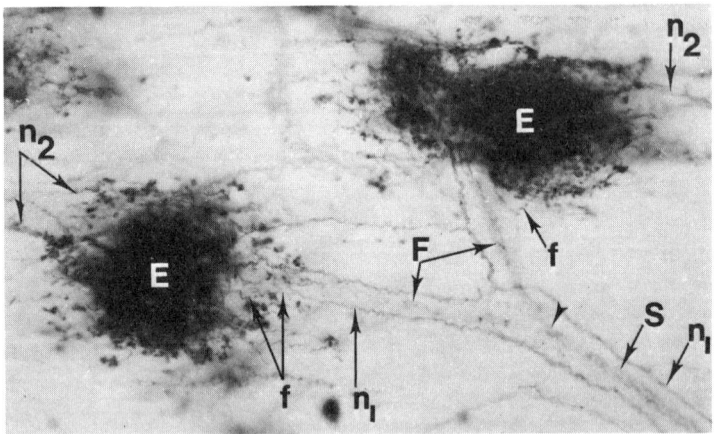

Fig. 2.11. Sheet preparation of atrial endocardium taken at the entrance of the superior vena cava and stained for cholinesterase. A thick nerve fibre (S) divides (at arrowhead), and each branch (F) gives rise to circumscribed end-organs (E). The thick nerve fibres are accompanied by thin cholinesterase-positive nerves (n_1) on to the end-organs where they split into fine fibres (f). Several thin fibres are seen around the end-organs, and nerves (n_2) coming from other directions also join the end-organs. Magnifications: 200:1. (From Tranum-Jensen, 1979.)

Electron microscopy

receptor. The morphology of the protrusions and their relations to collagen fibrils have a close similarity to structures in other mechanoreceptors, e.g. Golgi tendon organs (Schoultz & Swett, 1972).

Accumulations of numerous mitochondria were a prominent feature in all the varicosities. Similar accumulations of mitochondria have been found so frequently in several other types of mechanoreceptors, that they appear to be characteristic of such endings. There is a high level of cytochrome oxidase activity in the mitochondria of other sensory endings (Hanker,

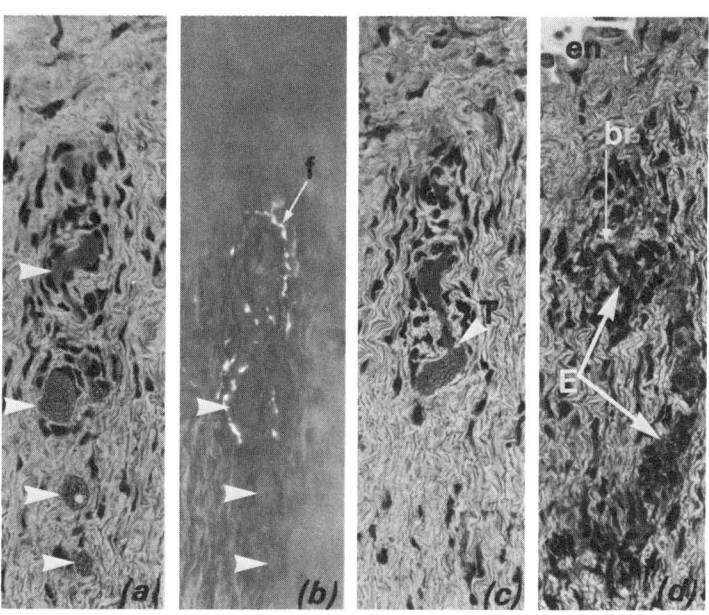

Fig. 2.12. Series of 4 μm sections cut from a block taken at the entrance of the right inferior pulmonary vein, freeze dried, and processed for the demonstration of catecholamines. (a)–(c) are cut in series and show fragments of a thick fibre (arrowheads) surrounded by several thin fluorescent fibres (f). At (T) the myelin sheath of the thick fibre terminates. A few sections revealed an end-organ (E) at the end of the thick fibre. A larger branch (br) of the thick fibre can be seen inside the end-organ. For correct topography the lower edge of (d) should be placed on top of (c). Tangentially sectioned endothelium (en) at upper left. The endocardium was slightly curved and the end-organ could not be seen full face in one section. Magnification: 305:1. (From Tranum-Jensen, 1979.)

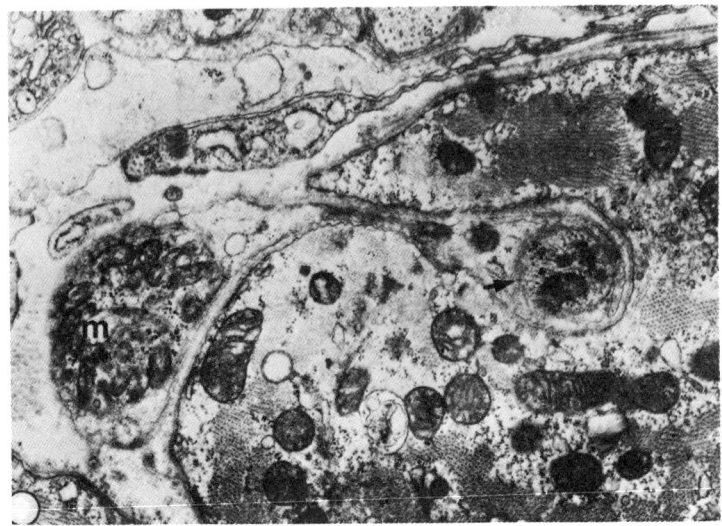

Fig. 2.13. Sensory nerve terminal with numerous mitochondria (m) and abundant glycogen stores penetrates into a profound invagination of the sarcolemma of the nodal cell (↗). Only a few vesicles are visible. Magnification: 19000:1. (From Moravec-Mochet et al., 1977.)

Dixon & Moore, 1973) suggesting that they are metabolically very active. Another prominent feature of many of the varicosities is that they contain a large number of glycogen granules and this has also been observed in other mechanoreceptor endings. Glycogen granules and numerous mitochondria have also been found during electron microscopic studies of the pacemaker structures of the heart, e.g. in the atrioventricular junction of the rat heart, Fig. 2.13 (Moravec-Mochet et al., 1977); these structures have also been considered to be afferent endings. The glycogen granules were often found closely associated with the profiles of smooth endoplasmic reticulum, which may appear as complexes of concentric or parallel cisterns with numerous glycogen particles between the cisterns. Glycogen granules are often present in large quantities around such complexes and similar complexes, but without associated glycogen, have been associated together with laminated bodies; and it is likely that they represent the degenerative end stage of these complexes. Complexes without associated glycogen and with no signs of degradation have occasionally been observed at some distance from the end-organ but Tranum-Jensen (1975) suggests that these findings indicate that the complexes are transported from the perikarya of the thick fibre to the terminals where they exert a function in glycogen synthesis and then degenerate. Glycogen associated with profiles of smooth endoplasmic reticulum was found in all the end-organs studied, but highly ordered complexes were found in only a few. Morphologically identical membrane complexes with associated glycogen particles have been found in perikarya in spinal ganglia (Pannese, 1969) and recently in cardiac ganglia (Ellison & Hibbs, 1974). This type of complex is not very common anywhere but has been observed in other nerve endings and Tranum-Jensen (1979) speculates as to whether the findings in spinal ganglia, cardiac ganglia and atrial end-organs are in some way related.

The degeneration process was constantly observed in the end-organ. Often varicosities were found which were completely filled with residual bodies and what appeared as entire, fully degenerated nerve branches were occasionally seen. Likewise, single scattered cells of the end-organs had a degenerated appearance. Similar degenerative phenomena have frequently been observed in other mechanoreceptors (Cauna, 1959). Tranum-Jensen (1979) considered that in a variety of mechano-receptors, e.g. Meissner's corpuscles, there was a considerable turnover of the neural material within nerve terminals and that not only was there a turnover of organelles but also there was sometimes a 'turnover' of terminals. Tranum-Jensen (1979) is of the opinion that the above findings in the end-organs of hearts of young animals suggests that the receptors are subject to a continued replacement of the neuro material throughout life, and that a slow remodelling of the end-organs may take place continuously.

Conclusion

From the results of light microscopy it seems that unencapsulated nerve endings are to be found mainly in the region of the atrio-venous junctions and a nerve 'end-net' is found throughout the atrial endocardium. The unencapsulated endings are receptors discharging into afferent fibres in the vagi and it seems that much of the nerve net consists of efferent sympathetic nerve fibres.

From the histological structure of the unencapsulated endings as shown in Figs. 2.1, 2.3 and 2.4 it can be seen that these endings are three dimensional, e.g. some of the components of the endings seen in Fig. 2.4 are out of focus, these being at different depths in the endocardium from those photographed in focus. Such a formation is easily observed on the microscope stage as the optics are racked up and down. From the above findings it is suggested that the receptors are stimulated by any deformation of surrounding tissue causing changes in tension in any direction and thus are well suited to respond to changes in stretch of the walls of the atria.

Electron microscopy confirms the unencapsulated end-organ as a receptor and, together with phase contrast and fluorescent studies, shows that efferent sympathetic nerve fibres course with the thick afferent fibre to end near the receptor ending, suggesting a sympathetic efferent component to the receptor end-organ. An exciting finding, but as yet, no function has been ascribed to this efferent sympathetic nerve.

3 ELECTROPHYSIOLOGY OF ATRIAL RECEPTORS

Though, as seen in Chapter 2, there is histological evidence of only one receptor end-organ in the atria, there is electrophysiological evidence which points to the existence of the three groups of receptors within the atria, and this evidence will be discussed in this chapter: receptors which discharge into myelinated fibres in the cervical vagi (e.g. Paintal, 1963a); receptors which discharge into non-myelinated fibres in the vagi (e.g. Thorén, 1976a); receptors which discharge into the sympathetic nerves (e.g. Malliani, 1979).

Receptors which discharge into myelinated fibres in the vagi

As reported in Chapter 2, the receptor end-organ most commonly observed histologically in the atria is the unencapsulated ending found in the endocardium, and located mainly at the vein–atrial junctions. These complex unencapsulated nerve endings which discharge into the myelinated fibres in the vagi, will be referred to as the Paintal-type atrial receptors and will be described first. Paintal has described various aspects of these receptors in a series of reports (Paintal, 1953a, b, c, 1963a, b, 1972, 1973a).

The earliest records of action potentials in these afferent vagal nerves originating from the great veins and the atria were presented by Amann & Schaefer (1943). Over the next ten years these observations were extended (Walsh & Whitteridge, 1944; Jarisch & Zotterman, 1948; Whitteridge, 1948; Dickinson, 1950; Neil & Zotterman, 1950). For instance, Jarisch & Zotterman (1948) attempted to locate the source of activity observed in branches of the vagal nerves in the chest by probing inside the walls of the atria; they commented 'a mere touch with a wooden pin on the regions around and between the caval orifices on the right side and the pulmonary veins on the left side produces a very marked discharge of large spikes'. Nevertheless there remained an element of controversy regarding their origin and particularly the precise relationship between the pattern of activity in these nerves and the atrial events of the cardiac cycle.

In an attempt to resolve this controversy Paintal (1953a), to his great credit, adopted a new technique of locating the origin of the receptor endings. He recorded action potentials from vagal fibres in the cat. Having first obtained a single fibre in which the trains of impulses were related to the various waves in the atrial pressure pulse, he rapidly opened the chest and by successively increasing the pressures within the atrial chambers was able to locate the origin of the receptor endings to the atrial walls; remarkably the functioning nerve fibre was not lost during the surgical intervention.

As a result of these investigations, Paintal (1953a) concluded that there were two basic patterns of discharge in these vagal fibres, one which occurred mainly during atrial systole and another which occurred during the phase of atrial filling. The afferent endings from which these nerves originated were designated type A and type B atrial receptors respectively (Fig. 3.1). However, subsequent observations (e.g. Neil & Joels, 1961) indicated that all the vagal afferent fibres which originated from the veins and atria did not fall precisely into these two categories, with the result that modifications were made to the original classification (Paintal, 1963a). The situation is further complicated by the observation that a proportion of these receptors, which discharge into vagal afferent fibres with atrial patterns of activity, do in fact originate from areas other than the atrial endocardium, e.g. two receptors in this category, one in the left main bronchus and one in the oesophagus, were described by Coleridge, Hemingway, Holmes & Linden (1957); for further comment on this point see later in the chapter.

The following patterns of activity (based on Paintal, 1963a) are recognised as originating in Paintal-type atrial receptors (Fig. 3.1):

(I) type A: these receptors discharge mainly during atrial systole (i.e. in time with the 'a' wave of the atrial pressure pulse) with occasional 'spikes' (two or less)

Receptors discharging into myelinated fibres

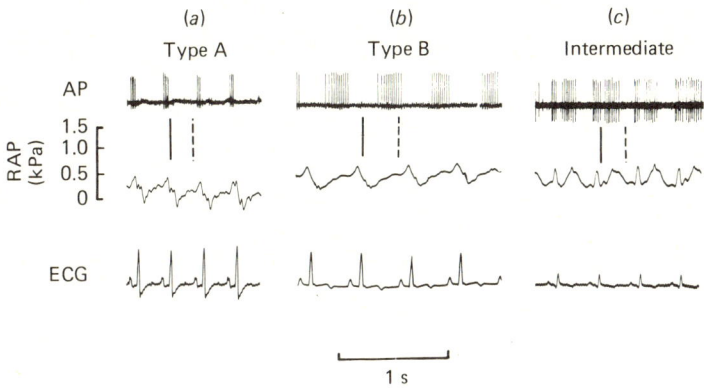

Fig. 3.1. Types of atrial receptors in the dog. From above downwards record of action potentials (AP), right atrial pressure (RAP) and electrocardiogram (ECG). The vertical lines are drawn to show the temporal relationship between bursts of action potentials and waves of the atrial pressure pulse. The continuous line indicates the end of the 'a' wave and the interrupted line indicates the end of atrial filling (peak of the 'v' wave of the atrial pressure pulse). (a) a record of a type A unit in which a high-frequency burst of action potentials coincided with the 'a' wave. (b) a record of a type B unit in which the burst of action potentials coincided with the 'v' wave. (c) a record of an intermediate unit which possessed both type A and type B activity. These three units were located to the atrial endocardium. (From Kappagoda et al., 1977b.)

during atrial filling (i.e. in time with the 'v' wave of the atrial pressure pulse).
(II) type B: these receptors discharge during atrial filling.
(III) intermediate type: these receptors discharge during both atrial systole and atrial filling.

Receptors originating from areas other than the atrial endocardium but having Paintal patterns of discharge, will be noted in inverted commas as 'type A', 'type B' and 'intermediate type' depending on the pattern of discharge; these clearly are not atrial receptors.

Paintal (1973a) has suggested that the different patterns of discharge from the atrial receptors were the result of basic differences in the 'natural stimulus' to each type of receptor. Implicit in this suggestion is the possibility that these receptors subserve different physiological functions and such an inference has led some authors to suggest a separate role for type A receptors (e.g. Arndt, Brambring, Hindorf & Röhnelt, 1971). Arndt et al. (1971) were of the opinion that type A receptors formed a component of a feedback system for the control of heart rate. As evidence in support of this hypothesis they presented a positive correlation between the heart rate (beats·min^{-1}) and the average frequency of the discharge of the receptors (spikes·s^{-1}). Such a relationship is hardly surprising in view of the inherent cardiac rhythm of the receptors. However, in order that these receptors function as a negative feedback component of a control system, the central nervous system must clearly be in a position to integrate over a period of time the afferent input from the receptors.

Such a conclusion is at variance with the hypothesis of Ledsome & Linden (1964b) who suggested that stimulation of atrial receptors by distension of balloons at the pulmonary vein–atrial junctions resulted in an increase in heart rate (see Chapter 6). The two contradictory points of view can be reconciled only if it is shown that distension of the pulmonary vein–atrial junctions in the manner of Ledsome & Linden (1964b) resulted in a reduction of the frequency of the discharge of type A receptors. However, Kidd, Ledsome & Linden (1966, 1978) showed that the technique increased the frequency of the discharge in atrial receptors although no specific comment was made by them about the type A receptors probably due to the relative paucity of type A receptors in the dog. In another investigation, Kappagoda, Linden & Sivananthan (1979) observed that distension of the vein–atrial junctions with small balloons stimulated both type A and type B receptors (Fig. 3.2). Thus the conclusions of Arndt et al. (1971) could be sustained only if it is argued that distension of the pulmonary vein–atrial junctions resulted in a disproportionate increase in the discharge of type B receptors which in turn would 'suppress' the discharge from the type A receptors. Such an event remains an unlikely possibility.

A different finding was reported for type B receptors by Zucker & Gilmore (1976); they found an inverse relationship between heart rate and the number of impulses per cardiac cycle, when pacing the heart. This investigation does emphasise, when considered with that of Arndt et al. (1971), discussed above, and with others who claim the adequate stimulus to type B receptors

Receptors discharging into myelinated fibres

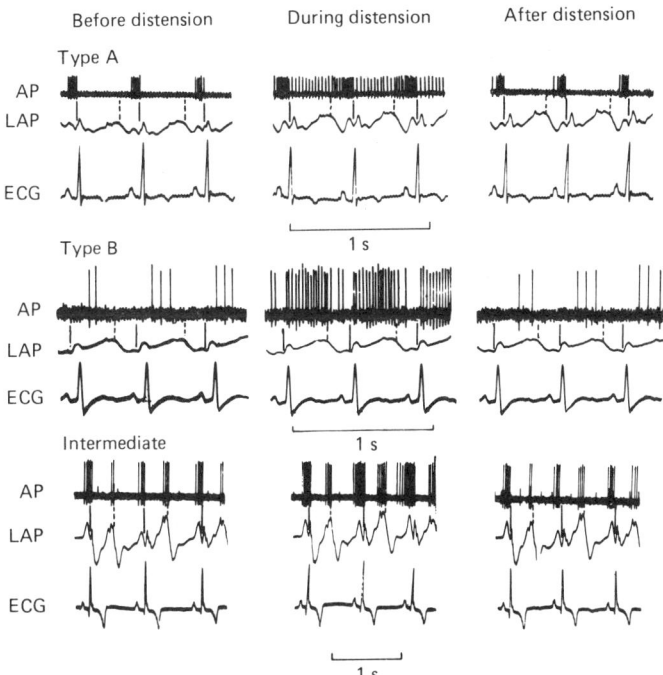

Fig. 3.2. The three Paintal types of atrial receptors and the effect of distension of balloons located at the pulmonary vein–left atrial junctions. In each panel from above downwards: records of action potentials (AP), left atrial pressure (LAP) and electrocardiogram (ECG). Vertical lines are drawn between action potentials and atrial pressure waves to indicate the temporal relationship between both. The continuous line indicates the end of the 'a' wave and the interrupted line indicates the peak of the 'v' wave of the atrial pressure waves. (From Kappagoda, Linden & Sivananthan, 1979.)

involves rates of change of atrial pressure and volume (Homma & Suzuki, 1966; Lloyd, 1975), that the adequate and effective signal to the second-order neurones in the CNS is unknown. In this regard, the evidence of Zucker & Gilmore (1976), that during the simple increase in heart rate the number of impulses in unit time entering the CNS is unchanged, may contribute. But it must be remembered that usually, physiologically, when the heart rate increases there is a concomitant increase in blood flow through the atria, no reduction in atrial volume, and an

Electrophysiology of atrial receptors

increase in the rate of change of pressure and volume up to the peak of the 'v' wave, events which would ensure an increased number of impulses in unit time.

However, the question of whether these atrial receptors can be divided into two groups on evidence other than their patterns of discharge obtained randomly is still a controversial issue, and so will be discussed at length here under several headings, pertaining to the following sources of evidence: histological structure, conduction velocities of their afferent fibres, receptor discharges in isolated tissues, spontaneous and invoked patterns of discharge of receptors and the natural stimulus to receptors.

Histological studies

Complex unencapsulated nerve endings have been demonstrated in the atrial endocardium of many mammalian species (see Chapter 2). In the dog these nerve endings are mainly found at the vein–atrial junctions (e.g. Nonidez, 1937; Miller & Kasahara, 1964) and in the atrial appendages (Floyd et al., 1972). An important conclusion from histological studies is that these nerve endings possess a 'spectrum' of histological appearance (Floyd, 1979; Tranum-Jensen, 1979) ranging from a very diffuse nerve ending occupying a relatively large area (400 μm diameter), to a small compact ending (see Chapter 2). However, Tranum-Jensen (1979) (see Chapter 2) found some end-organs located close to the myocardium and some farther away in the endocardial connective tissue and considered this could form the basis of an explanation of a variation in the time of discharge. It is not thought that this is an adequate explanation of the difference between type A and type B discharge (see later in this chapter).

Coleridge et al. (1957) in a combined histological and physiological study, attempted to study the histological appearances of the receptor endings which gave rise to the characteristic patterns of discharge in vagal nerves. In spite of the fact that both types of discharge were encountered no specific differences were noted in the histological appearances as defined by light microscopy. Thus so far, on morphological grounds the evidence does not support the proposition that these are two basic types

Table 3.1

	Receptors	No. of fibres	Conduction velocity (m·s⁻¹)	
			Range	Mean ± S.E. of mean
Paintal (1953c, 1963a, 1972)				
Cat	Type A	24	12–27	18 ± 0.8
	Type B	37	8–29	18 ± 1.0
Kappagoda, Linden & Mary (1977b)				
Dog	Type A	8	13–42	24 ± 3.6
	Type B	88	12–65	23 ± 1.0
	Intermediate	14	15–45	27 ± 2.3

of receptors. It would be necessary to examine the detailed structure of dendrite-tissue coupling and presumably then, quantitative data would be required.

Conduction velocities

The range of conduction velocities in afferent vagal fibres originating in atrial receptors has been examined in the cat (Paintal, 1953c, 1962). Paintal found that there was a considerable overlap in the conduction velocities of the fibres exhibiting type A and type B patterns of discharge. More recently, Kappagoda, Linden & Mary (1977b) have arrived at the same conclusion based upon the study of conduction velocities in the dog. The findings in both animals are summarised in Table 3.1. Conduction velocities in eight myelinated fibres from atrial receptors in the dog were studied by Coleridge et al. (1973) and they obtained a mean value of 22 m·s⁻¹ (range 12.7 to 27.0); presumably because no difference between types A and B were found they grouped the results together.

There is thus no evidence that the conduction velocities of the two groups of neurones are different.

Isolated tissues

Arndt, Bramring, Hindorf & Röhnelt (1974) examined the pattern of discharge of atrial receptors in the cat during sinusoidal

Electrophysiology of atrial receptors

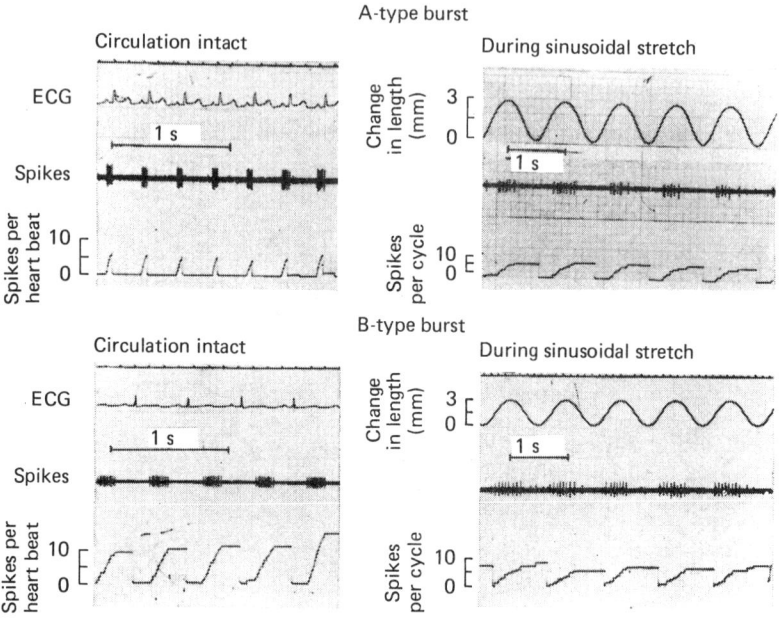

Fig. 3.3. Comparison of the discharge patterns of A- and B-type fibres with intact circulation and during sinusoidal stimulation of the receptor area *in situ*. Note the similarities in discharge with sinusoidal stimulation (right-hand part of the figure). (From Arndt *et al.*, 1974.)

stretch of strips of the atrial wall. Sinusoidal changes in length were imposed *in situ* on the strips of atrial tissue containing atrial receptors and recordings were made from slips of the cervical vagus. The responses were evaluated in terms of (i) the number of spikes per stimulus period, (ii) the average discharge rate, (iii) the instantaneous frequency, and (iv) the phase lag between the forcing function and the instantaneous frequency. The responses obtained from both types of receptor endings were identical (Fig. 3.3). This finding is also consistent with the conclusion that there is only one basic type of receptor.

Spontaneous patterns of discharge

These patterns of discharge of atrial receptors have been extensively studied by several investigators, particularly because of an additional controversy regarding the relative occurrence

Receptors discharging into myelinated fibres

of the various types of receptors. For instance, Coleridge *et al.* (1957) observed that in the dog there were relatively few receptors exhibiting a type A pattern of discharge but Paintal (1963a) claimed that in the cat the two patterns of discharge occurred in relatively equal proportions. These two conflicting views led to considerable speculation regarding the 'true' ratios of the various types of receptors in a given species of animal.

Before attempting to resolve this problem it is necessary first to discuss the experimental methods in some detail. Most investigators define atrial receptors on the basis of the patterns of discharge in fibres of the cervical vagus. However, there are several reports in the literature which have clearly indicated that there are receptor endings in the mediastinum and lung which not only discharge into myelinated vagal fibres but also possess atrial patterns of activity; these fibres account for approximately 10 % of fibres nominally described as atrial receptors (Coleridge *et al.* 1957; Coleridge, Coleridge & Kidd, 1964b; Kappagoda, Linden & Mary, 1976, 1977a, b). The investigation of Kappagoda *et al.* (1976, 1977a, b) showed that five out of the thirty receptors examined in cats and three out of thirty in dogs which were located outside the atrium, were pure 'type A' and thus mimicked atrial receptors. These receptors were found in a variety of sites in the mediastinum. Thus any meaningful comment on the incidence of the various types of atrial receptors can be made only after careful punctate location of the site of origin of the receptor ending. Since the location of a receptor involves sacrificing the animal, the only practical solution to this problem would appear to be location of the *first* receptor encountered with an atrial pattern of discharge during a systematic dissection of the vagi. Provided a sufficiently large number of atrial receptors, i.e. animals, are examined, it should be possible to decide the ratio of the receptors involved. Because of the mounting body of evidence (see later) which indicates clearly that the pattern of discharge in a given receptor can be altered (i.e. converted from one pattern to another) by procedures which alter the pressures and volumes within the atria, care must be taken to maintain an 'adequate' haemodynamic state.

Bearing these considerations in mind Kappagoda *et al.* (1976, 1977a, b) conducted a series of investigations in the cat, dog and rabbit. In all three species, which were investigated under

Electrophysiology of atrial receptors

Table 3.2.

	No. of fibres	Type A	Type B	Intermediate	Number converted
Dog	27	1	16	10	20
Cat	25	2	15	8	16
Rabbit	9	2	1	6	5

anaesthesia with pentobarbitone, they observed atrial nerve fibres exhibiting the three patterns of discharge as described by Paintal (1973a). The ratios of the three types are summarised in Table 3.2.

From these studies, three main conclusions could be drawn at this stage: (a) type A receptors are rare, (b) intermediate type receptors are common and (c) conversion is a relatively frequent occurrence because it was observed in over half the receptors including *all* the type A receptors. The significance of the last finding will be discussed in greater detail later but here it is important to comment that in the absence of a proper technique for the location of the sites of origin of the discharge a significantly different ratio could have been obtained.

Recently, Gupta (1977a) has reported a study in cats which yielded results which were significantly different from those observed by Kappagoda *et al.* (1976) in that a much larger proportion of type A receptors were obtained. A close examination of the data indicates that there may be several explanations for this difference. Gupta (1977a) does not state the precise criteria accepted in the definition of type A receptors and it is possible that his population included many that could be classified as intermediate types. Some support for this proposition is contained in the fact that the type A receptors and the intermediate receptors together formed approximately the same proportion in both studies i.e. 40% as reported by Kappagoda *et al.* (1976) and 41% as reported by Gupta (1977a). It is also not clear whether Gupta (1977a) located the first atrial receptor which he encountered. The possibility of selection has to be considered seriously for two reasons. First, it was not explicitly stated that only one fibre was examined in each cat, and secondly, no receptors located in extra cardiac sites were encountered. Since such receptors have been consistently observed to account for up to 10% of apparent atrial receptors in at least three large series (e.g. Coleridge et al., 1964b; Kappagoda et al., 1976, 1977a, b) it makes the series reported by Gupta (1977a) the exception rather than the rule.

There seems to be no evidence, from an examination of the spontaneous discharge of atrial receptors, that there are two groups of receptors or that there are any great species differences to suggest two groups in some animals and not in others.

Invoked changes in pattern of discharge

The unique nature of the type A and type B receptors has been challenged by a series of reports showing that one pattern of discharge can be converted to another.

There have been several such sporadic reports in the literature (e.g. Henry & Pearce, 1956; Coleridge et al., 1957; Neil & Joels, 1961) but in spite of these observations, Paintal (1972) has tended to minimise their significance by pointing out that these conversions were in fact observed under 'abnormal haemodynamic' conditions. To quote Paintal (1972), 'The type A receptors studied by Arndt et al. (1971) are noteworthy because in all 16 of them a 'v' burst of impulses was not produced by infusion, bleeding or injection of adrenaline. This is not unexpected in the cat but it is important to mention this point because it is sometimes held that conversion of one type of pattern (e.g. A type) into another is a *common occurrence*.' It is worthy of comment on the work of Arndt et al. (1971) that this sequence of infusion *before* bleeding and the injection of adrenaline was not used in this 'test' procedure. In fact their Fig. 1 (Arndt et al., 1971) clearly shows that the sequence started with haemorrhage. Such a test procedure requiring haemorrhage *before* infusion and injection of adrenaline is usually inadequate to convert type A discharge into an intermediate type. In monkeys, Zucker & Gilmore (1977) commented that type A receptors did not increase their discharge during infusion but no indication is given that any of the receptors were located. However, no specific attempts were made to convert these receptors.

Because of the extreme importance of this finding to the

definition of the natural stimulus, Mary (Kappagoda et al., 1976, 1977a, b) re-investigated this problem in cats, dogs and rabbits with the specific intention of determining precisely the proportion of receptors which could in fact be converted from one type to another. The techniques used for converting the patterns of discharge were similar to those adopted by other workers in the field – namely (i) infusion of dextran up to 20% of estimated blood volume, (ii) haemorrhage up to 10% of estimated blood volume, (iii) administration of adrenaline, (iv) prolonged inspiration, (v) prolonged expiration, and (vi) partial occlusion of the aorta and the pulmonary artery. At the conclusion of each experiment the chest was opened and the site of origin of the discharge was located precisely in the manner of Coleridge et al. (1957). From these studies several significant findings emerged.

Of twenty-five *atrial fibres* investigated in the cat (Kappagoda et al., 1976) it was possible to alter the pattern of discharge (i.e. convert from one type to another) in sixteen. These included two type A receptors, ten type B receptors and four intermediate type receptors (see later). Since this investigation yielded only two type A receptors both of which were converted, a further study was undertaken selectively to examine the type A receptors. This study yielded five type A receptors which were located to the atria and all were converted. The other interesting feature of this study was the finding that there was a group of receptor endings which discharged with a 'type A' pattern but which could not be converted. These units were *all* located at sites other than the endocardium. The fact that some 'type A' receptors were not located in the atria had previously been reported. For instance Coleridge et al. (1957) using precise punctate localisation found two 'atrial' receptors; one in the left main bronchus and one in the oesophagus. Another receptor, discharging in time with atrial systole with a discrete burst of activity typical of a type A receptor, was located in the right branch of the pulmonary artery behind the superior vena cava (Coleridge & Kidd, 1960). One must agree with their comment that 'a receptor cannot be assigned with certainty to a particular great vessel or chamber of the heart by inspection of the discharge and its relationship to the e.c.g.; it must be located by appropriate means in the animal with open chest'. In the

Receptors discharging into myelinated fibres

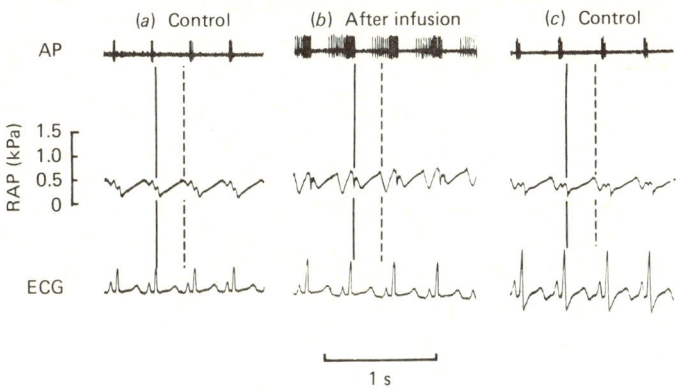

Fig. 3.4. 'Conversion' of the pattern of discharge in a left atrial type A receptor. From above downwards records of action potentials (AP), right atrial pressure (RAP) and electrocardiogram (ECG). The vertical lines are drawn to show the temporal relationship between bursts of action potentials and waves of the atrial pressure pulse. The continuous line indicates the end of the 'a' wave and the interrupted line indicates the peak of the 'v' wave of the atrial pressure pulse: (*a*) initial control record, (*b*) records obtained after infusion of dextran (25 cm^3, i.v.); (*c*) final control record. During the initial control period this receptor possessed a type A pattern of discharge. Following infusion of dextran, the pattern of discharge was that of an intermediate type unit. During the final control period this receptor regained its initial pattern of discharge, i.e. type A. (From Kappagoda, Linden & Mary, 1976.)

subsequent study in the dog and rabbit, Mary (Kappagoda, Linden & Mary, 1977*a*, *b*) obtained findings which were qualitatively similar to those observed in the cat.

From these two investigations, it was possible to draw certain conclusions regarding the procedures which were successful in effecting a conversion of the pattern of discharge of a given receptor. Conversion of receptors with type A patterns of discharge into type B or intermediate type patterns (i.e. appearance of spikes during atrial filling, or the disappearance of those occurring during atrial contraction) was achieved by procedures which increased atrial pressure and hence probably atrial volume – e.g. infusion, partial occlusion of aorta and the pulmonary artery (Fig. 3.4). Conversion of receptors with type B patterns of discharge into type A or intermediate patterns i.e. appearance of spikes during atrial contraction or the

Electrophysiology of atrial receptors

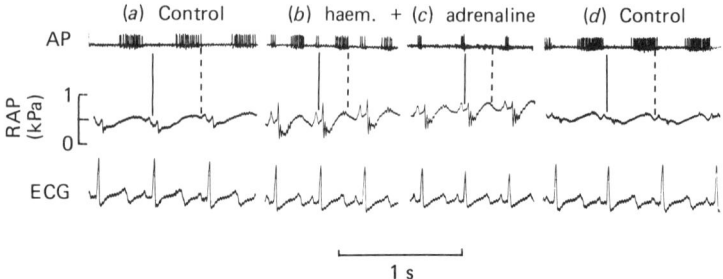

Fig. 3.5. 'Conversion' of the pattern of discharge in a left atrial type B receptor. The abbreviations and the position of the vertical lines are as in Fig. 3.4. (a) Initial control record; (b) and (c), two parts of a continuous recording taken during an attempt at conversion of the pattern of discharge i.e. bleeding (haemorrhage, 13 cm³) and administration of adrenaline (1.0 μg, i.v.); (d) final control record. During the initial control period this receptor exhibited a burst of activity during the 'v' wave of atrial pressure pulse, i.e. type B. (b) and (c) shows the same receptor discharging as an intermediate type and as a type A unit. During the final control period the receptor discharged as a type B unit again. (From Kappagoda et al., 1976.)

disappearance of those occurring during filling) was achieved by procedures which decreased atrial pressure and/or atrial volume, e.g. haemorrhage and administration of adrenaline (Fig. 3.5). Thus any hypothesis which seeks to explain the natural stimulus to the atrial receptors must clearly be able to explain these observations relating to conversion of the various patterns of discharge (see later).

The evidence in this section does not support the proposition that there are two groups of atrial receptors.

Natural stimulus to atrial receptors

Many reports have considered the possible natural stimuli to the atrial receptors and on the basis of their conclusions have claimed to sustain the proposition that this division of the receptors into type A and type B could support a functional division. These reports will be discussed here.

There is a considerable body of evidence that the stimulus to atrial receptors is mechanical in nature (see Paintal, 1972). There are, however, several reports in the literature which suggest that these receptors may also be stimulated by a variety of chemical substances such as veratridine, pituitrin, germitridine (Paintal, 1953b, 1955, 1957; Neil & Joels, 1961), but not by changes in plasma osmolality (Gilmore & Zucker, 1974a). Since many of these reports suffered from the absence of (a) precise location of the origin of the nerve endings (Paintal, 1955, 1957) and (b) simultaneous recordings of pressure within the cardio-vascular system, any conclusions regarding a direct effect of chemicals on these receptors must be viewed with some scepticism. There is no doubt that injection of these substances intravenously (Neil & Joels, 1961) or intra-atrially (Paintal, 1964) increases the rate of discharge in fibres carrying atrial patterns of discharge, but any further extrapolations from these findings is clearly unwarranted. It is emphasised that these exogenous chemical substances were employed merely as a means of stimulating the receptors, and not as a suitable technique for demonstrating that the receptors were true chemoreceptors (Dawes & Comroe, 1954). To show the latter would clearly require the demonstration of responses related to changes in physiological chemical agents such as pO_2, pCO_2 and pH.

Among these other possible chemical stimuli for atrial receptors, arterial pO_2 and pCO_2 have been considered (Paintal, 1973a). The former seems unlikely as atrial receptors do not alter their activity in a way predictable for chemoreceptors but continue to discharge in response to mechanical stimuli for a considerable period after cessation of the circulation (e.g. Coleridge et al., 1957) and evidence in favour of the latter is not available.

Thus, on evidence, it would be appropriate to consider the 'natural' stimulus for the atrial receptors to be related to mechanical events in the heart as opposed to chemical factors. Further, in view of the extent of the controversy surrounding the proposition that there are functionally different types of receptor, each of the two main types of atrial receptor will be considered separately.

Type B receptors. The pattern of discharge of type B receptors is closely related to the 'v' wave of the atrial pressure pulse – developing typically in a crescendo fashion. In spontaneously breathing animals it is also found that the frequency of discharge (spikes per cycle) increases with inspiration and diminishes with expiration. These changes are reversed in animals which are artificially ventilated but it must be appreciated that these changes merely reflect the changes in transmural atrial pressure which are known to occur during the respiratory cycle.

Langrehr (1960) suggested that the discharge from these receptors is related to the pull exerted on the atrial wall due to ventricular contraction. In his study, Langrehr (1960) found a significant correlation between the impulse frequency in the receptors studied and the mean pressure in the atrium. He was also able to demonstrate a significant relationship between impulse frequency and the force of ventricular contraction as expressed by the ratio stroke volume/systolic time. From these results, he concluded that ventricular contraction caused a pull on the atrial wall which in turn distorted the receptor ending. Considering the experimental techniques and the records published in the paper (Langrehr, 1960) it is apparent that no attempt was made to locate the receptors studied, and the pattern of discharge would also not satisfy the commonly held criteria for atrial receptors, e.g. the receptor shown in Fig. 2 of his paper (Langrehr, 1960) appears to have most of its discharge during ventricular systole.

To provide evidence with which to resolve this controversy, Paintal (1963b) attempted to define the natural stimulus to the type B atrial receptors by correlating the various components of the atrial pressure pulse with the frequency of the discharge. He found that there was an almost linear relationship between the mean atrial pressure and the frequency of the discharge – an observation which has also been reported by several other investigators (e.g. Dickinson, 1950; Langrehr, 1960; Kappagoda, Linden & Snow, 1972b). Paintal (1963b) defined mean atrial pressure as the average of the pressures at the peak of the 'v' wave and at the initial part of this wave of the atrial pressure pulse. He then proceeded to investigate the relationship between the frequency of the discharge and two components of the 'v' wave of the atrial pressure pulse – namely the amplitude ('initial pressure to peak') and the peak. Infusion resulted in parallel changes in amplitude, peak pressure and discharge of atrial receptors; bleeding resulted in parallel changes only in amplitude

Receptors discharging into myelinated fibres

and discharge. Paintal (1963b) suggested that the adequate stimulus for atrial receptors was a pulsatile increase in atrial volume and that the relationship to ventricular events was a secondary phenomenon.

Hakumäki (1970) also investigated this problem and suggested that the impulse activity in type B receptors was related to the so-called 'pressure impulse' which was defined as the product of the gradient of the upstroke of 'v' wave and its duration. This value in fact will be equal to that at the height of the 'v' wave. Thus the relationship depicted in Fig. 5 of this paper (Hakumäki, 1970) between the number of impulses and the 'pressure impulse' in individual cardiac cycles is similar to that shown by Paintal (1963b).

Gilmore & Zucker (1974b), in dogs, have also studied the effect of changes in atrial pressure on the discharge pattern of type B atrial receptors. The atrial pressure was altered either by infusing isotonic saline or by the withdrawal of blood. They related the frequency of the discharge (spikes per cycle) to two components of the atrial pressure pulse, namely the peak pressure of the 'v' wave and the amplitude of the 'v' wave (cf. Paintal, 1963b). The discharge of the receptor exhibited hysteresis; the discharge during the increase in atrial pressure (i.e. both the peak and the amplitude of the 'v' wave) was different from that during the decrease in pressure (Fig. 3.6). It was claimed that there was no alteration in the compliance of the atrial muscle. The technique for measuring atrial compliance is open to criticism, but the conclusion that changes in atrial pressure affect the degree of discharge of type B receptors is inescapable. If it is accepted that the compliance of the atrial muscle does not change, then the frequency of discharge of a type B receptor reflects the volume of the atrium during atrial filling (e.g. Linden, 1973); in addition since ventricular systole is relatively constant, the number of impulses per cardiac cycle and the frequency of discharge will be related to the rate of filling, and thus reflect inflow, venous return and cardiac output (Linden, 1973).

In a further investigation examining the response of type B atrial receptors, again in dogs, Zucker & Gilmore (1976) have shown that with an increase in heart rate brought about by pacing the right atrial appendage, the number of impulses per

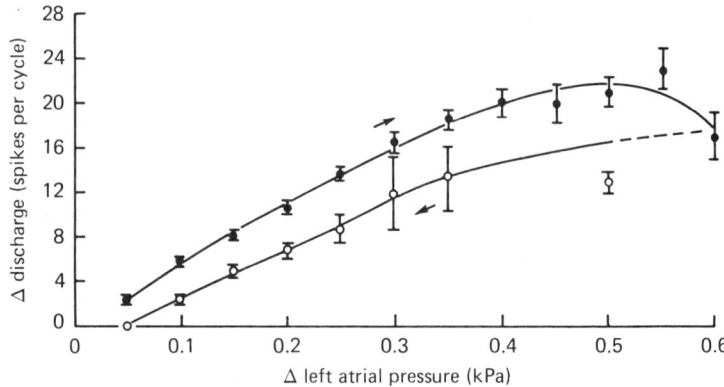

Fig. 3.6. Mean data of the hysteresis recorded from 24 type B atrial receptors. The changes in left atrial pressure have been grouped for each 0.05 kPa change. ●, expansion; ○, haemorrhage. Vertical bars indicate S.E. of mean. (From Gilmore & Zucker, 1974b.)

cycle exhibited an inverse relationship with the heart rate over the range 90–240 beats·min^{-1}. There were concomitant reductions in atrial pressure and the number of impulses per cycle was reduced. Though these relationships may vary, depending on the blood volume, they suggest that there is a relationship between atrial volume and the discharge of type B atrial receptors.

However, it is apparent from these investigations that there is no evidence to suggest other than that the adequate stimulus to type B atrial receptors is a change in tension in the atrial wall brought about by a change in volume in the atrium.

Type A receptors. The discharge of the type A receptors coincides with the 'a' wave of the atrial pressure pulse. In an attempt to define the natural stimulus for these receptors, Arndt *et al.* (1971) tried to relate the frequency of the discharge (spikes per cycle) to several components of the 'a' wave. They found no correlations between the frequency and the pressure at the commencement of the 'a' wave, or between the slope of the 'a' wave and the amplitude of the 'a' wave. In general it was found that in a total of sixteen type A receptors studied, the number of spikes per cardiac cycle remained 'more or less' constant (Fig. 3.7) when atrial mechanics were altered by cardiac pacing,

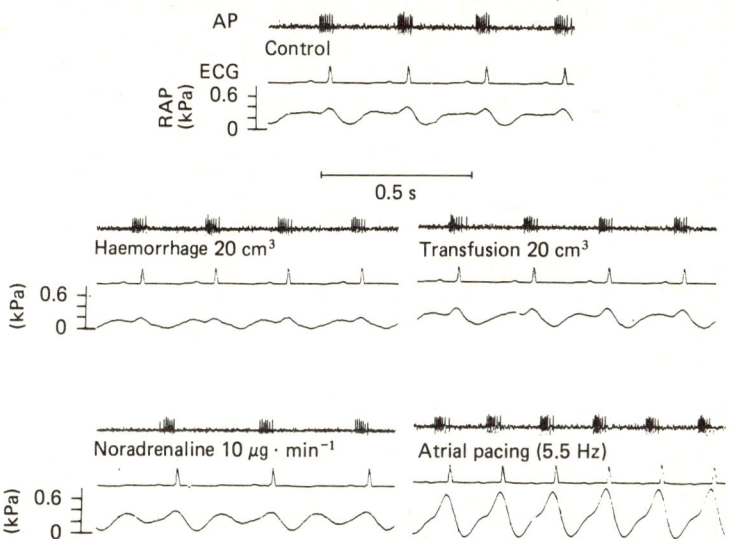

Fig. 3.7. Atrial type A burst. Representative example of the discharge pattern of an atrial type A burst with changing atrial mechanics. Note that the number of action potentials remains more or less constant despite wide fluctuations in the pressure components of the atrial 'a' wave. AP, action potentials; RAP, right atrial pressure; ECG, electrocardiogram. (From Arndt et al., 1971.)

changes in blood volume (bleeding 10–30% of estimated volume) and by infusion of noradrenaline (4, 7.5 and 10 μg·min^{-1} respectively). None of these receptors was located. Therefore doubt must be cast on the conclusions because some so-called 'type A' receptors have been found in sites other than the atria and true type A receptors can all be converted to intermediate receptors by techniques similar to the above (see earlier in this chapter and Kappagoda et al., 1976, 1977b). However, again it is apparent that the adequate stimulus to type A atrial receptors could be an increase in tension in the wall of the atrium brought about by atrial contraction.

Whilst these results revealed little about the natural stimulus for these receptors, Arndt et al. (1971) were of the opinion that the type A receptors formed a component of a feedback system for the control of heart rate.

Electrophysiology of atrial receptors

From the evidence discussed in this section there is, again, only evidence which allows a hypothesis that there is a single adequate stimulus to both types of atrial receptor, and no support for the proposal that there are two groups of receptors.

An alternative hypothesis. An alternative description of the natural stimulus to the atrial receptor can be based on the location of the atrial receptors at the vein–atrial junctions.

In the investigations described by Kappagoda *et al.* (1976, 1977*b*) all the receptors that could be converted were eventually located to various sites in the atrial endocardium. It was also observed that the precise location of a receptor in the atrial wall could have a bearing on the pattern of its discharge. For instance, in the cat (Kappagoda *et al.*, 1976) all the type A receptors were located in the atria relatively close to the flexures at the entrances of the veins (Fig. 3.8). The type B receptors were found in positions remote from the flexures at the vein–atrial junctions, i.e. in the pulmonary veins more distally than the location of type A receptors and along the lateral walls of the atria. No type A receptors and no intermediate receptors were found on the lateral walls of the atria or in the distal parts of the veins.

In the dog, receptors with type A and intermediate patterns of discharge were also found at the vein–atrial junctions (Kappagoda *et al.*, 1977*b*). Receptors with type B patterns were found at the vein–atrial junctions and sites remote from the vein–atrial flexures such as the distal parts of the pulmonary veins and the lateral atrial walls. All the type B receptors which could not be converted were located in the lateral walls of the atria or the distal regions of the pulmonary veins as had been found in the investigation in the cat (Fig. 3.8). This information about the location of the receptors is incorporated in a hypothesis which seeks to explain the natural stimulus to the atrial receptors. The argument leading to this hypothesis can best be developed by first considering two aspects of the problem: the mechanical stresses known to affect the discharge from atrial receptors and the movements of the atrial walls.

With respect to the mechanical stimuli to the atrial receptors, it has been demonstrated that the discharge from left atrial receptors is a function of the wall tension. Kidd *et al.* (1966,

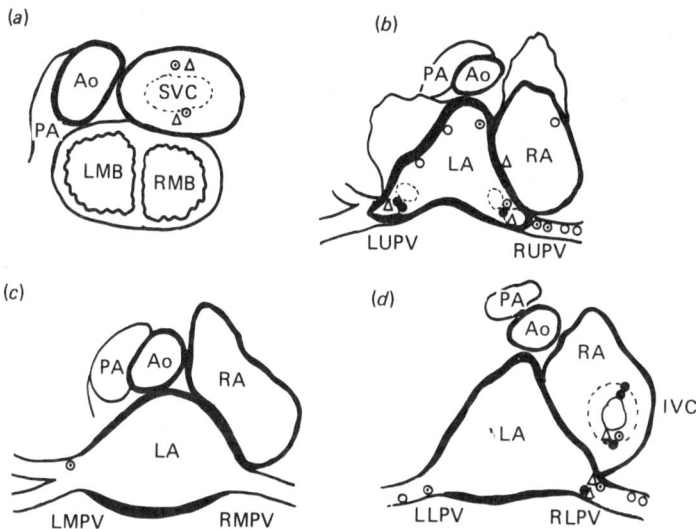

Fig. 3.8. A schematic diagram drawn from transverse sections made at four levels in the heart of a cat to demonstrate locations of 33 atrial receptors in the endocardium of the vein–atrial system. The levels of the sections were as follows: (a) 1 cm above the entrance of the superior vena cava (SVC) into the right atrium (RA); (b) entrances of upper pulmonary veins (L and RUPV) into the left atrium (LA); (c) entrances of the middle pulmonary veins (L and RMPV) into the left atrium; (d) entrances of lower pulmonary veins (L and RLPV) into the left atrium. ●, type A units, all of which were converted; ○, 'type B' units, which could not be converted; ⊙, type B units which could be converted; △, intermediate units. All the type A receptors were located at the entrance of the veins into the atria whereas all type B receptors which could not be converted were located in the pulmonary veins distal to their entrances into the left atrium or on the lateral walls of the atria. RMB, right main bronchus; LMB, left main bronchus; Ao, aorta; PA, pulmonary artery; and IVC, inferior vena cava. (From Kappagoda, Linden & Mary, 1976.)

1978) investigated the activity of these receptors under two experimental conditions: first, with the receptors located in a pouch prepared from part of the left atrium and perfused using pulsatile pressures and secondly, with the same receptors in the wall of the intact atrium and subjected to the pulsatile atrial pressure pulses. When the threshold pressures for the activation of the receptors under the two conditions were compared it was found that the threshold pressure for a receptor either type A or type B, in an intact atrium, was considerably smaller than that of the same receptor when studied in an atrial pouch. Considering the Law of Laplace (tension = radius × distending pressure), and roughly applying it to the atrium, it is apparent that the same wall tension can be achieved when the radius is small (in the pouch) as when the radius is large (in the whole intact atrium), but only at a greater pressure. Thus the findings of Kidd *et al.* (1966, 1978) are entirely consistent with the behaviour of receptors which respond to changes in wall tension.

Also there is support for this thesis from experiments in which the changes in frequency of discharge of atrial receptors have been related to the atrial pressure in animals of various sizes and thus with various sizes of atrium. Zucker & Gilmore (1975) contrasted the relationship between the change in discharge (spikes per cycle) and the change in left atrial pressure between the dog (average weight, 18 kg) and the rhesus monkey (average weight, about 5 kg). They found that for the same change in pressure there was a much smaller change in discharge of the atrial receptors in the monkey than the dog. Zucker & Gilmore (1975) have a complicated explanation for the difference between the rate of discharge in the primate as opposed to that in the dog; the explanation is based on 'the evolution of an upright or semi-upright posture' and they 'speculate that a less sensitive atrial receptor mechanism may be homeostatically appropriate in the primate'. However, this explanation is most unlikely; instead it is probable that it is really the comparable sizes of the atria in the two species that are of importance, the chamber of the atrium being much smaller in the smaller animal. Such an explanation would fit the hypothesis proposed above. There is also some support for this explanation from results obtained in the course of other investigations (Linden & Mary, unpublished). During investigations in which infusions of dextran in the dog and rabbit were given, the change in discharge (spikes per cardiac cycle) of atrial receptors was related to changes in atrial pressure, in the manner of Zucker & Gilmore (1975). In the event an average value of the change in discharge of about 3 impulses per cardiac cycle per 0.1 kPa pressure change was recorded in the dog, which was greater than that in the rabbit (about 0.2 impulses per cardiac cycle per 0.1 kPa). The results obtained in the dog are almost identical to those of Zucker &

Receptors discharging into myelinated fibres

Gilmore (1975); those they observed in the primate (about 0.7 impulses per cardiac cycle per 0.1 kPa) fall between those of the dog and the rabbit. The most likely explanation of the differences between all the animals is that proposed above which related the 'sensitivities' of the various atrial receptors directly to the sizes of the atria in which they are situated, and is fully explained by relying on the Law of Laplace.

Regarding the movement of the atrial wall, there is evidence which indicates that during atrial contraction there are parts of the atria which undergo extensive mechanical distortion. For instance in the left atrium, during atrial systole, the posterior wall is relatively fixed while the free lateral walls tend to move 'centripetally' (Gribbe, Lind, Linko & Wegelius, 1958). Such a movement would result in the junctional region around the pulmonary vein–atrial orifices being the area subjected to the greatest degree of mechanical distortion. Also, this relatively fixed posterior portion of the atrial wall would tend to diminish in area when the atrium is smaller (i.e. after haemorrhage) and to increase when the atrium is larger (i.e. after infusion) with corresponding movements of the points of inflexion at its periphery. In addition, there are other inflexions, with conclastic and synclastic curvatures, on the atrial wall at the entrances of the pulmonary veins and the relative positions of these would also be shifted as the size of the atrium is altered. In the case of the right atrium, it is suggested that during atrial systole, the points of inflexion change in a similar manner at the junctions of the superior and inferior venae cavae and the atrium (Kjellberg & Olsson, 1954; Lind & Wegelius, 1956). Thus the regions immediately adjacent to the caval orifices will be subject to mechanical distortion. These considerations become of major importance when related to the fact that the atrial receptors are found mainly at the vein–atrial junctions (see Chapter 2 for histological, and this chapter for electrophysiological, evidence).

With these two considerations in mind, it is easy to understand that a type B discharge would result from a rise in wall tension during filling. Such a discharge would increase during infusions and diminish during haemorrhage. On the other hand, it is suggested that a type A discharge would occur as a result of a localised rise in wall tension (i.e. stretch) brought about by atrial contraction, which in turn would occur due to one of two mechanisms. First, a contraction of atrial muscle would cause a simple 'tug' on a relatively fixed portion of atrial wall such as a vein–atrial junction and secondly, atrial contraction itself would change the points of inflexion at the flexures of the vein–atrial junctions which could stimulate the receptors by mechanical distortion rather than by simple linear increase in tension.

If such a hypothesis is correct then four findings must be confirmed. Firstly, there should not be any type A units on the lateral walls of the atria and in the distal regions of the great veins. Secondly, the type A (and intermediate) units should be confined to those regions which are subject to such distortions as those described above, i.e. they should be located around the relatively fixed posterior wall of the left atrium or near the flexures at the vein–atrial junctions. Thirdly, conversion should be effected by measures designed to alter the volume of the atria and hence the area of the relatively fixed posterior wall. Thus receptors located at the edge of the fixed region or on the flexures at the vein–atrial junctions would be moved relative to their former position at these points of great mechanical distortion (Fig. 3.9). Finally, no type B units that could not be converted should be located in the regions containing type A receptors but instead should be positioned on the lateral walls and in the distal regions of the pulmonary veins. The findings in the two investigations described by Kappagoda *et al.* (1976, 1977*b*) are not in conflict with these propositions and support the hypothesis that the pattern of discharge of atrial receptors is explained purely in terms of the mechanical events in the atria and the anatomical position of the receptors in relation to the vein–atrial junctions.

In the context of this hypothesis, it is interesting to consider recent publications by Recordati and his colleagues (Recordati, Lombardi, Bishop & Malliani, 1975, 1976). In the cat, they observed (Recordati *et al.*, 1975) that the discharge from type B receptors was dependent on the tension and the rate of change of tension in the atrial wall, tension being calculated from the Law of Laplace. Evidence was also presented to indicate that an inotropic change in the atrial muscle exerted an influence through changes in wall tension which resulted from alterations

Receptors discharging into myelinated fibres

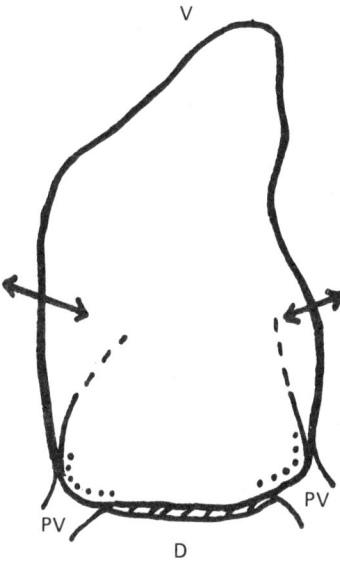

Fig. 3.9. A schematic diagram of the left atrium demonstrating movements of the atrial walls associated with changes in atrial size. The interrupted lines indicate the position of the lateral walls during atrial contraction. V, ventral, D, dorsal. During contraction the dorsal wall remains relatively fixed and the free lateral walls move inwards; the borders of the dorsal wall, at the entrances (dotted lines) of the pulmonary veins (PV), are subjected to the greatest degree of distortion during atrial contraction.

in atrial volume and pressure. In a subsequent investigation, Recordati *et al.* (1976), using a method of recording instantaneous changes in dimension of the right atrial wall of the cat, Recordati, Lombardi, Malliani & Brown (1974), studied the effect of inotropic interventions on type A receptors. They concluded that the systolic discharge from type A atrial receptors is a function of active tension developed by atrial muscle during contraction. This observation is consistent with the hypothesis outlined above in that a positive inotropic effect would result in a more forceful atrial contraction and hence a greater mechanical distortion of the receptor during systole – provided the receptor was located at a site which renders it likely to be so distorted, i.e. it is a type A receptor. Thus in a type A receptor, the discharge could be increased by inotropic changes independent of changes in volume, a finding which was confirmed by Recordati *et al.* (1976). Changes in volume independent of inotropic changes merely resulted in an alteration of the discharge during filling, i.e. conversion to intermediate type. This finding led the authors to conclude that only type A receptors may display an intermediate pattern of discharge.

Examining only type A and intermediate receptors in cats Recordati (1978) has confirmed the results of Kappagoda *et al.* (1976, 1977*b*) in that the responses of the receptors during atrial systole were mainly dependent upon the state of contraction of atrial muscle. The evidence of the location of the receptors examined by Recordati (1978) fits the hypothesis proposed here.

An investigation conducted in rabbits (Kappagoda *et al.*, 1977*b*) also lends further support to this hypothesis. In the rabbit there is a relative preponderance of receptors which show a discharge during atrial contraction (i.e. type A and intermediate type). In comparison with the dog and the cat, the rabbit clearly possesses a smaller atrium. Since the sizes of receptors are not significantly different in the three species (Miller & Kasahara, 1964), and since it is likely that the atrial movements are likely to be qualitatively the same, it could be argued that a relatively larger proportion of atrial receptors will be distorted during contraction of the smaller heart; hence the preponderance of intermediate and type A units. A similar explanation may be put forward to explain the preponderance of type A receptors observed in the Rhesus monkey (Zucker & Gilmore, 1977) although, as the receptors were not located, it is not known how many true type A receptors were being examined.

Conclusions. The evidence so far suggests that there is only one basic type of Paintal-type atrial receptor that responds to changes in wall tension. Such changes in wall tension could occur from atrial filling or from distortion during atrial contraction. Depending on the position of the receptor in the endocardium it could be affected by one or both of the above mechanisms. Thus if a classification of atrial receptors based on the pattern of discharge is to be maintained Paintal type B should form one group and Paintal intermediate type the second group. The latter would contain all those receptors within the atrial endocardium which on first examination appear to have either a type A or an intermediate pattern. All true 'type A' receptors (i.e. could not be converted to intermediate) were found not to be in the atrium but to reside in other structures outside the heart.

In terms of reflexes demonstrable under experimental conditions, the techniques used for stimulating these receptors (see Chapters 4–10) are clearly capable of stimulating all types of atrial receptors. There is as yet no evidence to indicate that the responses observed can be attributed to the stimulation of any one of the types of atrial receptor described in this chapter. However, this discussion does not constitute an argument for or against the idea that these different patterns of discharge form the basis for the existence of different biological roles for these receptors.

Receptors which discharge into non-myelinated fibres in the vagi

The second group of atrial receptors worthy of comment are those which, when stimulated, discharge into non-myelinated fibres in the vagi. Though their existence has long been suspected from the stimulation experiments of Oberg and his colleagues (see Chapter 7), these fibres were first recognised as originating in the atria of the dog by Sleight & Widdicombe (1965) and Coleridge *et al.* (1973). As pointed out in Chapter 2, the receptors have not been recognised histologically. Most of the investigations of activity in C fibres with receptors in the heart have been concerned with ventricular receptors and brief reference to these investigations will be made to form a background against which to judge the function of atrial receptors discharging into non-myelinated fibres.

Spontaneous discharge

In their electrophysiological examination of ventricular receptors, the majority of the receptors (ten out of fourteen) investigated by Sleight & Widdicombe (1965) discharged into non-myelinated fibres in the vagi and had conduction velocities less than $2 \text{ m} \cdot \text{s}^{-1}$. A cardiac rhythm was an unusual feature of these receptors. Ten years previously Paintal (1955) had

Electrophysiology of atrial receptors

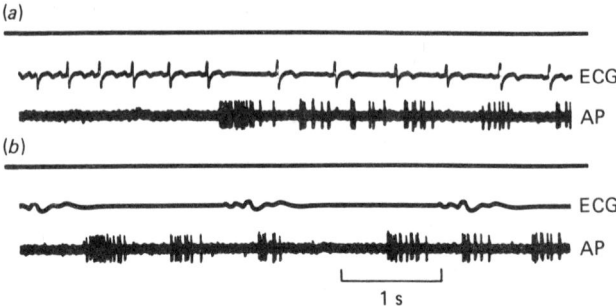

Fig. 3.10. Ventricular receptor with an irregular discharge (right vagal nerve). From above downwards, in each panel, datum line; electrocardiogram (ECG); action potentials (AP). (a) Veratridine, 7 μg·kg^{-1} injected into the left atrium 4 s before the beginning of the record; note cardiac slowing. (b) Bursts of impulses produced by stroking the ventral epicardial surface of the left ventricle after the animal had been killed, the heart opened and the endocardium pared away from this part of the ventricular wall. (Part of a figure from Coleridge et al., 1964b.)

described in the cat a group of ventricular receptors which discharged into vagal fibres and these receptors were also activated by intra-atrial injections of veratridine. These fibres possessed a cardiac rhythm and were estimated (on the basis of spike height) to have conduction velocities of the order of 10–20 m·s^{-1}. The situation regarding the receptors in the ventricle was clarified further by the experiments of Coleridge et al. (1964b) who demonstrated in the dog the existence of both types of ventricular receptors and in their hands only the ones which had an irregular discharge (Fig. 3.10) were activated by veratridine. For various reasons little useful comment can be made about the ventricular receptors showing a pulsatile discharge in time with the heart beat (see Fig. 4 in Coleridge et al., 1964b); they are few in number and little else is known about them. As Paintal (1972) has suggested, the 'coronary artery' mechanoreceptors of Brown (1965, 1966) really belong to this group of receptors and are not 'coronary' receptors. However, because Brown showed that stimulation of these receptors caused bradycardia and hypotension they can probably be included in the large group of systemic and pulmonary baroreceptors known to have this response.

Receptors discharging into non-myelinated fibres

The first substantial electrophysiological description of activity in C fibres appeared in 1973 (Coleridge et al., 1973). In this paper a group of afferent nerve endings supplied by C fibres or the smallest myelinated fibres was described in both dogs and cats. Most of the endings showed only a sparse discharge under normal conditions but they were stimulated by substances such as capsaicin, phenyldiguanide or veratridine injected into the blood stream. A certain proportion of the fibres they described undoubtedly originated from the atria. In fact, their distribution overlapped the areas of origin of the myelinated fibres illustrated in Fig. 3.11. They also showed that these atrial fibres responded to increases in atrial pressure produced by distension of balloons in the atrial lumen. More recently Thorén (1976a) examined trains of impulses in fibres in the vagi of cats and showed that the activity in the nerve endings, subsequently located in the atrial wall, did in fact respond to changes in atrial pressure. The mean spontaneous rate of discharge from the fourteen receptors examined was 1.4 spikes$\cdot$s^{-1} at a mean control pressure in the right atrium of 0.4 kPa and in the left of 0.9 kPa. The highest spontaneous discharge noted was 3.7 spikes$\cdot$s^{-1}. Generally there was no cardiac rhythm to the discharge but three receptors were usually activated during the 'a' wave, and two during the 'v' wave, of the atrial pressure pulse. Changes in atrial pressure brought about by infusion or bleeding the animal resulted in changes in activity in the fibres from both right and left atria (Fig. 3.12). The investigations of Thames (Thames, Donald & Shepherd, 1977; Thames, 1979) confirmed in the cat, with closed chest, breathing spontaneously, these results of Thorén (1976a). Three out of eight left atrial receptors discharging into non-myelinated fibres (mean conduction velocity, 1.2 spikes$\cdot$s^{-1}) were silent under testing conditions; the discharge of the remaining fibres was irregular. Atrial receptors discharged with a cardiac rhythm during end inspiration and early expiration.

In the course of differentiating, by vagal cooling, between the function of atrial myelinated fibres and C fibres, Kappagoda, Linden & Sivananthan (1979) examined twelve atrial receptors which discharged into non-myelinated (C) fibres in the vagi of the dog. Ten of the receptors possessed an irregular discharge and did not exhibit any cardiac rhythm. The activity in two fibres possessed a cardiac rhythm during the control period and

Electrophysiology of atrial receptors

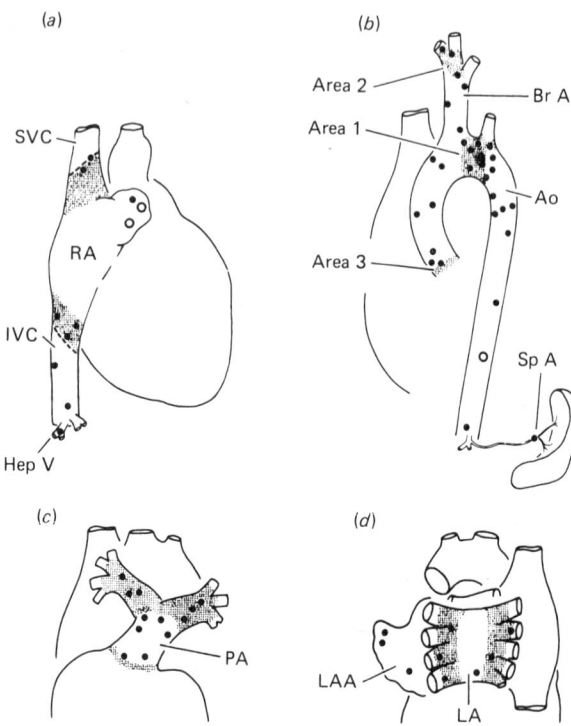

Fig. 3.11. Distribution of vascular endings compared with distribution of atrial and arterial mechanoreceptors supplied by large myelinated vagal fibres. (a) Right lateral view of heart and great veins; the broken lines indicate the attachment of the pericardium to the venae cavae. (b) Ventral view of the aorta. (c) Ventral view of the pulmonary artery. (d) Dorsal view of the left atrium. Each of the 61 solid circles represents a vascular ending whose potentials were recorded and whose location was determined accurately by punctate stimulation. Each of the three open circles represents a group of vascular endings whose impulses were recorded from a multifibre vagal strand. The stippling represents the main areas in which the endings of large myelinated vagal fibres are located (see text). (a) right atrio-venous receptors; (b) aortic baroreceptors; (c) pulmonary arterial baroreceptors; and (d) left atrio-venous receptors. Ao, aorta; Br A, brachiocephalic artery; PA, pulmonary artery; Sp A, splenic artery; RA, right atrium; LA, left atrium; SVC, superior vena cava; IVC, inferior vena cava; Hep V, hepatic veins; and LAA, left atrial appendage. (From Coleridge et al., 1973.)

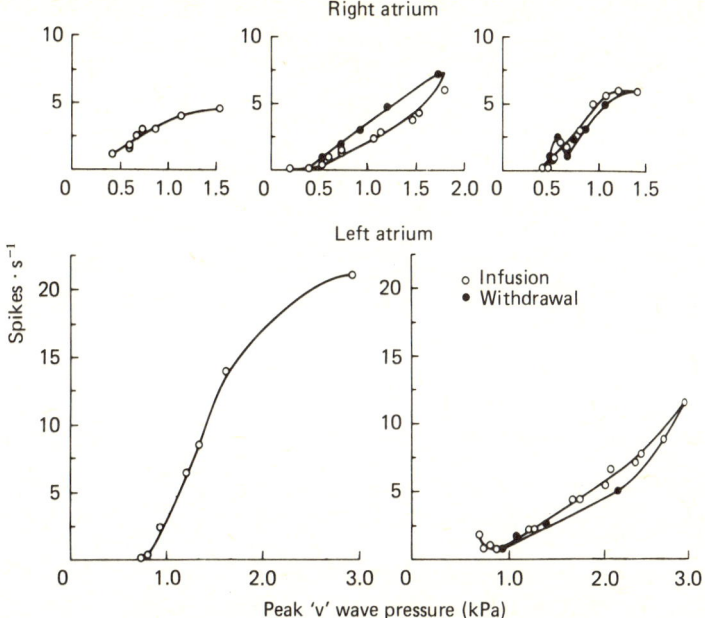

Fig. 3.12. Receptor activity in atrial C fibres (three right atrium; two left atrium) plotted against peak 'v' wave pressure during graded increase and decrease in blood volume (lines are drawn by inspection). (From Thorén, 1976a.)

during distensions. Fig. 3.13 shows, in several fibres, the responses to distension of small balloons placed at the left pulmonary vein–left atrial junctions. Fig. 3.13(a) illustrates the response obtained in two fibres; one of the fibres (with a conduction velocity of $1.2 \text{ m} \cdot \text{s}^{-1}$) had an initial spontaneous discharge of 10.7 spikes·s^{-1} which increased to 30 spikes·s^{-1} during distension of the balloon and returned to 8.3 spikes·s^{-1} during the final control period. In contrast Fig. 3.13(b) shows a fibre (conduction velocity $1.6 \text{ m} \cdot \text{s}^{-1}$) which had no spontaneous activity. The activity increased to 7.4 spikes·s^{-1} during distension of the balloon and the receptor ceased to discharge during the final control period. Of the twelve fibres examined, eight were similar to that in Fig. 3.13(b) and had a control discharge of 0.7 spikes·s^{-1} (mean; range 0–1.8) rising to 6.5 spikes·s^{-1} (mean; range 1.3–12.5) on distension of the balloons. The remaining

Electrophysiology of atrial receptors

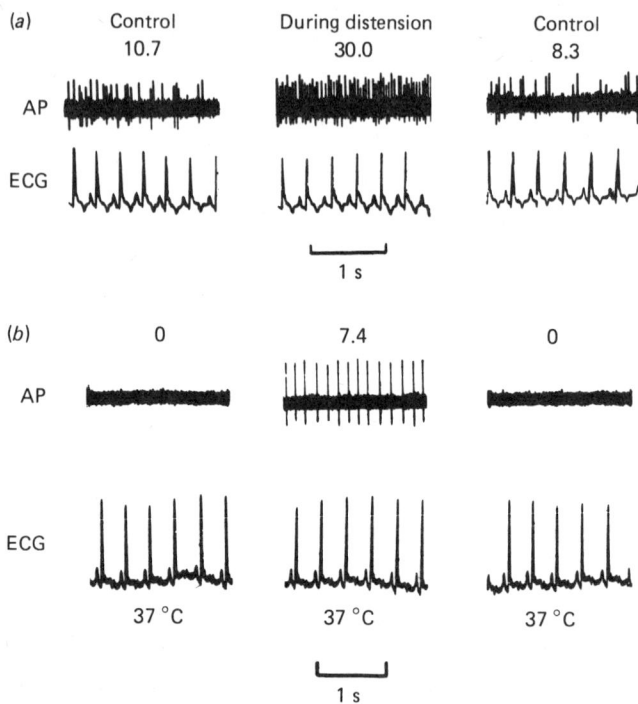

Fig. 3.13. The effect of distension of a balloon on the response in a vagal non-myelinated fibre attached to a receptor (a) with a high control discharge rate and (b) not discharging during the initial control period. The figure shows portions of experimental records with the vagus at 37 °C. Each record shows the action potentials (AP) and the electrocardiogram (ECG). The number above each tracing is the mean frequency (spikes·s^{-1}) calculated over 1 min.

four were similar to that in Fig. 3.13(a) having a control discharge of 7.9 spikes·s^{-1} (mean; range 0.1–11.8) rising to 28.5 spikes·s^{-1} (mean; range 23.1–33.6) on distension of the balloons. This apparent division into two groups bears a superficial resemblance to that observed by Sleight & Widdicombe (1965) who studied the response of ventricular receptors to veratridine; they found that receptors could be classified into two groups depending on their frequency of discharge. Also commenting on the behaviour of ventricular receptors discharging into vagal C fibres, Coleridge (Baker, Coleridge & Coleridge, 1979), in an excellent review of the topic, pointed out the possibility of the existence of two groups of these receptors depending on whether the adequate stimulus was mechanical or chemical; but he emphasised the non-homogeneity of this group of C fibres. However, in the study of C fibres emanating from atrial receptors reported above (Kappagoda, Linden & Sivananthan, 1979), the finding of two groups of fibres may well be an artefact; ligatures were tied around the various cannulae and balloon catheters in the pulmonary veins and appendage which may create local lines of increased tension near and around the balloon, which, in turn, could easily lower the threshold of some of the atrial receptors in the vicinity.

Natural stimulus

Very little is known about the behaviour of the vagal C fibres with receptors in the atria; much more evidence has been accumulated about ventricular receptors discharging into vagal C fibres. More than thirty years ago Amann & Schaefer (1943) and Jarisch & Zotterman (1948) recorded impulses in vagal afferent nerves whose receptors were in the ventricles of the cat heart. Since then Coleridge *et al.* (1964*b*), Sleight & Widdicombe (1965), in the dog, and Oberg & Thorén (1972*a*), in the cat, have recorded activity from single C fibres (see Fig. 3.10). Subsequently, more investigations (for an extensive presentation and discussion of recent findings see Coleridge *et al.*, 1973; Baker, Coleridge & Coleridge, 1979; Coleridge, Coleridge & Kidd, 1979) have described the behaviour of ventricular C fibres and some extrapolation from these data to the behaviour of atrial receptors discharging into C fibres can be made with care. Thus the question of what is the natural stimulus to these ventricular receptors has been debated at length (e.g. Baker *et al.*, 1979; Coleridge *et al.*, 1979; Sleight, 1979; Thorén, 1979*a*). After a carefully presented review Coleridge (Coleridge *et al.*, 1979) concludes there may be various adequate stimuli in that some of the receptors are mechanoreceptors capable of signalling changes in the inotropic state of the ventricles, or changes in volume; others are chemosensitive, and respond to substances produced within the myocardium, e.g. prostaglandins; and a few may be conventional chemoreceptors responding to changes in pO_2, pCO_2 and pH. Sleight (1979) proposed a hypothesis to suggest that the 'major stimulus for ventricular receptor excitation is a rise in intramyocardial tension in the wall of the left ventricle'. Several primary events may affect tension in the myocardium, including an increased catecholamine concentration resulting in a smaller heart contracting vigorously or an increase in ventricular volume.

It is to be hoped that these proposed explanations of how the ventricular receptors are stimulated naturally will be tested in the near future. But it is not surprising that the natural stimulus to receptors in the atria, which discharge into non-myelinated fibres in the vagi, is also unknown. However, Thorén (1976a) examining C fibres emanating from the atria of the cat concluded that the receptors were activated mainly by distension of the atria and the receptor discharge was related usually to the 'v' wave of the atrial pressure pulse, particularly during increased atrial volume caused by infusion. He also concluded that these changes in discharge could occur over a range of atrial pressures within the physiological range. Similar conclusions were drawn by Thames (Thames et al., 1977; Thames, 1979) who recorded activity from eight left atrial receptors with non-myelinated vagal afferent fibres in spontaneously breathing cats and found a linear relationship between the rate of discharge and the atrial transmural pressure similar to that observed in left atrial type B (Paintal) receptors.

More care must be taken when interpreting, and extrapolating from, the findings in the rat. The characteristics of atrial C fibres with vagal afferents, in the rat, have recently been examined (Thorén, Ricksten & Noresson, 1978; Thorén, Noresson & Ricksten, 1979) and it was found that all the atrial fibres had a conduction velocity of between 0.4 and 1.2 $m \cdot s^{-1}$ indicating they were C fibres.

Thorén (1979a) commenting on these results says, 'Interestingly enough, no receptors with medullated afferents were found in the rat heart. Moreover, it was not possible to identify any receptors with non-medullated afferents in the left ventricle.' Considering also that many of these receptors discharged at higher frequencies with patterns similar to those characteristic of Paintal-type atrial receptors there is a distinct possibility that many of these may, in fact, be myelinated fibres which were examined. The rat vagus nerve is short, making the estimate of conduction velocity difficult; this difficulty was compounded in the experiments of Thorén (Thorén *et al.*, 1979) because he stimulated the receptor site, i.e. not the nerve but endocardium and muscle, to evoke the impulses from which the recording of conduction velocity was calculated.

Recently Thorén (1979*a*) has brought together all the information pertaining to C fibres with receptors in the heart; he has postulated that this receptor group (C fibres) 'throughout the entire cardiopulmonary region constitutes the major part of the afferent vagal input to the vasomotor centre. These receptors respond mainly to increased volume of the heart, but ventricular C fibres can also increase their activity upon an increased ventricular contractility.'

Thus it appears that with reference to these receptors acting as mechanoreceptors some measure of agreement is being reached; it is proposed that the adequate stimulus to ventricular receptors discharging into C fibres is an increase in wall tension caused by either greatly increased forceful contraction or an increased diastolic distension. By analogy and from the work of Thorén (1976*a*) it appears atrial receptors also discharging into C fibres respond to similar stimuli. It is possible they are all part of the same afferent system. However, the propositions have still to be put to the test.

Receptors which discharge into the sympathetic nerves (so-called sympathetic afferents)

Recently attention has been drawn to the possibility of reflexes from the heart which have their afferent nerves going directly into the spinal cord through the sympathetic nerves, the existence of which was first suggested by Edgeworth (1892). Subsequently evidence of afferent fibres in sympathetic nerves with sensory endings in the heart was provided by Woollard (1926), Nettleship (1936), Nonidez (1939), Hirsch & Orme (1947), Khabarova (1963) and Hirsch, Nigh, Kaye & Cooper (1964). Recently Casati, Lombardi & Malliani (1979) recorded action potentials in 'sympathetic' non-myelinated afferent nerves from the ventricles with the receptors not exhibiting cardiac rhythms but being sensitive to mechanical events, not to distension or

Electrophysiology of atrial receptors

asphyxia, and they make a special plea that 'the unmyelinated cardiac sympathetic afferents should not be considered purely nociceptive in function'. Recent reflex interest on this topic was started by Brown (1967) who observed experimentally the excitation of afferent sympathetic nerves during myocardial ischaemia, following his finding that 'sympathetic' afferent fibres from the heart could be excited by mechanical and chemical stimuli (Brown, 1964).

Since then, there has been considerable interest in such possible cardiac reflexes mediated by 'sympathetic' afferent fibres (for reviews see Coleridge, Coleridge & Kidd, 1979; Hainsworth, Kidd & Linden, 1979). Although many of these reflexes cannot be directly traced back to the atria it is necessary to review the evidence in detail.

The electrophysiological evidence for the existence of afferent sympathetic fibres from the atria will be reviewed here and the reflexes involving these fibres will be discussed in Chapter 7. Uchida and his colleagues have, over the past few years, published a series of reports relating to activity in these fibres (see Uchida, 1979, for review). Uchida & Murao (1974c) were able to record the action potentials from the left second and third rami communicantes in anaesthetised dogs (see Fig. 3.14). The origin of these fibres was established by tapping the surface of the left atrium. The conduction velocities of these fibres were also measured. A proportion of these fibres had conduction velocities in the range $8-23$ $m \cdot s^{-1}$ suggesting that they were myelinated A fibres while the remainder had conduction velocities less than 2 $m \cdot s^{-1}$ and hence were considered to be C fibres. The receptor fields of the former were said to be circumscribed (3–5 mm in diameter) while those of the latter were more diffuse (4–10 mm in diameter). These values must be approached with caution since they were probably defined by tapping on a beating atrium and the possibility that the receptor endings are multiterminal in nature must be borne in mind in view of the evidence of Holmes & Torrance (1959) and Coleridge, Coleridge & Kidd (1979). Some of the fibres in both categories exhibited spontaneous activity. The discharge from all the receptors discharging into A fibres which showed any spontaneous activity was synchronous with the waves of the atrial pressure pulse. The discharges into some of the C fibres were also related to the 'a' wave of the atrial pressure pulse.

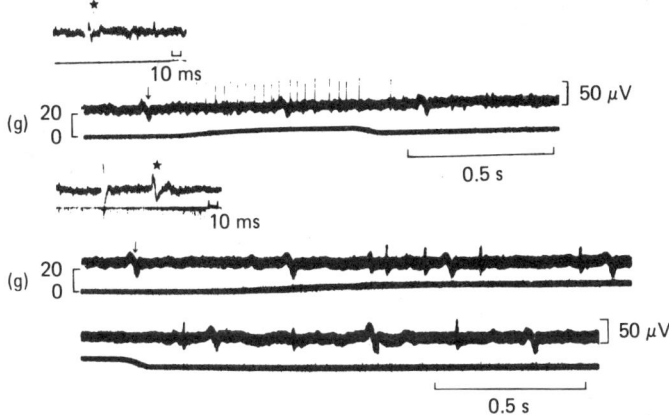

Fig. 3.14. First (top) trace: electrically evoked action potential of A fibre (labelled with star). Conduction velocity = 10.5 m·s⁻¹, voltage threshold = 1.4 V. Second trace: action potentials evoked in same nerve filament by tapping left atrial wall. Pressure to wall measured by strain gauge and expressed in grams. Downward arrow indicates QRS of electrocardiogram. Third trace: electrically evoked action potential of C fibre. Conduction velocity = 1.6 m·s⁻¹; conduction time = 480 ms; voltage threshold = 10.5 V. Fourth and fifth traces: action potentials evoked in same nerve filament by tapping left atrial wall. Magnification of action potential is the same for all photographs. (From Uchida & Murao, 1974c.)

A group of receptors having essentially the same characteristics as those described above were later demonstrated in the right atrium of the dog (Uchida, 1975). Once again the recordings were made from the second and third rami communicantes. These receptors which discharged into both myelinated and non-myelinated nerves also responded to changes in pressures in the right atrium. These changes were well within the physiological range.

In an attempt to elucidate the physiological stimulus to these receptors and following the investigation of ventricular receptors discharging into fibres in the sympathetic rami, Hess, Zuperku, Coon & Kampine (1974) and Kostreva, Zuperku, Purtock, Coon & Kampine (1975) studied the effect of changes in cardiac pressures on the discharge from the receptors in the atria. The experiments were performed in anaesthetised dogs maintained on a total cardiopulmonary bypass and recordings of action potentials were made from the second and third rami communicantes. The receptors were stimulated by distending, in a pulsatile manner, a balloon positioned in the right atrium. The pressure in the right ventricle was held constant during the stimulation (Fig. 3.15). It was found that the activity in the fibres was affected by changes in atrial pressure within the physiological range; the effect was enhanced by maintaining the pressure in the right ventricle at a relatively high level. Since the activity in these fibres was modulated by changes in pressure in both the atria and the ventricles in this manner, it could be argued that the receptors involved are of the multiterminal variety. These authors also observed that the activity was maximal when the balloon pulsations coincided with atrial diastole. This observation was interpreted by the authors as evidence in favour of these receptors being displacement receptors.

Another group of workers who have promulgated excellent work in this difficult area and who have mainly been concerned with attempts to elicit reflexes involving these 'sympathetic' afferent nerves (see Chapter 6), have been centred around Malliani in Milan. They also have recently (see Malliani, 1979) provided evidence of 'sympathetic' afferent fibres with receptors in the atria and shown several examples of their irregular spontaneous discharge with changes resulting from injection of saline, mechanical probing, etc.; an example from their work is shown in Fig. 3.16. They found activity in phase with 'a' (particularly 'a' – these fibres emanating from receptors in the pulmonary veins) and 'v' waves of the atrial pressure pulse and respiratory variations in discharge probably resulting from secondary changes in atrial pressure. Previously, Malliani, Recordati & Schwartz (1973) had reported evidence of afferent cardiac 'sympathetic' fibres with atrial endings, describing their spontaneous discharge and responses to various haemodynamic stimuli.

The investigations reviewed so far have indicated beyond any doubt that there is a group of atrial receptors which have their afferent paths in the upper thoracic rami communicantes. Holton, Kidd & Koley (to be published; Holton, 1977) confirmed the existence of receptors in the atria, ventricles, pericardium and pleura which discharge into afferent fibres in the sympathetic rami communicantes. It was also shown that distension of

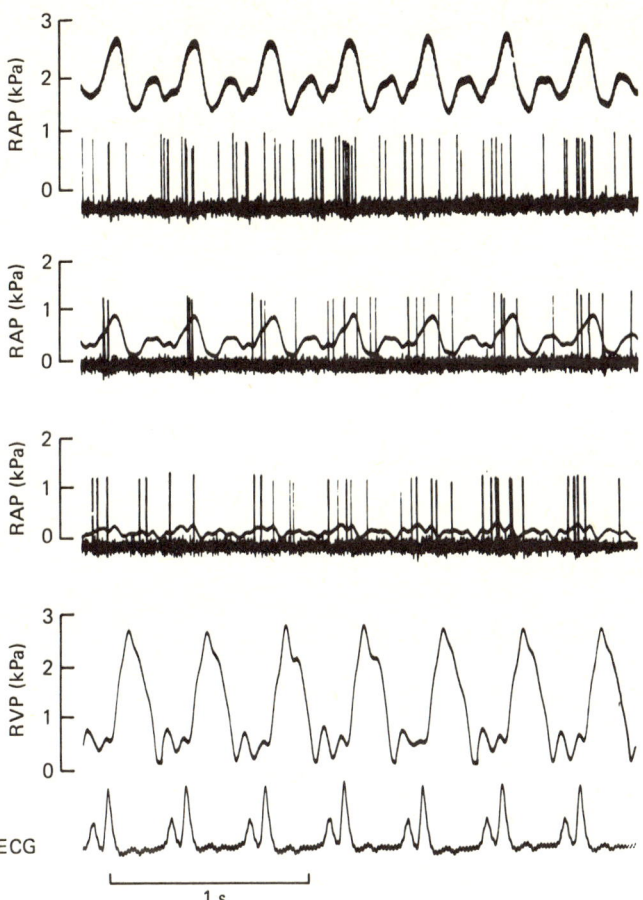

Fig. 3.15. Representative sympathetic afferent nerve activity in a multifibre preparation in dog; receptor responds to changes in right atrial systolic pressure with right ventricular systolic pressure held at 2.7 kPa. Signal-to-noise ratio was enhanced electronically. Spike amplitudes are approximately 50 μV. ECG belongs to bottom two traces. RAP, right atrial pressure; RVP, right ventricular pressure; ECG, electrocardiogram. (From Kostreva *et al.*, 1975.)

balloons in the left atrial appendage and in the pulmonary vein–atrial junctions caused an increase in discharge in sixteen single fibres in sixteen dogs; the receptive sites of four of these fibres were located in the left atrial wall. Four other fibres were

Electrophysiology of atrial receptors

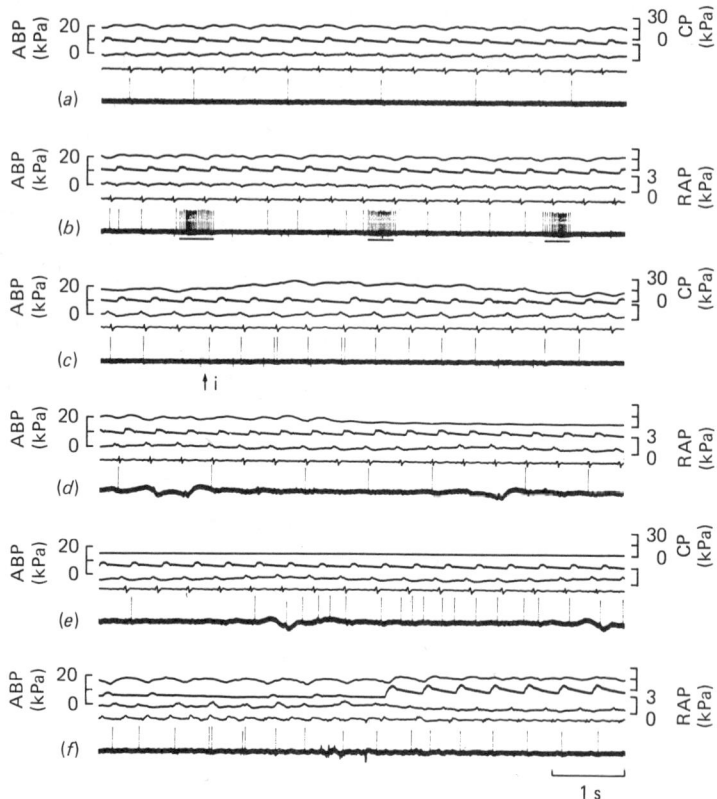

Fig. 3.16. Activity of a sympathetic fibre with left atrial endings during various haemodynamic stimuli and during interruption of left coronary artery perfusion. (*a*) spontaneous activity; (*b*) mechanical probing of an area of the left atrium performed on the beating heart; (*c*) fast injection (i) of 2 cm³ of saline into the inflow coronary tubing; (*d*) interruption of left coronary artery perfusion (indicated by the decrease of coronary inflow pressure); (*e*) starts 52 s after the end of the preceding record. 10 s after the end of (*e*) the coronary perfusion is instituted again; however, the ventricles do not contract efficiently (beginning of (*f*)). (*f*) The heart recovers during the second half of the record. Tracings from top to bottom, represent the coronary inflow pressure (CP), the arterial blood pressure (ABP), the right atrial pressure (RAP), the ECG and the nervous recording. (From Malliani *et al.*, 1979.)

located in the left ventricle and the remaining eight in tissues outside the heart. Only the atrial receptors consistently increased and sustained their discharge in response to distension of the balloons. As pointed out in Chapter 2 there is no histological evidence describing these receptor endings. Indeed it is not known in which tissue of the wall of the atrium or ventricle they are to be found, though from the reactions of the receptors to stimulation with blunt probes it would appear that they may be present throughout the thickness of the wall.

What is apparent about the receptor endings discharging through 'sympathetic' afferents is that the receptive fields are relatively large and about half the fibres have many receptor endings, i.e. they are multiterminal. Holton (1977) examined 105 'sympathetic' afferent fibres in 39 dogs and found that the receptive fields were large, the distance between discretely sensitive points within the receptor areas being from 3 to 150 mm, after paying particularly careful attention in the methodology, to the criteria for acceptance of the recording of a single fibre and to the area of distortion to very light mechanical stimulation. Again, examining as much tissue as possible, Holton (1977) observed that half the fibres had many terminal sensory sites and six had more than four. It must also be accepted that in such a study the exploration for multiterminals cannot be complete and that an unknown number of the other 'single' terminal fibres probably could have exhibited multi-terminal endings. This report confirms what was originally found by Holmes & Torrance (1959) who examined single afferent fibres in the thoracic rami of sympathetic nerves and applied discrete mechanical stimuli at many sites. They observed that stimuli applied to an area of several square centimetres evoked responses in the same afferent fibre. Also the sensitive areas were between organs or in more than one organ, e.g. one fibre had a receptive field defined by stimulating the pleura overlying the aorta, pulmonary artery and oesophagus. These findings of multiterminals were expanded by Banzett, Coleridge, Coleridge & Kidd (1976), who reported in cats and dogs that discrete receptor sites could be found within large receptive fields located on the aorta, left subclavian artery, pulmonary artery, pulmonary vein, left atrium, left ventricle, bronchi, trachea, lung, pericardium, oesophagus and pleura. They found

Electrophysiology of atrial receptors

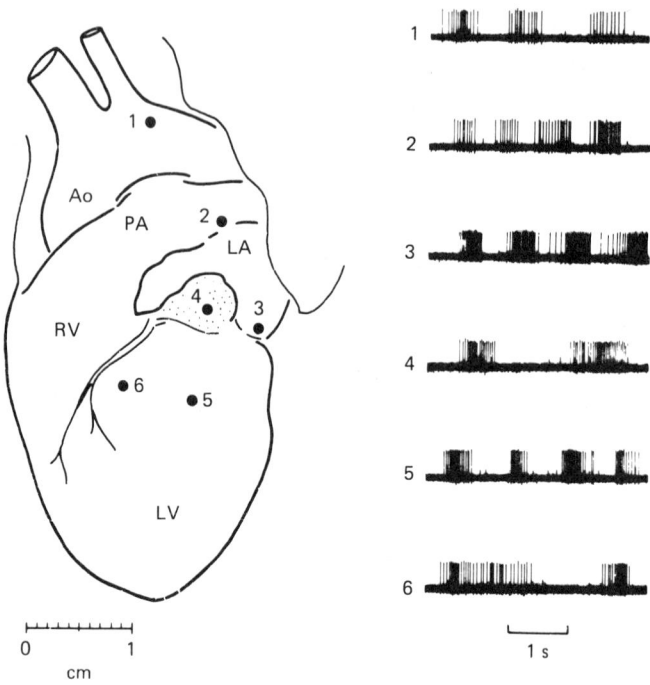

Fig. 3.17. Impulse activity recorded in the cat from a single afferent sympathetic fibre (third left thoracic ramus) with six discrete mechano-sensitive areas on the aorta, pulmonary artery, left atrium and left ventricle. The six records on the right are responses to stroking the sensitive spots (1–2 mm diam) on the external surfaces with a fine bristle. Stimulation away from these discrete areas was without effect. The location of the spots was confirmed by probing the non-beating heart at the end of the experiment. (Coleridge, Coleridge & Kidd, unpublished experiments.)

that of 98 single afferent fibres examined in these tissues, more than 50% had multifocal sites of origin; 16 fibres innervated two or more thoracic structures and had very large receptive fields; one fibre, for instance, had receptor sites on the aorta, left ventricle and left atrium (Fig. 3.17). The implications of such multi-receptor sites, particularly involving the atrium, will be referred to in Chapter 7, but it is worth emphasising here the enormous difference between the receptive fields of these receptors, extending large distances and over different organs, and those of Paintal-type atrial receptors where there are fewer end-organs per fibre (mean, 1.74 per fibre; see Chapter 2), a much smaller receptive field ($< 350\ \mu$m in largest dimension) and whose response to probing with a fine probe extends only to a spot less than a square millimetre.

The natural stimulus to many of these receptors is claimed to be mechanical (e.g. Malliani, 1979) but the clear relationship of the precise distortion, in relation to pressure, which effectively stimulates the receptors has not yet been defined. The significance of reactions to large changes in the circulation, such as in haemorrhage or to the injection of chemicals (e.g. Uchida & Murao, 1975) is unknown.

However, it may be concluded for the purposes of subsequent explanation of the function of atrial receptors that 'sympathetic' afferents with receptors in the atria exist and are stimulated by mechanical means such as a rise in atrial pressure or local distension of balloons.

4 METHOD OF ESTABLISHING REFLEXES FROM ATRIAL RECEPTORS

As stated in Chapter 1, one of the main objects of this monograph is to consider the reflex effects of stimulating nervous end-organs, or receptors, in the atria. Also in Chapter 1 an acceptable definition of a reflex effect was presented and criteria to be used in experiments designed to establish the presence of a reflex were defined. In this chapter it is intended to elaborate on the practical effects of applying these criteria. It will then be possible to use this information as a background against which to judge the quality of the investigations, reviewed in subsequent chapters, which claim to have established reflex cardiovascular responses emanating from atrial receptors. Particular attention must be paid to the examination of each of the component parts of the reflex as described in Chapter 1, and in as much detail as possible. The study of reflexes in experimental animals inevitably involves the use of procedures which will influence the results. Hence, in interpreting experimental results, and in comparing results from different laboratories, it is essential to consider in detail all aspects of the methods used.

Therefore, in this chapter an attempt will be made to delineate the nature of the evidence sought and the practical manner in which such information is obtained in the attempt to establish the reflex effects of stimulating atrial receptors.

The stimulus – the manner of its application

The endocardium of the mammalian heart contains three types of nerve endings (see Chapters 2 and 3), the complex unencapsulated receptors (Paintal-type atrial receptors) which are attached to myelinated fibres in the vagi, receptors which discharge into non-myelinated fibres in the vagi and receptors which discharge into 'sympathetic' afferent fibres.

Application of the stimulus

Since the original demonstration of the 'Bainbridge Reflex' (Bainbridge, 1915) there have been many attempts at devising a method of stimulating receptors in the atria (for more detailed discussion see Chapter 5). One of the earliest was that used by Bainbridge himself who used infusions of blood and saline in quantities sufficient to increase the pressure in the great veins to demonstrate a 'reflex' increase in heart rate. This procedure, not surprisingly, resulted also in significant changes in systemic arterial pressure.

Another procedure for stimulating receptors in the low pressure areas of the circulation which in recent years has gained some acceptance is a technique involving the immersion of the subject up to the neck in water. Since this procedure results in an accumulation of blood in the thorax and since it also results in an increase in the rate of urine flow it has been advanced as a procedure for investigating the reflex regulation of extracellular fluid volume (e.g. Epstein, 1976). But such redistribution of blood will obviously cause changes in the discharge of many receptors throughout the circulation, and not only to those receptors within the chest; a brief account of the various functions of those receptors is given in Chapter 7. Immersion up to the neck increases the central blood volume, the central venous pressure and the volume of the heart (see Epstein, 1976). It also results in a concomitant increase in cardiac output (up to 30%) and in the mean systemic pressure (Arborelius, Balldin, Lilja & Lundgren, 1972; Levinson, Epstein, Sackner & Begin, 1977).

The two experimental techniques quoted above as examples are inadequate to provide any insight into the nature of any specific reflex responses – particularly those involving the atrial receptors; it is not possible to claim that any particular receptors are being stimulated, and only those receptors.

The atrial receptors are located mainly at the junctions of the veins and the atria (Figs. 2.1 and 4.1, see also Chapter 2) and they respond to changes in atrial pressure (Chapter 3). Knowing these anatomical sites of the atrial receptors with unencapsulated endings, three methods of discretely stimulating some of the areas of atrial wall containing the receptors were evolved in Leeds; first, small balloons were inserted into the left pulmonary vein–atrial junctions and distended with no effects on blood flow

Method of establishing reflexes

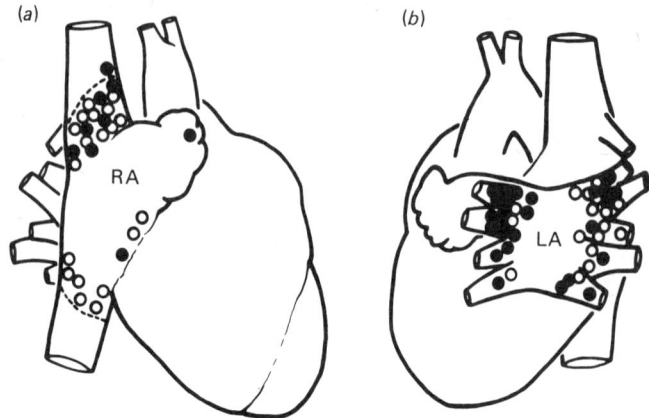

Fig. 4.1. Diagrammatic representation of the position of 92 cardiac receptors, each of which had been located by electrophysiological means. Each receptor is indicated by a circle: ○, afferent fibre in right vagus; ●, afferent fibre in left vagus. (a) Right lateral view of the heart; (b) posterior view. The receptors were distributed as follows: (a) right atrio-venous region, 28; (b) left atrio-venous region, 45. In (a) the interrupted line indicates the attachment of the pericardium. RA, right atrium; LA, left atrium. (From Coleridge et al., 1964.)

through the left atrium; secondly, larger balloons were inserted into the superior caval–right atrial junction and the blood flow from the head bypassed to the femoral vein; and thirdly, a temporary pouch of the left atrium which contained the atrial receptors was created and perfused, with no haemodynamic changes in the remaining part of the atria. These preparations are described below.

Left atrial receptors, small balloons

Ledsome and Linden (1964b) devised a method of stretching the left pulmonary vein–atrial junctions in a manner which did not interfere with the remainder of the circulation. Small latex balloons attached to surgical grade nylon tubes (I.D. 1.0 mm) were inserted into the left pulmonary veins and advanced to the pulmonary vein–atrial junctions. The balloons were secured in position and the left lung was ligated (Fig. 4.2). Subsequent distension of the balloons with warm saline (1 cm^3 in each),

Right atrial receptors

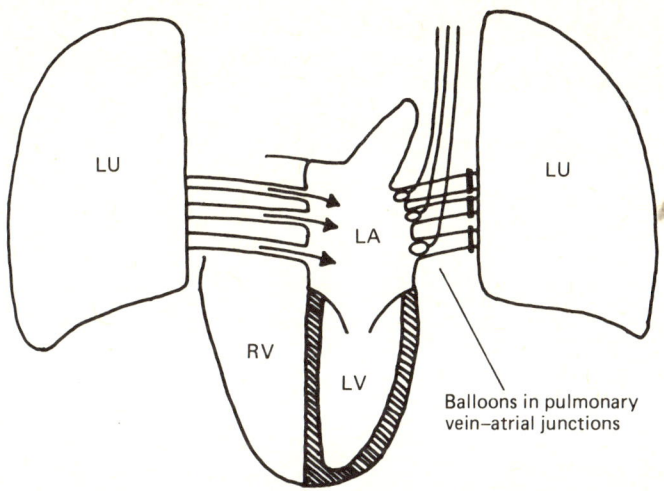

Fig. 4.2. Diagram of preparation used to stimulate left atrial receptors. LU, lung; LA, left atrium; RV and LV, right and left ventricles. Diagram illustrates left lung root tied off, small balloons at pulmonary vein–atrial junctions and total venous return passing through right lung. Therefore it is possible to distend balloons and stretch junctions without altering flow through the heart or atrial pressure. (From Linden, 1972.)

attaining the shape of a sphere about 0.8 cm in diameter, stretched the vein–atrial junctions and thereby activated the receptors. Ligation of the left lung root distal to the point of insertion of the balloon catheter, prevented any obstruction of the pulmonary circulation by distension of the balloons *per se*; the evidence that such an obstruction did not occur in these experiments was provided by the absence of significant changes in atrial pressure during distension of the balloons.

Right atrial receptors, balloon and bypass

Kappagoda, Linden & Snow (1972*a*, *b*) used a larger balloon to stimulate the right atrial receptors located at the junction between the superior vena cava and the right atrium. A cannula containing two balloons was inserted into the superior vena cava and positioned as shown in Fig. 4.3. The proximal balloon A, when distended, occluded the superior vena cava. The blood

Method of establishing reflexes

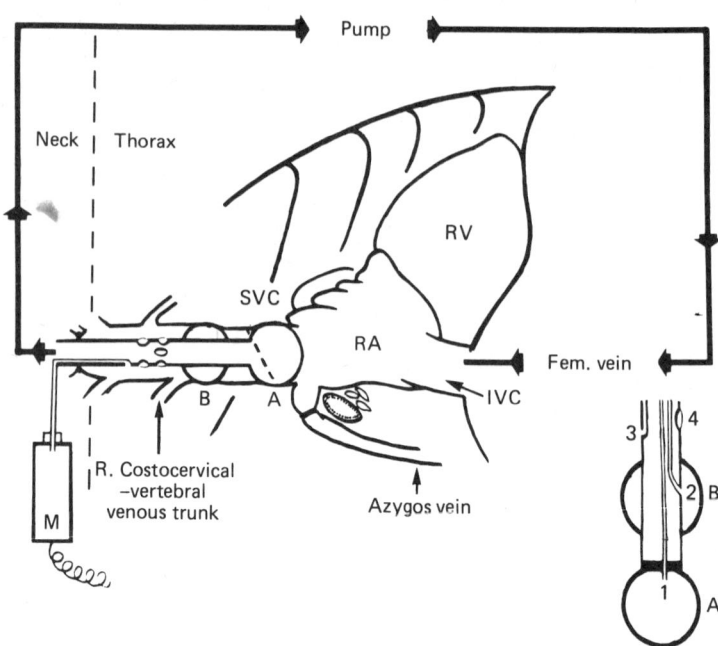

Fig. 4.3. Diagram of experimental preparation: SVC and IVC, superior and inferior venae cavae; RA and RV, right atrium and ventricle; M, strain-gauge manometer. A cannula incorporating two balloons (A and B) is inserted into the superior vena cava through the external jugular vein. Inset is a diagram of the end of the cannula to show orifices to balloon A (1), to balloon B (2), for recording of pressure in superior vena cava above the point of occlusion (3) and one of several orifices in the cannula through which the blood is aspirated (4). The balloon B acts as a cuff which occludes the superior vena cava. The blood accumulating in the superior vena cava is pumped away through the cannula and returned to the animal via the femoral vein. The junction between the superior vena cava and the right atrium may then be stretched by distending the terminal balloon A without interfering with venous return to the heart. The balloon B must be located caudal to the entrance of the right costocervical–vertebral venous trunk in order to ensure that the venous return is not obstructed when the balloon A is distended. The interrupted line across the superior vena cava indicates the reflexion of the visceral pericardium at the parietal surface visible in the preparation as a pale line. (From Kappagoda, Linden & Snow, 1972*b*.)

accumulating in the vena cava was drawn through the cannula and returned to the inferior vena cava by a roller pump. Once the 'by-pass' was established, distension of the distal balloon stretched the junction between the superior vena cava and the right atrium and activated the atrial receptors in the endocardium of this region. Once again, stretching the vein–atrial junction *per se* did not result in any further obstruction to venous return as indicated by the absence of significant changes in pressures in the superior vena cava and the right atrium.

Left atrial pouch

Ledsome & Linden (1967) created an isolated pouch out of the left lateral part of the left atrium in anaesthetised dogs. The pulmonary veins were dissected free and ligatures placed around the three main left pulmonary veins as close to the lung tissue as possible. A cannula directed towards the atrium was inserted into each of the three pulmonary veins, to be used later in the experiment for recording pressure (cannula in middle lobe vein) and inlet and outlet (upper and lower lobe veins) channels from, and to, the perfusion pump which caused the pulsating pressure changes in the pouch. The left lung root was clamped off as far lateral to the entry of the cannulae as possible. With the left lung retracted to the left, the apex of the heart was lifted and gently pulled over to the right, under direct vision the *right* pulmonary veins were dissected free from the oesophagus behind. Especial care was taken not to damage the connective tissue adjoining the *left* pulmonary vein–atrial junctions as these were adjacent to the atrial receptors later to be stimulated. The dissection was carried upwards almost to the main pulmonary artery. A stainless-steel clamp was made with two thin blades opposed and at right angles to the handles. The blades were 8 cm long and had a convexity to the right (radius of curvature 9 cm). The posterior blade of the clamp was introduced up the dissected channel behind the left atrium with the anterior blade resting on the anterior wall of the left atrium lateral to the atrial appendage. When closed, the tip of the clamp lay posterior to the pulmonary artery almost in contact with the arch of the aorta; the posterior blade rested solely on the oesophagus behind, and in front was applied to the wall of the left atrium

Method of establishing reflexes

at the left edge of the entrance of the right pulmonary veins into the left atrium. The atrium was thus clamped so as to form two chambers; one chamber into which the right pulmonary veins opened and which acted as a channel to the left ventricle; the second chamber which was a pouch made up of the left part of the left atrium, the left pulmonary vein–atrial junctions and the three pulmonary veins each containing a cannula. A record of systemic blood pressure was observed throughout the insertion of the clamp and the fact that systemic arterial blood pressure did not fall was taken to mean that the flow through to the left ventricle was not significantly obstructed. The pouch was immediately perfused with Ringer–Locke solution by means of a Dale–Schuster pump. The solution was kept at 38 °C (± 1 °C) and a mixture of 5% CO_2 in O_2 continuously bubbled through it; heparin (Pularin, Evans Medical Ltd) was added to give a concentration in the solution of 5000 IU·litre^{-1}.

Thus, the isolated left atrial pouch could be distended without causing changes in flow through, or pressure in, the remainder of the left atrium.

Monitoring atrial pressure

Whilst all these procedures permitted localised regions of the atria to be stretched without obstruction to the flow of blood through the atria, they also emphasised the great importance of recording pressures in the atria during the course of these experiments. Recording these pressures provides firm evidence that the stimulus (distension of the balloons or pouch) causes no further obstruction to the flow of blood. Owing to the relatively small size of the atria, the addition of small volumes of saline into the balloon (e.g. more than 3 cm^3 into the left atrium) could compromise the flow of blood through the atria. Occasionally, using three small balloons, even the addition of a total of 3 cm^3 may cause a small rise in left atrial pressure; in such circumstances either less volume has to be injected, e.g. by using two balloons instead of three, or the preparation has to be adjusted. Thus, even when using small balloons positioned at the left pulmonary vein–atrial junctions the animal should be tilted slightly to the right to prevent the heart over-hanging the balloons. Such an arrangement, if not corrected, could also lead to the heart being stimulated 'externally' during distension of a small balloon in the atrial appendage leading to ectopic beats; in this case, care must be taken to see that during distension the outside wall of the appendage does not rub against the ventricular tissue. Equally, an excessive tilt could lead to pressure on the venae cavae and consequent obstruction to venous return. The routine monitoring of atrial and other cardiovascular pressures and the electrocardiogram serves to draw attention to these changes in the circulation during periods of stimulation and thus permits adjustments to the preparation to avoid the consequences. In the absence of such measurements, assessment of experimental results is transformed into an exercise in interpretation, or at worst, guesswork. For instance, in two publications by Edis & Shepherd (1969) and Edis, Donald & Shepherd (1970), the distension of balloons located at the left pulmonary vein–atrial junctions was shown to result in a response that was related to the magnitude of the initial heart rate, i.e. at low initial heart rates the manoeuvre resulted in an increase in the heart rate, and at high initial heart rates, a decrease (see Chapter 7 for further details). These findings are clearly in conflict with those reported in other investigations reviewed later in this book. In their investigation (Edis & Shepherd, 1969), the stimulus was provided by three balloons each of which was distended with 3 cm^3 of saline. The atrial volume in the dog is of the order of 7–10 cm^3 (18–20 kg dog), and it could reasonably be expected that distension of such balloons would result in a partial obstruction of the flow of blood through the mitral valve, an adequate explanation of the results. The argument could be resolved only by analysing the changes in left atrial pressure but the latter were not measured in these experiments. Thus, the problem remains unsolved, but emphasises yet again that it is necessary to measure the pressure in the left atrium in this type of experiment.

The stimulus – its nature

In demonstrating reflex paths in experimental animals, it is often not possible to apply a stimulus which is wholly 'physiological'. Indeed, on many occasions, the physiological stimulus to the receptors under study may not be known. Thus it has been

Method of establishing reflexes

suggested that stimulation of receptors in the heart by distension of balloons bears little relevance to 'normal physiology' (e.g. Heymans & Neil, 1958). Therefore it is appropriate to consider in detail the effect of this stimulus on the atrial receptors themselves.

Attempts to grade the stimulus

Because of the peculiar geometry of the vein–atrial junction it has not proved possible to obtain a graded increase in the stimulus by varying the volume of warm saline injected into each balloon. The balloons were so designed that with the volumes of saline injected in the earlier experiments (0.5–1.5 cm^3) the pressure within the balloons was very high (about 27 kPa) compared with that in the atria (1.3 kPa) and surrounding tissue, but each balloon would, therefore, attain a spherical shape of predetermined size. However, although the object was to distend to a predetermined volume so as to stretch the pulmonary vein–atrial junction it was suggested that excessive force was used to distend the tissues. Therefore, in four dogs the pressure within each balloon was measured at each distension volume under two conditions; first, during the experimental periods during which the heart rate response was observed, and secondly, when the balloons were free in air post mortem. The pressure within the balloon gives no indication of the degree of stretch imposed on the tissues; but an indication of the 'stretching force' may be obtained from a consideration of the difference in pressure in the balloon in the two positions (pressure measured in the balloon during experimental distension *in vivo* minus the pressure in the balloon free in air post mortem). During all these experimental distensions the heart rate increased. No relation between the difference in the pressure (the so-called 'stretching force') and the increase in heart rate was observed. In some experiments as the volume of the balloons was increased from 0.5 to 1.5 cm^3, the 'stretching force' decreased in value. For instance in one dog the balloons were distended successively with 0.5–1.5 cm^3 of saline; the increase in heart rate with distensions was 10 and 21 beats·min^{-1} respectively, but the three balloons showed differences in pressure ('stretching force') of 1.3, 2.0 and 4.0 kPa during

Nature of the stimulus

distension with 0.5 cm³ saline, but 0.9, 1.1 and 2.1 kPa during distension with 1.5 cm³ saline. It is probable that with a small balloon in this situation the difference between the pressure within the balloon *in vivo* post mortem does not give a reasonable measure of the force which stretches the surrounding tissue. It may be that one explanation of this phenomenon is that, on distension, the balloon may slip slightly in relation to the particular tissues such that the receptors opposed to one part of the balloon during a small distension may be opposed to a different part of the balloon, possibly with less stretch, when the balloon is stretched to a greater volume.

The problem of grading the stimulus was approached another way by inflating one, two and three balloons sequentially and so recruiting more atrial receptors (see Chapter 6).

Electrophysiology

In Chapter 3 it was shown that stimulating atrial receptors can result in an increase in the trains of impulses in myelinated fibres in the vagi. That the three means of stimulating left and right atrial receptors under discussion, resulted in increases in the discharge of these receptors within the physiological range, was shown using techniques of recording action potentials similar to those referred to in Chapter 3.

In the case of the left atrial receptors, Kidd *et al.* (1966, 1978) have shown that distension of small balloons located at the junctions between the pulmonary veins and the left atrium increases the discharge from atrial receptors (Fig. 4.4) located in the region. Distension of the small balloons in six dogs led to the discharge from six atrial receptors being recognised in slips of vagal nerves; each of these was located to the atrial endocardium. These findings have been confirmed more recently by Kappagoda, Linden & Sivananthan (1979). The response of an increase in discharge to distension of the balloons, sometimes after an initial small decrease from a peak discharge, has been shown to continue as long as the balloons are distended; for up to 1 min, Kappagoda, Linden & Snow (1972b); up to 2 min, Kidd *et al.* (1978); up to 30 min, Linden & Mary (unpublished, Fig. 4.5); also evidence that the inhibition of activity in efferent renal nerves, in response to stimulation of atrial receptors, is

83

Method of establishing reflexes

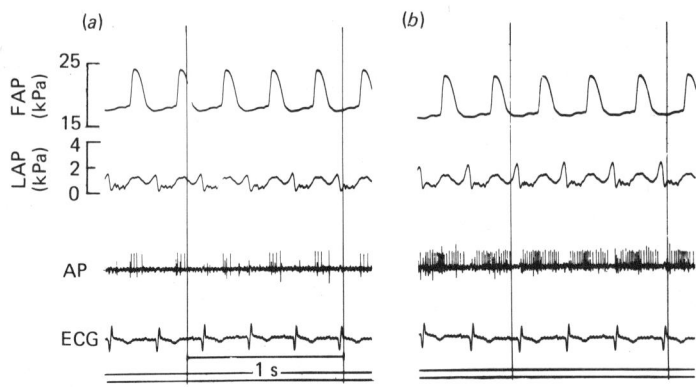

Fig. 4.4. Effect of distension of balloon on discharge of action potentials from left atrial receptor. From above: femoral arterial pressure (FAP) in kPa; left atrial pressure (LAP) in kPa; action potentials (AP) from slip of vagal nerve; ECG; two datum lines. (a) Before distension of the balloon; (b) during distension of the balloon with 1 cm^3 of warm saline. Time between vertical lines in each panel is 1 s. Note (1) the sparse (3–4 spikes per beat) pulsatile discharge in a single fibre with balloon not distended; (2) the great increase (about 20 spikes per beat) in the pulsatile discharge during distension of the balloon. Location of receptor proved at post mortem to be in the endocardium of left upper pulmonary vein–atrial junction. (Linden, 1973.)

maintained for 30 min, was obtained by Linden, Mary & Weathcrill (1980a).

The question of the rate of adaptation of atrial receptors may now be considered. For instance Kappagoda, Linden & Snow (1972b) recorded action potentials in slips of a vagal nerve and studied the effect of stretching the junction between the superior vena cava and the right atrium for 1 min; no change in the initial discharge rate was observed in four of six fibres examined. Gilmore & Zucker (1974b) showed that there was no change in the discharge rate of atrial receptors with a type B pattern of discharge, for a period of 15 min during distension of a balloon in the left atrial appendage which also caused an increase in left atrial pressure. Arndt et al. (1974) confirmed that the average discharge rate remains constant during stretch of atrial strips containing receptors having any of the three patterns of discharge. Gupta (1977b) showed in the cat that atrial receptors having any of the three patterns of discharge adapt only very slowly over

Nature of the stimulus

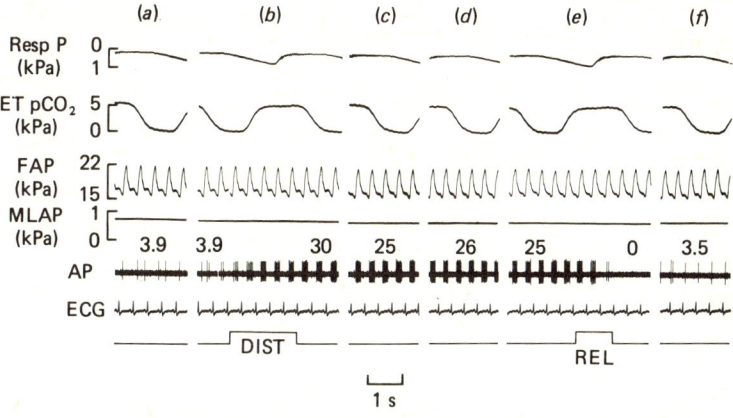

Fig. 4.5. Parts of a continuous experimental record showing the effects of distending a small balloon with 1 cm³ saline for 30 min, at the left upper pulmonary vein–atrial junction, on the discharge from a type B atrial receptor. From above downwards, tracheal pressure (Resp P), end-tidal pCO_2 (ET pCO_2), femoral arterial pressure (FAP), mean left atrial pressure (MLAP), action potentials (AP), electrocardiogram (ECG) and event marker. Changes in event marker signals the distension (DIST) and release of distension (REL) of the balloon. Records were obtained during control (a), and distension (b), 10 (c), 20 (d) at 30 (e) min after distension, final control (f). The numbers above the records of action potentials are mean frequencies (spikes·s^{-1}).

a period of 40 s. He studied isolated atria in which the pressure was elevated by the injection of saline. In fact even the slow decrease in the number of impulses generated could be a result of a decrease in atrial pressure as is evident in Figs. 1–3 of his report (Gupta, 1977b). Paintal (1953b) also reported slow adaptation in left atrial receptors having a type B pattern of discharge, following saline infusion in the isolated left atrium of the cat, but no information on the level of pressure in the left atrium was given. Care has to be taken when considering whether some of the above experiments were capable of demonstrating true adaptation of the receptor. As pointed out by Kidd et al. (1978) the reduction in activity during distension of small balloons may not entirely represent adaptation, as is usually described for receptors, because the balloon moves in relation to the wall containing the receptors and the receptors

Method of establishing reflexes

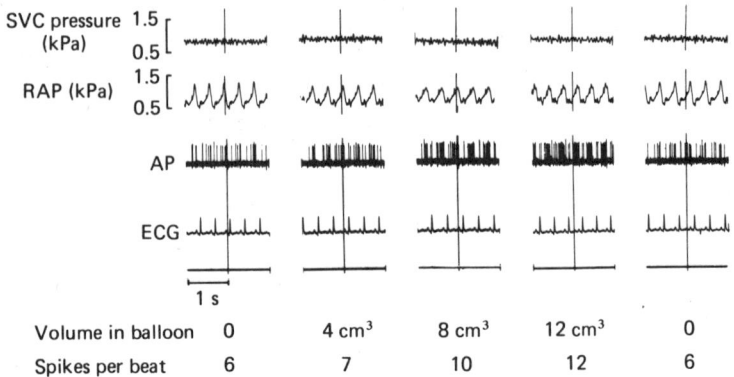

Fig. 4.6. Effect of stretching the junction between the superior vena cava and the right atrium on a single unit in the cervical vagus. Each panel of experimental record shows from above downwards the superior vena cava (SVC) pressure, right atrial pressure (RAP), action potentials (AP) from a slip of the right cervical vagus and electrocardiogram (ECG). As the volume in the terminal balloon A was increased in increments of 4 cm³ (i.e. as the superior vena caval–right atrial junction was stretched) the impulse frequency (spikes per beat) increased from 6 per beat to 12 per beat. The impulse frequency returned to the control value after the release of the distension. This particular single unit showed a discharge during atrial filling and during atrial systole. (From Kappagoda, Linden & Snow, 1972b.)

are exposed to a dynamic stimulus; evidence for this statement is produced in their Fig. 1B.

It is possible to compare the increase in discharge of atrial receptors caused by distending the small balloons with that caused by increases in atrial pressure resulting from infusions. Thus it is possible to go some way towards assessing 'physiological relevance'. For example, Kappagoda, Linden & Sivananthan (1979) examining the effect of distension of small balloons at the pulmonary vein–atrial junctions, have shown that distension of a balloon at a pulmonary vein–atrial junction resulted in a mean increase in the discharge of type B receptors from about 4 spikes per cycle to about 12 spikes per cycle. When this change is viewed against the effect of infusions (e.g. Gilmore & Zucker, 1974b) it is clear that this increment could be brought about by a relatively small alteration in mean atrial pressure, e.g. of the order of an increase of 0.3 kPa, from about

Nature of the stimulus

0.5 kPa to 0.8 kPa (Gilmore & Zucker, 1974b). In addition the pattern of action potentials involved in the increase resulting from distension of either balloon system (large or small) is similar to that observed from the normal atrium, e.g. Fig. 4.4 and Kidd *et al.* (1978); Fig. 4.6 and Kappagoda, Linden & Snow (1972b). Thus though the balloon has a steady pressure within it, the movement of the heart throughout the cardiac cycle converts the stimulus into a phasic one, and, therefore, the central second-order neurones in the reflex pathways are receiving a physiological pattern of activity from the primary afferent neurone (Kidd *et al.*, 1978).

In relation to right atrial receptors, it has been shown by Kappagoda, Linden & Snow (1972b) that distension of balloons at the junctions between the superior vena cava and the right atrium also stimulated the atrial receptors located at this site (Fig. 4.6). Again to assess the relevance of this stimulus, it is necessary to examine the relative effects of increments in atrial pressure and of balloon distension on the discharge from the atrial receptors. In the case of the right atrial receptors, Kappagoda, Linden & Snow (1972b) have shown that small increments in mean atrial pressure (from about 0.5 kPa to 1.0 kPa) which resulted from infusions of fluid caused an increase in the activity of the receptors (from 4 spikes per cycle to 13 spikes per cycle) which was comparable to that which occurred following distension of the balloons (from 0 to 10 cm^3) and which resulted in an increase in discharge from about 6 spikes per cycle to 13 spikes per cycle (Fig. 4.7 and Kappagoda *et al.*, 1972b); the same interpretation may be made from the work of Dickinson (1950).

Action potentials in slips of vagal nerves were also recorded whilst pressure in the left atrial pouch changed (Kidd *et al.*, 1966, 1978). The same receptor was also studied in the whole atrium by removing the medial clamp and allowing the receptor to be stimulated by the normal changes in left atrial pressure. In this investigation strict criteria for accepting the fibre for investigation were used. As each nerve strand was examined changes in activity in afferent vagal fibres were observed and the activity in the single functional preparation was studied further only if it satisfied certain criteria: the application of pulsatile pressures to the pouch should induce consistent increases in

Method of establishing reflexes

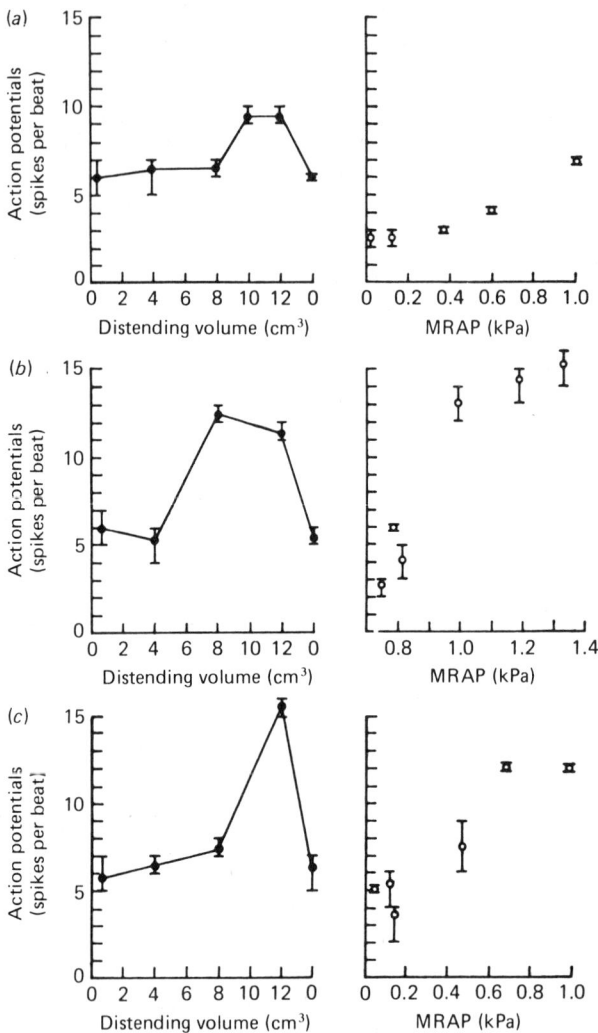

Fig. 4.7. Comparison of the effect of stretching the superior vena caval–right atrial junction (●) and changing the mean right atrial pressure (MRAP, ○) on three single units ((a), (b), (c)) in the right cervical vagus. Impulse activity (spikes per beat) is plotted against distending volume (cm³) and against mean right atrial pressure (kPa). The bars represent ranges of responses. (From Kappagoda, Linden & Snow, 1972b.)

Nature of the stimulus

discharge from the receptors; the steady distension by the balloon or pouch should induce a sustained increase in discharge maintained throughout the period of distension; and activity in the fibres should not be markedly influenced by changes in the stroke of the respiratory pump and should not have the characteristics of a pulmonary receptor. In 13 dogs, five receptors which responded consistently and in a maintained fashion to distension of the pouch, were located in the atrial endocardium.

Anticipating the discussion about the small reflex changes in heart rate observed during distension of the pouch (Chapter 5) it should be noted that high pressures of the order of about 5–7 kPa in the pouch were required in the heart rate study (Ledsome & Linden, 1967) to evoke a moderate reflex increase in heart rate of 10.3 beats·min^{-1} (mean; range 3–27). Also similar high pressures in the pouch of the order of 2.5–5 kPa were required to induce a moderate increase in discharge of impulses from atrial receptors, up to 8–12 impulses per pump pulse at similar rates of pulsation. Differences in the response of receptors (Fig. 4.8) in the pouch compared with the 'open' atrium (clamp removed) are compatible with the explanation previously advanced for the high pouch pressures required to elicit a small increase in heart rate (Ledsome & Linden, 1967). It is suggested that when the pouch was created the radius of the distended part of the atrium diminished and, in accordance with the Laplace relationship, a proportionately greater pressure would be required to guarantee the same circumferential tension in the atrial wall; the interpolation of the appropriate values for the radius of the atrial wall without the clamp predicted that the changes in pressure required to induce similar wall tensions were of the same order of magnitude as those which were applied in the action potential study to induce equivalent changes in impulse activity.

Therefore, in terms of the input to the CNS the effect of distending balloons, at the vein–atrial junctions, or a pouch of the left atrium on these receptors closely mimics the effect of increases in atrial pressure within the physiological range.

Method of establishing reflexes

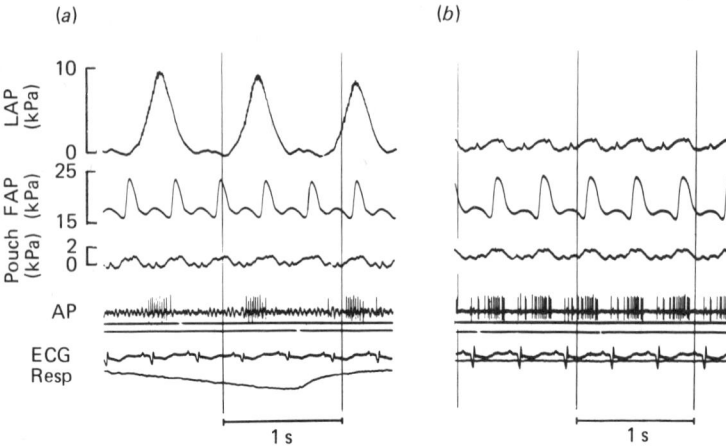

Fig. 4.8. Action potentials and pressure from an atrial receptor when in wall of pouch and in the 'open' atrium. From above down: pressure in pouch (kPa); FAP, femoral arterial pressure (kPa); LAP, left atrial pressure (kPa); AP, action potentials from receptor; ECG, electrocardiogram; Resp, tracheal pressure (inflation downwards). (a) Clamp across left atrium and pressure pulse applied to pouch. (b) Activity from same receptor when clamp removed to restore pouch to original size ('open' atrium) and after infusion of 200 cm³ 0·9 % sodium chloride solution. When this section of record was taken, inflation was briefly interrupted. (From Kidd et al., 1978.)

Specificity of the stimulus

The endocardium of the atrium contains at least two histologically distinct forms of nerve endings, i.e. the complex unencapsulated nerve endings and the end-net (see Chapter 2). The complex unencapsulated nerve endings have been shown to discharge into myelinated fibres in the cervical vagus. The precise nature of the end-net remains a matter for investigation.

However, there is electrophysiological evidence that other receptors originating in the atria discharge into non-myelinated fibres in the vagi and yet others discharge into the sympathetic afferent fibres in the rami communicantes (see Chapter 3). In terms of physiological responses in these fibres there is evidence to indicate that in the cat, the atrial nerve endings discharging into non-myelinated fibres in the vagi respond to relatively small changes in mean pressure in the left atrium (e.g. Thorén, 1976a). Responses similar to these have also been observed in nerve endings discharging into the sympathetic nerves (e.g. Kostreva *et al.*, 1975). Thus it is imperative to be certain of the nature of the receptor endings activated by the distension of the balloons even though the stimulus is applied to functional areas which contain a preponderance of the complex unencapsulated nerve endings. Recent investigations (see Chapter 3) have shown that such a stimulus (distension of small balloons at the pulmonary vein–atrial junctions) is capable of activating all three types of nerve endings, i.e. the nerve endings which discharge into both myelinated and non-myelinated vagal fibres (Kappagoda, Linden & Sivananthan, 1979) and the nerve endings which discharge into the sympathetic fibres (Holton, Kidd & Koley, to be published; Holton, 1977). Thus in the study of reflexes caused by the activation of atrial receptors, in addition to applying a small localised stimulus, it is necessary to devise additional procedures which permit a definite identification of the receptors involved in any particular response. Procedures necessary to establish precisely which receptors are being stimulated include electrophysiology, fine point location and histology, and the establishment of the particular afferent pathway and type of afferent nerve involved in any reflex response. These topics are covered in detail in Chapters 2, 3, 6 and 9 but an introduction to some of the means of establishing reflexes, particularly from atrial receptors, is given in the next section.

Reflex pathway

Once a response to a stimulus has been demonstrated, the reflex nature of the response can be established by examination of the particular afferent and efferent paths of the reflex. In most reflexes originating from the heart, such an examination involves the determination of the effect on the response of interfering with transmission in these pathways.

Method of establishing reflexes

Afferent pathway

On evidence presented in Chapter 3 the vagi and the sympathetic nerves contain afferent fibres from the atrial receptors; as pointed out there are receptors discharging into myelinated fibres in the vagi, receptors discharging into non-myelinated fibres in the vagi and receptors discharging into myelinated and non-myelinated fibres in the sympathetic rami communicantes. Usually the procedures for distinguishing whether these receptors and these afferent nerves are involved in the reflex responses under study involve either sectioning the nerves or blocking with anodal (e.g. Thorén et al., 1977) or cold blockade (e.g. Kappagoda, Linden & Sivananthan, 1979). Care has to be taken with each of these techniques and though cold blockade can be made to be sophisticated and accurate under specific conditions (Kappagoda, Linden & Sivananthan, 1979) there are doubts about the efficacy of, and difficulties with, anodal block of the vagus (e.g. Coleridge et al., 1973; Thorén et al., 1977; Hainsworth et al., 1979; Hopp, Zuperku, Coon & Kampine, 1980). Thus if both vagi are sectioned in the neck and the carotid and aortic regions are denervated and then a reflex response is obtained from atrial receptors it would be postulated that 'sympathetic' afferent nerves were involved, particularly if further section of the rami communicantes then abolished the response. Such a technique eliminates the atrial receptors discharging into the vagi as being responsible but does not distinguish between myelinated and non-myelinated in the sympathetic nerves. There is a separate question of whether complete denervation of the aorta and carotid sinus baro- and chemoreceptors can be accomplished surgically which cannot be fully discussed here (see Ito & Scher, 1973, 1974).

Section or complete blockade of the cervical vagal nerves, a common practice when investigating changes in heart rate, brings special doubts as to the efficacy of these manoeuvres to demonstrate specific reflexes; the vagi contain afferent fibres from several types of cardiovascular receptors, which are involved in many cardiovascular reflexes with various effects on the heart and circulation (see Chapter 6 for a brief report of reflexes from receptors, other than atrial receptors, in the chest). Many fibres in the cervical vagi originate below the diaphragm as well as within the chest. It is as well to remember that histological examination of the cardiac vagal fibres in the cat has shown that about 75% of the afferent nerve fibres are non-myelinated (Agostini, Chinnock, Daly & Murray, 1957), and the function of most of these fibres is unknown.

The fact that the reflex response is still observed after section of the vagi, allows the conclusion that neither the afferent nor the efferent pathway lies in the vagi. But if the reflex response is abolished then it is dangerous to conclude, solely from this evidence, that the afferent nerves for that reflex were in the vagi. Both efferent and afferent fibres have been sectioned and major changes in the background state of the animal, e.g. heart rate, degree of vasoconstriction from abolition of some baroreceptor reflexes, have taken place even to the extent that some reflex changes would not be observed. For instance, to examine the afferent path of a reflex which results in an increase in heart rate, it would not be sufficient to section the cervical vagi as this procedure would eliminate the tonic efferent vagal fibres and hence result in a high control heart rate; there will be changes in systemic arterial blood pressure and atrial pressures and these will be inversely related and may be higher or lower depending on the relative states of the blood volume and capacity of the vessels before vagal section. Against this background, of the great changes in the control state, it would be difficult or even impossible to demonstrate an increase in heart rate which is mediated by sympathetic efferent nerves.

Thus, considerable care should be exercised in designing experiments involving vagal fibres and particularly vagal afferent fibres. The problem of examining reflexes involving vagal afferent fibres will be dealt with in depth in Chapters 3, 5 and 6, where several means of completing this task are described and results obtained using new techniques are presented and discussed.

Efferent pathway

Usually procedures to allow examination of the efferent pathways of reflexes from the heart involve sectioning the efferent nerves or pharmacological blockade. Sectioning a sympathetic nerve to a limb vessel or blockade with an α-adrenoreceptor antagonist

Method of establishing reflexes

to abolish an effect are acceptable techniques. Also an investigation of a response of an increase in heart rate, where sympathetic nerves may be involved, allows the use of similar techniques with a β-adrenoreceptor antagonist or sectioning the ansae subclaviae. However, sectioning the vagi or using atropine to block the efferent vagal fibres alone are not reliable techniques on which to base conclusions about an efferent pathway. The vagi carry many afferent fibres (see above), there is a large tonic effect of the vagi on the heart rate and the use of atropine carries other disadvantages, e.g. there are effects on central neurones (Goodman & Gilman, 1970). Also it must not be assumed that the section or blockade of the vagi and/or sympathetic efferent nerves will result in equivalent effects whatever the state before blockade: effects of first stimulating one nerve then the other and then reversing the order indicate that the effects are not algebraically manipulated (e.g. Warner & Cox, 1962; Levy & Zieske, 1969) though a simple algebraic summation of effects can occur (e.g. Randall, Pace, Wechsler & Kim, 1969). Thus section of the vagi and/or sympathetic nerves will not have predictable relative effects under all conditions.

Care of experimental animals

It is virtually impossible to study physiological mechanisms in intact animals and man, because analytical dissection of the component parts is necessary. Therefore, in general, most cardiac reflexes are investigated in animals under specific experimental conditions; they are usually anaesthetised, artificially ventilated and prepared surgically.

The ability to obtain reproducible results in experiments on anaesthetised animals depends to a large extent upon the care with which the background state of the animal is established and maintained. Very little evidence exists as to the relative importance of the many factors involved and often what is important in a particular series of experiments only becomes apparent from the experience of failure. Most care evolves as individual laboratory folk-lore obtained from fairly lengthy experience, a point which cannot be too heavily emphasised. However, there is some evidence that the type and depth of anaesthesia, the temperature of the animal, the acid–base state and the gas composition of the blood are of importance in the particular type of reflex being discussed in this monograph.

Anaesthesia

The type of anaesthetic is important. For example, Biscoe & Millar (1966) showed that the three anaesthetics, cyclopropane, halothane and ether all depressed the reflex response of changes in heart rate and blood pressure to aortic nerve stimulation in the rabbit. Robertson, Swan & Whitteridge (1956) showed that the sensitivity of the carotid sinus baroreceptors in the cat was increased by inhalation of ether, chloroform or trichloromethylene. Van Citters, Franklin & Rushmer (1964) have shown that chloralose has only a minimal effect on the circulation compared with pentobarbitone which has a marked depressant action. Further evidence of the effects of anaesthetics on the circulation is given by Price & Cohen (1964).

The effect of chloralose and pentobarbitone anaesthesia on the acid–base state and oxygenation of the arterial blood has been studied in the dog by Ledsome et al. (1971). On induction of anaesthesia they found pentobarbitone caused a transient respiratory acidaemia and chloralose a small non-respiratory acidaemia. The non-respiratory acidaemia caused by chloralose was considered to be the result of the infusion of the unbuffered solution of the anaesthetic; this effect can be prevented by including a small amount of bicarbonate instead of chloride in the solution infused. Over a period of anaesthesia lasting up to eight hours all dogs tended to develop a small non-respiratory acidaemia.

No quantitative method of assessing the depth of anaesthesia is as yet available. Horvath (1969) was able to obtain an inverse correlation between the amount of anaesthetic given (a Dial–urethane mixture) and the variability of the amplitude of the cortical auditory evoked response. In a similar study involving the use of chloralose which is a common anaesthetic used in animal studies, Linden, Malpus, Saunders & Snow (1974) have shown that increasing the dose of chloralose results in the diminution of the reflex effects on the heart rate of stimulating atrial receptors. This depression was reversible. It is possible that the development of such methods will lead to a much needed simple and accurate method of assessing the depth of anaesthesia. At the present time the depth of anaesthesia when using pentobarbitone is usually assessed by observing the response of changes in heart rate and blood pressure to gross stimuli. When using chloralose an effective test is to observe the response to a sharp tap on the animal operating table; a resultant reflex contraction of the limb and trunk muscles and a transient increase in the heart rate and blood pressure is taken as indicating a light plane of anaesthesia. However, care and experience are required with this technique as there is, occasionally, little change in this response with large changes in the depth of anaesthesia. Of the two anaesthetics most commonly used in cardiovascular investigation, chloralose and pentobarbitone, it is considered that there are more advantages to be gained by using chloralose than pentobarbitone if cardiovascular reflexes are being studied.

In Leeds great care is taken to maintain a steady state of light anaesthesia so that control states before and after interventions are strictly comparable in terms of measured variables such as heart rate, blood pressure (mean, systolic, diastolic, waveform), easily elicited reflexes, e.g. reflex muscle contractions to table tapping, eye blinking, acid–base state, respiratory state, no twitching or involuntary movements etc. In earlier experiments following the initial intravenous infusion of a solution of α-chloralose (dose up to 100 mg·kg^{-1}, Etablissment, Kuhlmann, Paris), anaesthesia was maintained by further intermittent intravenous infusion of chloralose (approximately 10 mg·kg^{-1} every 10 min). In assessing the amount of the maintenance dose several points ought to be taken into consideration, including the rapidity with which the animal became unconscious during the infusion of the initial dose of anaesthetic at a constant rate of 6 cm^3·min^{-1}; the quantity of this initial dose necessary to obtain the required depth of anaesthesia based on clinical assessment; the decrease in heart rate on injection of the maintenance dose, and attempts should be made to keep this dose adequate to maintain the heart rate at mid-period constant; the maintenance dose should be adequate to prevent movement or attempts to breath 'against' the pump given that the acid–base state is within the normal range. The blood pressure should not change during the giving of the maintenance dose which should be given slowly.

To avoid any possible influence on the stability of the state of anaesthesia by such intermittent doses, a technique involving a continuous intravenous infusion of chloralose solution was eventually developed as has been reported (Kappagoda, Linden & Mary, 1979). The technique requires first the maintenance by thermostats of a solution of chloralose (1 g·100 cm^{-3} saline) at 57 °C to prevent precipitation or transformation into β-chloralose, and second the infusion of this solution at a temperature similar to that of the animal. A variable rate infusion pump (Braun, Infusomat) was used. The two requirements were met by keeping the assembly of the reservoir containing the solution and the infusion at 57 °C using heated water jackets and perspex housing. The tubing which led from the pump to the femoral venous cannula was maintained at 38 °C by a heated water jacket. Using this technique (Kappagoda, Linden & Mary, 1979) it was shown in dogs in which the temperature ranged from 37 °C to 38.5 °C, that the temperature of chloralose at the tip of the venous cannula varied from 37 °C to 38.8 °C at infusion rates from 0.5 to 2.5 cm^3·min^{-1}, the rate usually required in dogs ranging in weight from 10 to 35 kg. However, this technique requires periodic careful observation and close assessment of the depth of anaesthesia, using the above criteria: alterations of 0.5 cm^3 per 10 min of the infusing solution can change the depth detectably within a 30 min period.

Blood gases and the acid–base state

The profound effects of hypoxia and hypercapnia on the pulmonary and systemic circulations should make it apparent that the pO_2 and pCO_2 of the arterial blood must be measured and kept within normal limits. The effects of variation in blood pH are less well known. It has been shown that the response of the heart to stimulation of vagal nerves is increased during an acidaemia (Campbell, 1955; Linden & Norman, 1969). Also acidaemia reduces the response of an increase in heart rate to weak stimulation of the sympathetic nerves to the heart; such an increase in the heart rate of up to 40 beats·min^{-1} brought about by stimulating sympathetic nerves was prevented by

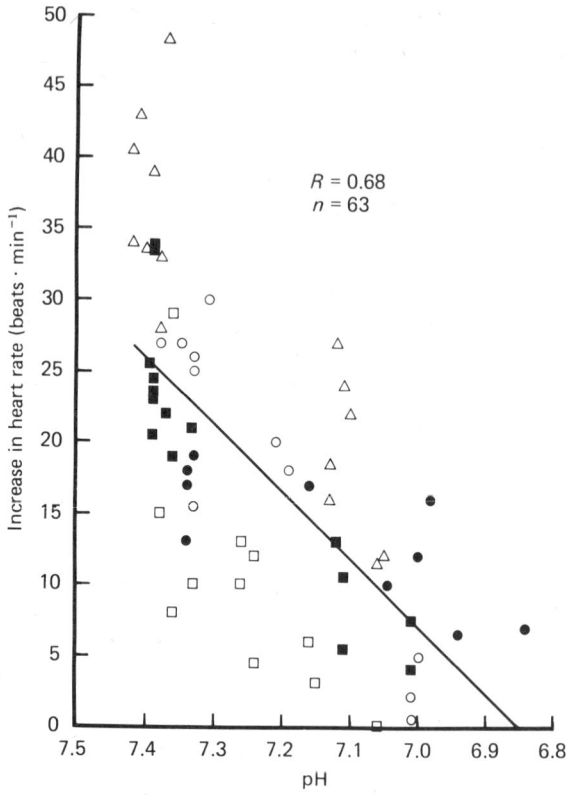

Fig. 4.9. The relationship between the increase in heart rate from stimulation of left atrial receptors and the pH of the arterial blood. Each symbol represents the responses from one dog. (From Harry et al., 1971.)

rendering the blood acidaemic (Linden & Norman, 1969). Also the depression of the reflex increase in heart rate from stimulation of left atrial receptors, which has a sympathetic efferent nervous limb, by acidaemia (Harry, Kappagoda, Linden & Snow, 1971), also demonstrates the importance of maintaining the acid–base state of the animal within normal limits in experiments which involve reflex changes in heart rate, especially if the efferent pathway involves the sympathetic nerves to the heart (Fig. 4.9).

Current methods of assessing the acid–base state require that at least two of the three variables, pH, pCO_2 and CO_2 content in the blood, be measured. The results are then usually plotted on a nomogram from which an estimate of any non-respiratory disturbances of the acid–base state may be obtained (e.g. Siggaard-Andersen, 1963; Kappagoda, Linden & Snow, 1970). A difficulty which arises with most nomograms is that they are based upon the behaviour of blood *in vitro* (e.g. Siggaard-Andersen, 1963) and there is now sufficient evidence available to show that such nomograms lead to significant inaccuracies when applied to changes in the whole animal (see Kappagoda *et al.* (1970) for a further discussion of this problem). Most nomograms have now been modified in an attempt to compensate for this anomaly (e.g. Siggaard-Andersen, 1971) but it is probably still wiser to monitor the acid–base state and relate the measured parameters (pCO_2 and pH) to an *in vivo* CO_2 titration curve as recommended by Kappagoda *et al.* (1970), Kappagoda, Stoker, Snow & Linden (1972) and Stoker, Kappagoda, Grimshaw & Linden (1972), than to attempt to predict either past or future loss of base as in the standard nomograms (e.g. Siggaard-Andersen, 1963, 1971).

In this laboratory the acidosis consequent on anaesthesia (see above), on surgery (Miller & Morris, 1961) and on long experiments is assessed from the relationship of pCO_2 to pH, based on whole animal studies (Kappagoda *et al.*, 1970), and prevented in dogs by various means: samples of arterial blood are taken initially and again as soon as the preparation is set up and analysed for pH, pCO_2 and pO_2. The respiratory pump has been simply modified to allow the control of the gas mixtures inspired including inhalation anaesthetics and air; oxygen is added to the intake and can be controlled to inspired concentration of better than 1%. The animals are ventilated with 40% oxygen in air maintaining a pO_2 in the arterial blood of about 26 kPa; more than that encourages collapse of parts of the lung. The pCO_2 in the alveolar air is continuously monitored, the alveolar–arterial gradient is initially established and the alveolar ventilation set to maintain a pCO_2 of about 5.3 kPa in the arterial blood; periodic checks of the gradient are made throughout the experiment and if it has changed the ventilation is reset. To prevent the appearance of the non-respiratory acidaemia a continuous infusion of a solution of sodium bicarbonate at a rate of about 1.2 mmol·kg^{-1}·min^{-1} in a concentration of 1 mmol·cm^{-3} (8.4 g $NaHCO_3$ per 100 cm^3) was

Method of establishing reflexes

recommended (Kappagoda et al., 1970). Using this technique in a recent series of ten dogs anaesthetised with chloralose the pH of arterial blood after 5–7 h of experimentation with varying degrees of trauma, mostly chest and abdomen open, has resulted in a non-respiratory pH (Kappagoda et al., 1970), which initially was 7.390 (mean; S.D. 0.017), and finally 7.384 (mean; S.D. 0.014); paired t-test of final against initial control value was not significant at $P > 0.1$ (Linden, R. J. & Mary, D. A. S. G. unpublished).

Thus, in the study of cardiac reflexes, the maintenance of a light degree of anaesthesia, adequate oxygenation, a normal pCO_2 and a normal pH of blood are important in eliciting reflex responses. Indeed, failure to have considered these aspects of experimentation in many investigations may well contribute an explanation of some of the conflicting experimental results previously reported.

5 REFLEX EFFECTS ON THE HEART, I: REVIEW OF PREVIOUS WORK

No previous review has limited its frame of reference to one which only includes an examination of the reflex effects of stimulating atrial receptors and observing effects on heart rate. However, there are reviews, which should be consulted by the interested reader, having some of this topic as part of a wider brief (e.g. Paintal, 1963a, 1972, 1973a; Coleridge & Coleridge, 1972; Linden, 1973, 1975, 1976; Sleight, 1975; Hainsworth, Kidd & Linden, 1979; Thorén, 1979a).

Heart rate and atrial pressure have been freely associated since Bainbridge published the report of his investigation in 1915. Since Bainbridge (1915) claimed that, 'The reflex acceleration of the rate of the heart which takes place when the venous inflow is increased in the normal animal is caused by impulses arising within the heart, and the effective stimulus is an adequate rise of venous pressure', there has been a tacit assumption that there is such a reflex as the 'Bainbridge reflex'. Heymans & Neil (1958) quoted evidence for and against there being such a reflex, but although stating there were those who did not believe in its existence (Jarisch & Zotterman, 1948; Wiggers, 1949) they themselves were 'firmly of the opinion not only that it exists but that it is important in conditions of increased circulatory activity'. They also pointed out that it was somewhat curious to consider that the Bainbridge effect is the one reflex from the heart itself which is known by every medical student.

During the period since Bainbridge first reported his investigation in 1915 there have been numerous investigations purporting to confirm or deny his conclusions. In this chapter it is hoped to review the literature relating the evidence to the discussion on the validity of techniques briefly described in Chapter 4.

As pointed out in Chapter 4 it is important to remember that investigators, claiming the demonstration of reflexes, should be able to give evidence indicating a receptor with an adequate stimulus, an afferent pathway, an efferent pathway and effector organs. Given these criteria for establishing reflexes it is possible to review the literature in sections, each one being dependent on the technique for the stimulation of possible receptors. The reported investigations will be commented upon in four groups: those investigations involving infusions, those involving perfusion techniques, those in which the stimulus is more discrete in which various parts of the heart are distended, and a miscellaneous group in which no attempts are made to stretch the walls of the heart.

Infusion experiments

Bainbridge (1915) accepted that in the normal animal 'plethora' resulted in a higher venous inflow, a higher venous pressure, a higher cardiac output and an increase in heart rate and he sought 'definite evidence as to the means by which the acceleration of the heart is brought about'. He therefore used the technique of intravenous infusion as a means of creating 'plethora' and a raised venous pressure in the right side of the heart. Implicit in this technique is the idea that any change noted in the cardiovascular system after such an infusion could be attributed to the stimulation of receptors within the right side of the heart.

Bainbridge (1915) described an increase in heart rate (e.g. Fig. 5.1) in response to intravenous infusions and he considered the increase in heart rate to be a reflex response brought about mainly by the withdrawal of vagal tone. This work of Bainbridge was widely accepted as a clear demonstration of a reflex response and was considered to be one of the main control mechanisms which prevented over-distension of the heart. Although Bainbridge did not locate the receptors involved in the response it was suggested by him that the receptors were located within the heart. However, over the next 50 years many workers have reinvestigated this phenomenon and obtained results which were either similar to those of Bainbridge (e.g. Meek & Eyster, 1922; Anrep & Segall, 1926; Tiitso, 1939; Ballin & Katz, 1941; Takino, 1951), or widely divergent (e.g. DeGraff & Sands, 1925; Coleridge & Linden, 1955; Jones, 1962; Ahmad & Nicoll, 1963;

Infusion experiments

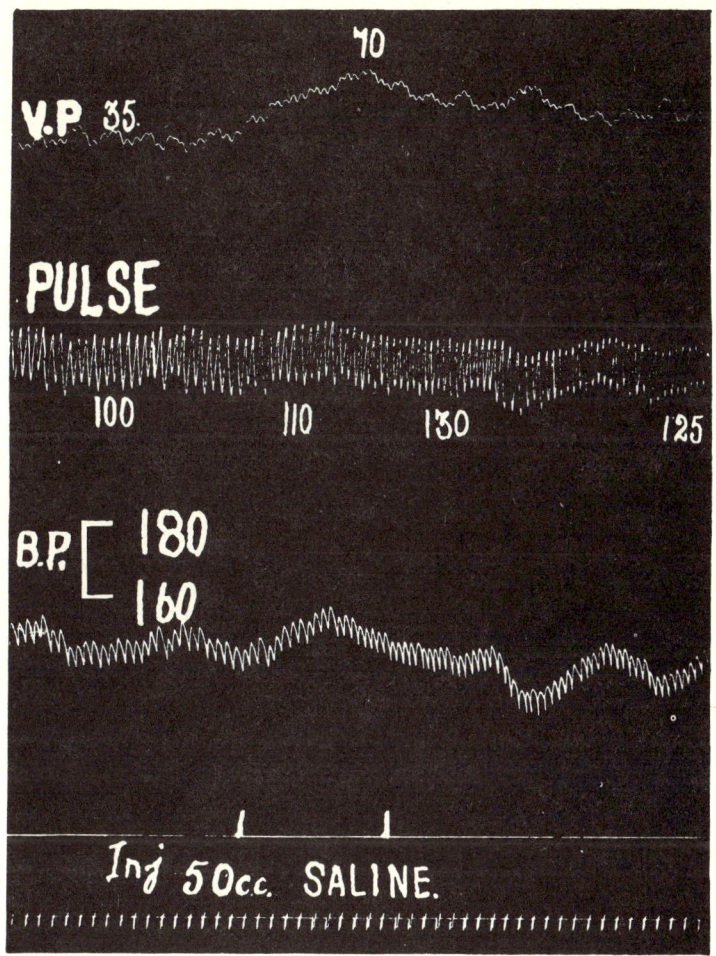

Fig. 5.1. Example of the results of a rapid injection of 50 cm³ saline. (From Bainbridge, 1915.)

Hirsch, Boyd & Katz, 1964; Blatteis & Horvath, 1964). In view of these discrepancies it is necessary to consider in detail the techniques used and the results obtained by Bainbridge (1915). His experiments were performed on relatively small animals (recorded weights range from 5 to 11 kg) and the amounts infused were large, of the order of 10% to 50% of the calculated blood volume (calculated on the basis of 80 cm³ of blood per kg).

Reflex effects on the heart, I

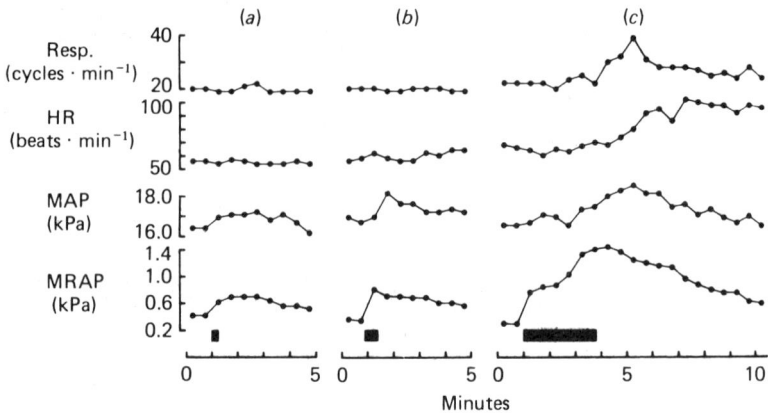

Fig. 5.2. Dog 21.2 kg; anaesthetic, morphia, Dial–urethane and sodium pentobarbital. The effect of three infusions of blood (solid blocks): (a) 50 cm^3 per 15 s; (b) 80 cm^3 per 30 s; (c) 400 cm^3 per 2 min 50 s. Period of 20 min between each infusion. From above downwards: Resp, respiration (cycles·min^{-1}); HR, heart rate (beats·min^{-1}); MAP, mean arterial pressure (kPa); MRAP, mean right atrial pressure (kPa). (From Coleridge & Linden, 1955.)

The infusions were made over periods of time ranging from 11 s to $3\frac{1}{2}$ min. It was apparent that the magnitude of the response was related to both the volume and the rate of infusion.

Bainbridge (1915) suggested that the stimulus for the response was an increase in venous pressure. Though this conclusion was arrived at mainly by a process of argument rather than a presentation of evidence, Bainbridge did point out that 'The quickening of the heart begins when the venous pressure has risen sufficiently to dilate the heart and to raise the diastolic pressure, and as the venous pressure falls the rate of the heart again diminishes;....' That the increase in heart rate does not always follow precisely the changes in atrial pressure can be seen from Fig. 5.2 (Fig. 2 from Coleridge & Linden, 1955), where it can be seen (Fig. 5.2(c)) that, particularly with the third and large infusion, the heart rate did not increase until after the end of the infusion whereas at that time the atrial pressure was at its highest and proceeded then to decrease, i.e. the atrial pressure was falling as the heart rate was increasing. Again it is extremely unlikely that a stimulus of this nature would have

Infusion experiments

increased venous pressure to the exclusion of changes elsewhere in the circulation. Indeed it is possible that changes in the systemic and pulmonary arterial pressures occurred and the former is apparent in some of the records published in the paper (Bainbridge, 1915) and from Fig. 5.1. The important observation that, during infusion, there is no strict relationship between venous pressure, usually measured as right atrial pressure, and heart rate has frequently been pointed out (e.g. Coleridge & Linden, 1955; Donald & Shepherd, 1963; Hirsch *et al.*, 1964) even though there is a relationship between the amount of infusion and right atrial pressure. Also there is no relationship between systemic arterial pressure and the heart rate (e.g. Coleridge & Linden, 1955; Hirsch *et al.*, 1964). It is not difficult to imagine that some receptors elsewhere in the chest or systemic circulation could be responsible for the increase in heart rate.

Vagal pathways

The evidence for the reflex nature of the response was based primarily on the effect of sectioning sympathetic nerves to the heart and of the administration of atropine sulphate on the response to an infusion. Both these procedures partially abolished the response although this effect was more evident with atropine sulphate. These observations led to the conclusion that the response was reflex in nature and that the efferent path of the reflex lay both in the sympathetic and vagal nerves.

Sectioning the vagi abolished the response and since one part of the efferent pathway was still intact he concluded that the entire afferent pathway lay in the vagi. The vagus is a mixed nerve containing many afferent and efferent fibres of unknown origin and function. Sectioning both vagi causes a major alteration in the base line values, such that it is doubtful whether the post vagotomy state can be regarded as a control state for experiments designed to show only the absence of a small group of previously active afferent fibres (see Chapter 4 for discussion on the hazards of vagal section in the determination of reflex responses). For instance it is possible to consider the possible effects of eliciting the reflex responses at different initial heart rates. In all the instances recorded by Bainbridge (1915) in which an increase in heart rate was obtained, initial heart rates ranged from 70 to 165 beats·min^{-1}. The two highest heart rates (165 and 140 beats·min^{-1}) were obtained after the administration of atropine sulphate. After sectioning the vagi the initial heart rates in four experiments quoted were 170, 150, 170 and 140 beats·min^{-1}.

It is relevant, therefore, to consider the initial heart rates in the experiments of other workers who have studied the effect of intravenous infusions on dogs without the vagi sectioned. DeGraff & Sands (1925) reported an increase in heart rate in only 50% of their experiments. In the two experiments in which no change in heart rate occurred the initial heart rates were 134 and 168 beats·min^{-1} and in the four experiments in which the heart rate fell, the initial rates ranged from 133 to 208 beats·min^{-1}.

The results of Coleridge & Linden (1955) showed that, although there was some overlap, with initial heart rates higher than 150 beats·min^{-1} the response to an intravenous infusion was a bradycardia. The initial heart rates in anaesthetised dogs quoted by Sassa & Miyazaki (1920) were between 69 and 138 beats·min^{-1} and in the two experiments quoted by Anrep & Segall (1926) were 114 and 93 beats·min^{-1}. The last two groups of workers consistently obtained an increase in heart rate following intravenous infusions. Ballin & Katz (1941) did not report initial heart rates in their paper. To return to the paper of Bainbridge (1915), it is therefore possible that the initial heart rates in the four experiments in which the vagi were sectioned may have fortuitously fallen into the 'transitional region', around 150 beats·min^{-1} in which an increase in heart rate may not have occurred anyway, or the change may have been very small in either direction. These findings therefore add to the doubt (see Chapter 4) about the validity of bilaterally sectioning the vagi as a test for determining the afferent path of a reflex involving heart rate.

To complicate the problem further Coleridge & Linden (1955) in anaesthetised dogs found that intravenous infusions resulted in either an increase or a decrease in heart rate or no change in heart rate depending on the size of the infusion and the initial heart rate. When the initial heart rate was high intravenous infusions caused a reduction in heart rate and when

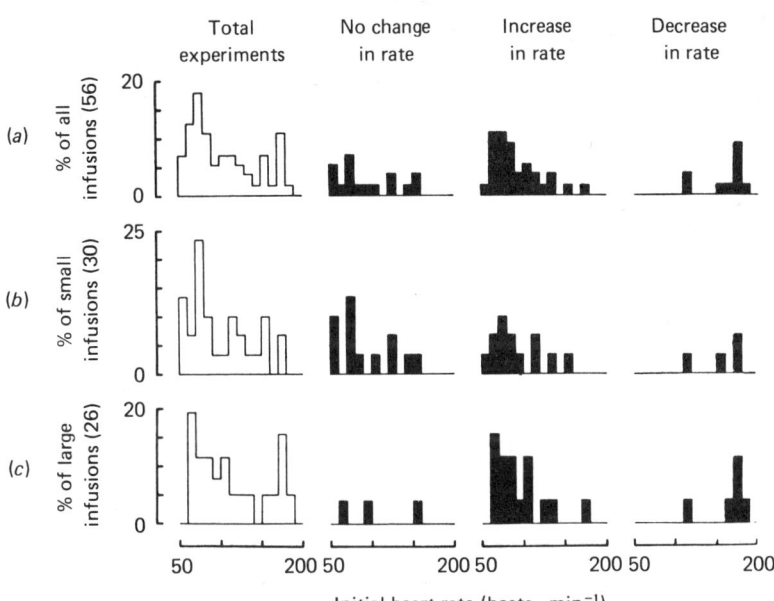

Fig. 5.3. Relationship between initial (pre-infusion) heart rate, alteration in rate and size of infusion in 56 experiments on dogs anaesthetised with morphia, Dial–urethane and sodium pentobarbital. (a) all infusions; (b) small infusions; (c) large infusions. Open blocks represent total experiments in each group; these are subdivided (solid blocks) according to whether there was no change, an increase or a decrease in heart rate in response to the infusions. All results are expressed as percentages of the group total: (a) 56 experiments; (b) 30 experiments; (c) 26 experiments. (From Coleridge & Linden, 1955.)

the initial heart rate was low intravenous infusions caused an increase in heart rate (Fig. 5.3). Results which were qualitatively similar to those of Coleridge & Linden (1955) have been obtained in the anaesthetised dog (Hirsch et al., 1964) and in the anaesthetised cat (Jones, 1962). Although the point at which the direction of the response changed was not very precise, an increase in heart rate did not usually occur if the initial heart rate was greater than 150 beats·min^{-1} and a decrease in heart rate never occurred with initial heart rates less than 110 beats·min^{-1} (Coleridge & Linden, 1955). These results also appeared to be consistent with an earlier claim by Sassa & Miyazaki (1920) that the increase in heart rate following intravenous infusions was greater in animals with a 'good vagal tone'.

In conscious dogs both Horwitz & Bishop (1972) and Vatner, Boettcher, Heyndrickx & McRitchie (1975) claimed that massive infusions (up to 3 litres) of saline always caused an increase in heart rate. By the use of atropine and β-adrenoreceptor blocking drugs these two investigations suggest that both sympathetic and parasympathetic efferent nerves are involved during these large scale 'volume loading' experiments. Similar volume loading by Hakumäki (1970, 1972) showed that there were increases in efferent sympathetic discharge in a cardiac nerve and decreases in efferent vagal nerves – although of course there can be no certainty that the efferent nerves studied were a sample of those affecting the heart. In none of these investigations was there any evidence that any particular receptors or afferent nerves were involved and only marginal evidence that a reflex might be involved. Recently in chloralose anaesthetised dogs, by examining changes in activity from the left atrial and arterial baroreceptors, Hakumäki (1979) did not find it possible to explain changes in heart rate caused by infusions. During the response of tachycardia changes in both efferent sympathetic and vagal nerves occurred, but during bradycardia only changes in sympathetic nerves occurred; during both responses increases in discharge of both aortic baroreceptor and left atrial receptors were observed. Such an investigation contributed nothing to an explanation of either the cause of any change in heart rate during infusions or an elucidation of the function of atrial receptors. It does seem that with massive infusions of saline almost any receptors in the body could be involved, both known and unknown, and including a possibility that some were not stretch receptors but chemoreceptors (e.g. Aviado & Schmidt, 1955).

It is concluded that there is no evidence of specific reflex responses emanating from the atria with afferent fibres in the vagi, as a result of investigations involving infusions.

Non-vagal pathways

Although Bainbridge (1915) failed to elicit a response following vagal section it has recently been suggested that part of the response of an increase in heart rate could be explained by spinal neural mechanisms (e.g. Gupta, 1975; Bishop, Lombardi, Malliani, Pagani & Recordati, 1976; Gupta & Singh, 1977). In anaesthetised dogs Gupta (1975) showed that he could obtain a tachycardia on infusion after β-adrenoreceptor blockade which was absent in dogs with combined β-receptor blockade and blockade of spinal autonomic afferent nerves; he suggested that the tachycardia resulting from infusions was partly a result of a reflex with its afferent pathway in the spinal cord and its efferent pathway in the vagal nerves. In a later investigation Gupta & Singh (1977), again using the infusion technique, suggested that the afferent pathway was predominantly on the right side, and that its entry into the spinal cord 'at T_1 may be via both dorsal and ventral roots'. Using infusions of blood in vagotomised cats with high spinal section, Bishop et al. (1976) produced a reflex tachycardia and hypertension which was abolished by section of the upper thoracic dorsal nerve roots.

Haemorrhage

Instead of an infusion to cause an increase in blood volume and pressure some investigators have used a haemorrhage to evoke a change in a stimulus. The classical response of the heart to haemorrhage is an increase in heart rate brought about by a fall in blood pressure causing less stimulation of systemic arterial baroreceptors (Heymans & Neil, 1958). However, such a simple explanation is questioned as being the full one by, for example, Aviado (1957) who showed that the tachycardia of haemorrhage was not necessarily related to changes in pressure: also, Gupta, Henry, Sinclair & von Baumgarten (1966) bled animals whilst keeping aortic blood pressure constant, and still obtained an increase in heart rate. It was, therefore, suggested that other receptors were involved. Different results were obtained in man more than 40 years ago by, for example, Eyster & Middleton (1924) who showed, in their Charts 1 and 2, that during rapid bleeding the heart rate first increased and then decreased. More recently similar experiments in animals (e.g. Oberg & White, 1970b) have reproduced these results. Responses of tachycardia and bradycardia were observed in different circumstances and they concluded that each of two groups of receptors, 'arterial baroreceptors and receptors with afferent fibres in the cardiac nerves, when operating in the absence of the other', was capable of producing tachycardia. In addition, 'rapid haemorrhages often produced bradycardia'. These experiments point to other receptors being involved but such assaults on the circulation do not assist the analysis of the function of any particular group of receptors, because (see Chapter 7) receptors with every conceivable function are to be found in the chest.

Direct action on the sinu-atrial node

It has been suggested that increased pressure in the right atrium stretches the sinu-atrial node having a direct effect on the node such that there is an increase in heart rate (Blinks, 1956; Pathak, 1958; Keatinge, 1959). In isolated hearts it has been shown that the frequency of discharge in the sinu-atrial node increased with an increase in atrial pressure until a certain critical value is reached beyond which the frequency decreased (Pathak, 1958; Keatinge, 1959). Isolated sinu-atrial nodes from the cat have been shown to increase their rates of discharge in response to stretch, a result which was unaffected by atropine and noradrenaline (Lange, Hsin-Hsiang, Chang & Brooks, 1966). Extrapolating from his observations to the whole animal Pathak (1966) has suggested that the dual response to intravenous infusions resulted from an alteration in the 'setting' of the sinu-atrial node. Pathak (1959) has also shown that intravenous infusions in dogs resulted in an increase, a decrease or no change in heart rate and that this response was unaffected by sectioning the vagi. Donald & Shepherd (1963) demonstrated that intravenous infusions resulted in an increase in heart rate in chronically denervated dogs. However, one must remember that it is difficult to demonstrate complete denervation, that re-innervation is fairly rapid, and that blood-borne agents, e.g. adrenaline, may change heart rate.

In an attempt to determine the role of the stretched atrial wall in the tachycardia of the Bainbridge effect Reitz, Dong & Stinson (1971) examined the effect of large infusions of saline in unanaesthetised dogs who had previously had cardiac autotransplants. In autotransplantation the atria are transected ventral to the venae cavae and pulmonary veins and the parts of the atria which remain (host atria) are innervated. The autotransplanted atria are extrinsically denervated. Infusions of

300–800 cm³ increased the atrial pressure which in turn caused an increase in heart rate only in the innervated host portion, not in the denervated portions of the heart. It was concluded that local stretch did not appear to be responsible for the tachycardia in the intact animal. However, these investigations involve large scale trauma to tissues with the possibility of rendering the relevant parts inactive. Some support for this suggestion comes from the work of Vatner *et al.* (1975) who found that there was no change in the heart rate with their large infusions following vagotomy and β-receptor blockade even though the atrial pressures were raised by massive infusion to as much as 3.5 kPa. It must be concluded that direct stretch of the sinu-atrial node or atrial muscle contributes little to the increases in heart rate usually observed in response to increases in atrial pressure; the stretch stimulus has to be excessive before a response is observed.

Conclusions

It appears that infusions either increase or decrease the heart rate or have no effect on the heart rate. The response appears to be related to the initial heart rate and, to some extent, the amount and rate of infusion. Though in some instances the effects are abolished by sectioning the vagal nerves there is some evidence that the response is not always affected by vagal section. It is unlikely that the effects of such infusions result from the response to stretch of the sinu-atrial node but there is a possibility that the changes in heart rate result from changes in a multiplicity of reflexes within the cardiovascular system.

The result of an infusion is never to stimulate only those regions of the heart containing atrial receptors as changes in systemic and pulmonary artery pressure also occur. Also when saline is used there are obvious changes in the composition of the blood; any increase in heart rate resulting from infusion has been attributed to chemoreceptor activity (Aviado & Schmidt, 1955). Therefore, all these experiments failed in their quest to elucidate the mechanisms involved in the Bainbridge reflex because no one group of receptors was discretely stimulated. It is also clear that infusion experiments do not shed any light on the effect of stimulating atrial receptors.

Aviado, Li, Kalow, Schmidt, Turnbull, Peskin, Hess & Weiss

(1951) drew a more general conclusion. They reported that a rapid infusion of blood (200 cm^3 in 5 s) for the first time frequently caused a temporary fall in blood pressure and bradycardia but repeating the experiments gave less clear cut effects even though the blood volume was unaltered. Slower infusions of the same volume of blood resulted in a simple rise in blood pressure accompanied by either a bradycardia or a tachycardia and they concluded 'we were unable to determine the factors responsible for these variations'. They also concluded 'that definitive results were unlikely to be obtained from such experiments and turned next to perfusion procedures as a means for securing better control over the variables involved'.

Considering all the numerous attempts to elicit the mechanisms by which infusions caused changes in heart rate we must agree with the conclusion in the first part of the last sentence – the next section will illustrate that the use of perfusion techniques fared little better.

Perfusion experiments

Isolating and perfusing the whole heart in an innervated perfused heart–lung preparation, Anrep & Segall (1926) claimed to have confirmed the observation of Bainbridge that an increased output of the heart gives rise to a reflex acceleration. They observed reflex acceleration of the heart even when atrial pressure did not change and after extirpation of the stellate ganglia. They concluded that the 'question of location of the receptor part of the reflex should still be left open and it is premature to regard venous pressure as being responsible for the reflex'. They were wise in this decision as the increase in heart rate resulting from stimulation of atrial receptors involves only sympathetic efferent nerves (see next chapter).

Following their conclusion that little information would result from infusion experiments Aviado *et al.* (1951) used large donor dogs; they used Dale–Schuster pumps to perfuse various parts of the circulation with either donor mixed venous or arterial blood, returning the blood to the donor. Essentially four preparations were used: (a) mixed venous blood was pumped into the right atrium, to perfuse the whole circulation, and blood was returned from the recipient venae cavae to the donor;

raising the pressure in the venae cavae did not cause any changes in heart rate, and raising the pressure in the right atrium of the recipient by increasing pump output caused bradycardia at the first attempt and diminishing bradycardia or tachycardia at subsequent attempts, vagotomy eliminating the bradycardia but not the tachycardia; (b) arterial blood was pumped into the left atrium, perfusing the left side of the recipient heart and systemic circulation, the blood being returned from the recipient's pulmonary artery; an increase in pressure in the right heart 'frequently' caused bradycardia which did not occur after vagotomy; (c) arterial blood was pumped into the abdominal aorta perfusing most of the systemic circulation, blood draining from the pulmonary artery as before – the results were identical to those described in (b); (d) the right side of the heart was isolated on a separate pump system and the left atrium perfused with arterial blood to maintain the systemic circulation of the recipient dog, essentially (a) and (b) combined; the characteristic effect of elevating the pressure in the right side of the heart by increased pump flow into the atrium or increased resistance to pulmonary outflow was bradycardia and hypotension.

The results depended on the vagi being intact but persisted after the injection of atropine and cardiac sympathectomy. The authors concluded that there was a 'reflex system' originating in the right atrium and pulmonary artery bifurcation apparently arising from stretch receptors and causing bradycardia and vasodilatation.

In all these experiments the stimulus was applied for relatively short durations (30 s) and judging from the published records it is possible to postulate either an increase or a decrease in both heart rate and blood pressure depending on the time from the onset of the stimulus at which the measurements are made. It is possible that the records merely served to emphasise the transient nature of the observed responses.

Quoting extensively from this paper emphasises the difficulty of this type of experiment. The extensive surgery required to insert the cannulae will obviously destroy many of the afferent and efferent nerves in and around the arch of the aorta and atria, the integrity of which is essential in order to be able to examine full nervous responses of the heart both to stimulation of receptors in the heart and to any potential changes in efferent nerves to the heart. It is also obvious that the design of these experiments makes it impossible to limit the stimulus to any one part of the circulation and it is clearly possible that the receptors in the ventricles such as those described by Coleridge et al. (1964b) may be involved in the responses obtained during the use of such perfusion techniques. It is essential to provide electrophysiological evidence of the effect of the perfusion on receptors in the perfused area said to contain the proposed receptors and on receptors outside but adjacent to the area. It is, therefore, not possible to accept, on evidence such as this, that there is 'a reflex system in the right auricle and pulmonary arterial bifurcation, apparently arising from stretch receptors and giving rise to bradycardia and vasodilatation'.

In experiments similar to those of Aviado et al. (1951) Barer & Kottegoda (1958) carefully cannulated the pulmonary artery in two directions and the right atrium of the anaesthetised cat. The right heart could then be distended either by increasing the flow to the right atrium or increasing the resistance to ejection from the pulmonary artery. Results similar to those of Aviado et al. (1951) were observed and the same criticisms apply.

Twenty-five years earlier Daly & Verney (1926) observed a bradycardia following a rise in pressure in the aorta whilst keeping the pressure in the vessels of the head and neck constant – they suggested the receptors were in the aorta, the left ventricle or the lungs. The following year Daly & Verney (1927) reported an investigation in which they changed the pressure in the left side of the heart by two means. First they used a cardiometer which enclosed the ventricles and the atria or just the ventricles. Secondly, they used a system of cannulation which allowed the outflow from the ventricle to be restricted whilst maintaining a constant pressure in the cerebral vessels. Reduction of pressure in the cardiometer surrounding the ventricles caused a slowing of the heart and the slowing was dependent on the integrity of the vagi. In the second series of experiments a rise in pressure in the left side of the heart was brought about by restricting the flow through the aortic cannula; the cerebral pressure remained constant throughout the observed slowing of the heart, which was again found to be dependent on the integrity of the vagi, and they concluded that the distension of the whole heart or only the ventricles caused a reflex slowing of the heart. From these experiments it is not possible to say exactly where the receptors involved in the proposed reflex were sited and indeed it is doubtful whether sectioning of the vagi establishes unequivocally the previous presence of a reflex (see Chapter 4). It is also important to point out, because the response to distension of the chambers was limited to bradycardia, that the surgery involved in placing cannulae in the root of the aorta and in the subclavian artery is extensive in an area in which both afferent nerves from the heart and efferent nerves to the heart are present. It is not possible to place cannulae in these vessels without destroying an unknown number of afferent and efferent nerves.

Goetz (1965) reinvestigated this problem using a right heart 'cul-de-sac' preparation; in this preparation the whole of the right side of the heart (i.e. atrium and ventricle) was distended and it was found that a rise in pressure resulted in an increase in heart rate. This increase in heart rate was unaffected by sectioning the vagi and by sympathetic blockade. Goetz (1965) therefore suggested that the effects were entirely due to stimulation of the sinu-atrial node. However, it is worth noting that the effects demonstrated were not quite so specific since it was also found that at a higher atrial pressure (> 4 kPa) there was a reduction in heart rate. This reduction in heart rate, unlike the bradycardia demonstrated by Aviado *et al.* (1951), was not abolished by sectioning the vagi. These results appear to support the earlier claims by Pathak (1958) and Keatinge (1959) that the sinu-atrial node exhibits such a dual response when stretched by increasing the pressure inside isolated right atria (see later in this chapter). Results broadly similar to those of Goetz (1965) have also been obtained by Vick (1963) using a modified Starling heart–lung preparation. Goetz (1965) finally concluded that distension of an area composed of the right heart and the great veins leads to an increase in heart rate. Further increases in pressure resulted in a reduction in heart rate, and both these responses were independent of the autonomic nerves of the heart. However, it must be pointed out that the experiments of Goetz (1965) do not provide evidence to support the hypothesis that the atrial receptors are not involved in cardiovascular reflexes affecting the heart rate. First there is no measure or discussion of the normal pressures or distensions in the right atrium within the normal ranges of activity of the heart; in this regard it is important to note the experiments of Kappagoda, Linden & Snow (1972a) where it was found that a much larger distension of the balloons was necessary to cause a small change in heart rate when the denervated sinu-atrial node was distended than when the reflex response was obtained. Again a criticism of the investigation of Goetz (1965) is that the surgery involved in the preparation of the cul-de-sac and the positioning of the ligature round the superior vena cava could have destroyed receptors, afferent nerves and efferent nerves.

Aviado & Schmidt (1959) vascularly isolated the left side of the heart in anaesthetised dogs. By the use of techniques such as increasing the inflow of blood to the left atrium or occluding the mitral orifice or the aortic orifice with a balloon, they observed a bradycardia and a hypotension. By adding and subtracting one experiment from another they concluded that the 'participating pressure receptors are believed to be in the walls of the left ventricle rather than the left atrium'. These so-called subtraction experiments are difficult to interpret because the control baselines vary from experiment to experiment. Also it does seem that this sort of experiment adds little to the knowledge of the function of any receptors in the atrium because in addition there would be the usual destruction of nerves caused by the dissection in and around the aorta and the atria.

In two controlled perfused preparations in the anaesthetised dog using cardiac bypass techniques Ross, Frahm & Braunwald (1961) attempted to 'localise these receptors within the heart'. The effects of increasing intracardiac pressures on the heart rate were variable and slight and 'the specific chambers in which pressures were elevated did not appear to influence' the results. Some changes in vascular resistance were observed. It is obvious that, with such gross disturbances as are caused during these sorts of experiment, it is not possible at all to attribute any of the responses to any receptors in any particular chamber, or, on not obtaining responses to conclude that such receptors, when stimulated by an increase in pressure, are not effective in causing changes in heart rate. Such investigations contribute little.

Abrupt changes in pressure in the left heart and pulmonary vessels of pump-perfused dogs caused a decrease in heart rate and a fall in blood pressure abolished by sectioning of the vagi (Lloyd, 1972). During experiments in which the mean aortic pressure was low, however, increases in both heart rate and blood pressure were observed. Lloyd (1972) presented his results as a relationship between changes in pressure in the left atrium and changes in heart rate and blood pressure. However, because the only attempt Lloyd (1972) made to show reflex mechanisms was to section the vagi which abolished the responses it is not possible to decide what contribution the atrial receptors made. Indeed it is possible that many reflexes were involved including those originating in the lungs, pulmonary arteries, left atrium, left ventricle and systemic arterial tree.

It is apparent from the above discussion that it is not possible to conclude from evidence in the literature that reflexes from specific groups of receptors have been identified: the stimulus during perfusion is not restricted to any one part of the heart. It is important therefore, in the next section, to discuss the group of experiments involving distension of parts of the heart.

Discrete distension of parts of the heart

Right atrium

Sassa & Miyazaki (1920) repeated the experiments of Bainbridge in frogs, rabbits, cats and dogs. After finding no increase in heart rate as a response to infusions in the frogs and rabbits, a small increase in heart rate and an increase in heart rate similar to that obtained by Bainbridge in the dogs, they assumed that the response described by Bainbridge was reflex in nature and attempted to locate the receptors and prove the reflex nature of the response in dogs. With the chest intact a metal tube with one end covered by a rubber membrane was passed down the external jugular vein and air was injected into a balloon to distend the right atrium or part of the superior or inferior vena cava. In another group of animals with the chest open a rubber balloon was placed through the atrial appendage and distended in the same way. Distension of the balloons in either atrium resulted in an increase in heart rate which was considered to be reflex in nature because it was abolished after sectioning the vagi. This reflex was believed to be initiated by impulses arising from the atria and from the veins close to the junctions of the veins with the atria. However, in their experiments no provision was made to prevent an obstruction to venous return and these results could be partially attributed to a reduction of venous return and a subsequent fall in cardiac output and systemic blood pressure resulting in less stimulation of arterial baroreceptors. Though full details of these experiments (Sassa & Miyazaki, 1920) were not given, such a reduction in blood pressure was said to occur in many instances.

In view of the obvious short-comings in the experiments of Sassa & Miyazaki (1920), Ballin & Katz (1941) re-investigated the function of the receptors at the junction between the superior vena cava and the right atrium by distending these regions without interfering with venous return. Two methods were used to distend the superior vena cava: first a modified Morawitz cannula was placed in the superior vena cava of an anaesthetised open chested dog such that a balloon extending along the outside of the cannula could be inflated through an air line allowing the lumen of the cannula always to be of constant size whether the balloon was inflated or not: the other specially designed cannula had an umbrella-ribbed expansile end and was inserted into the external jugular vein of an unanaesthetised animal under local anaesthesia so that the expansile tip of the cannula was placed at the junction of the superior vena cava and the right atrium, the position of the cannula being controlled by X-ray and checked at post mortem in each animal. With each technique an increase in heart rate was noted in only one instance; in the anaesthetised dog distension of the balloon caused the increase in heart rate even after bilateral vagotomy and also on occasion caused decreases in heart rate: in the unanaesthetised dog expansion of the metal umbrella so as to distend the superior vena caval–right atrial junction resulted in an increase in heart rate sufficient to be considered as a positive response on only one occasion during thirty attempts in eight dogs, and on this occasion the increase in heart rate was attributed to the fact that the dog became excited and displayed tachypnoea and dyspnoea. Ballin & Katz (1941) therefore concluded that there was no evidence to implicate receptors at the junction of the superior vena cava and the right atrium in the cardiac acceleration which followed intravenous infusions.

Discrete distension of parts of the heart

Blatteis & Horvarth (1964) distended the inferior vena cava near its entrance to the atrium and the right atrium directly by local stretching of these sites for 3 min using a balloon catheter in eight dogs and a specially designed prong-catheter (Blatteis & Tucker, 1961) in eight other dogs. During distension of the balloon reflex tachycardia was not observed in any of the preparations as the central venous pressure increased in the inferior vena cava or in the right atrium. Consequently during distension when the venous pressure central to the site of distension fell the heart rate in the intact dogs generally increased and this they showed to be a result of a lower cardiac output and thus of less baroreceptor stimulation. Prong-distension of the inferior vena cava or right atrium which did not obstruct but allowed a free flow of blood, caused a mean rise of about 0.3 kPa in the local venous pressure, but did not cause an increase in heart rate. They concluded that an increase in central venous pressure alone did not elicit a reflex increase in heart rate such as the Bainbridge reflex.

Recently, Greenwood & Kappagoda (1979) have resurrected this technique and in their experiments the 'junction between the superior vena cava and the right atrium was stretched by "expanding" a spherical wire cage mounted on a steel cannula': an increase in heart rate was obtained in eight dogs, though it was not shown that any atrial receptors were stimulated. From a subequent report (Greenwood & Kappagoda, 1980) it is concluded that it is likely that atrial receptors would be stimulated by this technique though again there is no evidence to that effect, or that other receptors outside the atrium would not also be affected. That mainly the Paintal-type atrial receptors were stimulated is suggested by the fact that the increase in heart rate was abolished by bretylium tosylate in exactly the same manner as in the investigation of left atrial receptors (e.g. Ledsome & Linden, 1964*b*; see also Chapter 6).

It is difficult to reconcile the various results in these investigations and impossible to be sure which receptors were being stimulated, though it is likely in the latter investigations to be atrial receptors. It is therefore apparent that the experiments described so far have failed to yield any conclusive evidence regarding reflexes from the right atrium.

Left atrium

Takino (1951) claimed that 'The reflex cardiac acceleration of the heart is proved beyond doubt by the rise of blood pressure in the pulmonary veins and their vicinity in the left atrium', following experiments in which he infused liquid through the external jugular vein and through the heart into the left atrium of the rabbit. In an attempt to stimulate the receptors in the pulmonary veins a small gummed balloon was inserted into the left auricle and then the end of this tube was moved from the auricle to the outlet of the pulmonary veins and their vicinity. It is difficult to believe that distension of this balloon with 1 cm^3 of air would directly stimulate the receptors at the pulmonary vein–atrial junctions of the small atrium of the rabbit; and indeed there is evidence in the figure of a decrease in arterial blood pressure on distension. The full results of this investigation are not presented but comments are made on the response to injection of 1 cm^3 of air into the balloon; a reflex cardiac acceleration is said to occur which was not completely abolished after cutting the left vagus in a rabbit which had previously had the right vagus sectioned six days previously. It is not possible to conclude from this investigation that stimulation of any particular receptors in the heart result in a reflex increase in heart rate because it is not possible to conclude that systemic arterial baroreceptors were not involved as a result of obstruction to blood flow in the left atrium.

Study of reflexes from the left side of the heart was helped by the development of methods for discretely stimulating left atrial receptors. Ledsome & Linden (1962, 1964b) inserted small balloons into the left pulmonary veins of the dog so that the balloons were precisely positioned at the vein–atrial junctions where it is known that there is a preponderance of atrial receptors (see Chapters 2 and 3). Distension of these balloons with small volumes of warm saline (1 cm^3) stretched this junction and resulted in a reflex increase in heart rate in every instance. Ledsome & Linden (1967) performed a second series of experiments in which a pouch was constructed consisting of the left atrium and the left pulmonary vein–atrial junctions and obtained similar results. These experiments unequivocally demonstrated a reflex increase in heart rate from distension of

Discrete distension of parts of the heart

the pulmonary vein–atrial junctions. This region contained the complex unencapsulated nerve endings (see Chapter 2) and it was likely that these receptors were involved in this reflex. These and further investigations using the same techniques for the discrete stimulation of atrial receptors are fully described, and the results discussed, in Chapter 6. Here it is sufficient to indicate that the topics involved are: left atrial receptors and the question of an inotropic response (Furnival, Linden & Snow, 1971), right atrial receptors and heart rate (Kappagoda, Linden & Snow, 1972a), atrial receptors in the appendage and heart rate (Kappagoda, Linden & Saunders, 1972b), and the recruitment of atrial receptors and increased responses (Kappagoda, Linden & Mary, 1975).

Edis *et al.* (1970) in anaesthetised dogs attempted to stimulate only the left atrial receptors by stretching the left pulmonary vein–atrial junctions using large balloons 1.5 cm long inserted into each of the pulmonary veins. During distension of balloons they observed a vasodilatation and a bradycardia or a tachycardia which was dependent on the initial heart rate. No attempts were made to show that these larger balloons did not stimulate other receptors. That these results were different from those obtained previously by Ledsome & Linden (1964b) could possibly be explained by the fact that much larger balloons were inserted in the pulmonary veins and atria, much larger volumes were injected into the balloons, there were falls in cardiac output and the increases in heart rate did not involve sympathetic nerves at all (e.g. the increases in heart rate were not blocked by propranolol); thus whatever receptors were being stimulated the reflex described by Ledsome & Linden (1964b), and claimed to result from stimulation of atrial receptors, was not involved. Possible explanations of the results of this investigation other than stimulation of Paintal-type atrial receptors are discussed in Chapter 6.

In two investigations Ledsome (Albrook, Bennion & Ledsome, 1972; Burkhart & Ledsome, 1974) inserted small balloons into the pulmonary vein–atrial junctions and showed that on distension of the balloons in the decerebrate dog there was increase in heart rate. The dogs were made decerebrate by electrical coagulation of the brain in the mid-collicular region. A further investigation (Burkhart, Funnell & Ledsome, 1977; Ledsome,

1979) using the same technique reported the results of decerebration at the level of the inferior cerebellar peduncle (rostral medulla). There was no apparent difference between the reflex increase in heart rate obtained in these decerebrate dogs and the heart rate responses observed in the intact dog. Though this does not preclude a hypothalamic influence being involved in the heart rate response, these very beautiful investigations suggest that the control centres for this reflex response reside in the brainstem region. Ledsome (1979) referred to Burkhart et al. (1977) who made 4 mm diameter lesions in the medulla of anaesthetised dogs, centred on the obex, dorsal to the hypoglossal nucleus. Following these lesions the reflex response to distension of the pulmonary vein–atrial junctions was almost abolished. They concluded that the afferent nerves from the atrial receptors synapse in the intermediate portion of the nucleus of the tractus solitarius close to the obex. Such a synapse had previously been suggested (Keith, Kidd, Linden & Snow, 1975) during experiments in which action potentials had been recorded in medullary neurones during stimulation of atrial receptors. The results of these experiments and the possibility of interaction between activity in afferent nerves from atrial receptors and activity in afferent nerves from arterial baroreceptors are discussed in Chapter 8.

Burkhart & Ledsome (1974) investigated the effect of distending the pulmonary vein–atrial junctions in the spinal animal supported by a constant infusion of noradrenaline. They claimed still to obtain an increase in heart rate on distension of the balloons which was abolished following vagotomy. Unfortunately following vagotomy the blood pressure fell during distension of the balloons which suggests that the balloons were obstructing the free flow of blood through the atrium. It is difficult to accept their conclusion that there is a vagal component to the reflex tachycardia obtained by stretching the pulmonary vein–atrial junctions and stimulating the atrial receptors (see Chapter 6 for fuller discussion).

Parts of the atria were stretched by various means by Brooks, Hsing-Hsiang, Lange, Mangi, Shaw & Geoly (1966), Koizumi, Ishikawa, Nishino & Brooks (1975) and Kollai, Koizumi, Yamashita & Brooks (1978). In anaesthetised dogs three means of distension were used: (1) small latex balloons were attached

Discrete distension of parts of the heart

to the tip of polythene tubes and the effect of 1–9 cm^3 distensions were observed, (2) two fixed rods were attached to the base of either the right or left auricle and a strong silk thread was then attached superficially half-way between the fixing bars and over the sinu-atrial node or the venous–atrial junction; the thread was then run over a pulley and weights were attached to the end to give a desired degree of stretch, and (3) the weight-bearing ligature was attached to the apex of the atrium so that the entire atrial myocardium could be stretched. Brooks *et al.* (1966) by applying techniques (2) and (3) obtained increases in heart rate during 254 out of 261 tests of the stretch effects. Tests after vagotomy produced variable results, sometimes giving a greater increase in heart rate than the control and sometimes less. With variable responses and such a crude means of stimulation it is not possible to conclude that any portion of these increases in heart rate were reflex in nature. Such a stimulus would result in secondary effects in other parts of the heart and other tissues and probably result in haemodynamic changes, in turn resulting in secondary reflexes. Such changes were reported by this group (Koizumi *et al.*, 1975): full details of these experiments are not given so it is not possible to conclude that discrete areas of the atrium containing receptors were stimulated. In addition in the records produced in the figures there is always a fall in blood pressure when the balloons were distended, suggesting that at least parts of the responses were due to a concomitant change in systemic baroreceptor stimulation which could explain some of the results involving both increases and decreases in heart rate. This investigation contributes nothing to increase the knowledge of the effects of stimulating atrial receptors. However, it is accepted that stretching of the sinu-atrial node can cause an increase in heart rate as had previously been shown by Blinks (1956), Keatinge (1959), Pathak (1959), Goetz (1965) and Pathak (1966) (see earlier in this chapter), which might, in part, explain their results. But it is probably simpler to ignore these investigations, where the nature of the receptor stimulus is unknown, where there is no evidence of atrial receptors, or for that matter any other receptors, being involved, and where there are several mechanical effects of the 'stimulus' on the circulation.

Stimulation by methods not involving distension

Little comment will be made on attempts involving methods other than distension of the chambers of the heart to evoke reflexes purporting to originate in receptors in the atria because these methods, electrical stimulation of nerves, blockade of tonic activity in the vagal nerves and the injections of chemical agents, are even less discriminating than perfusion experiments. It is difficult with stimulation and blockade of nerves even to be certain which set of which afferent fibres are involved (or even if they are afferent or efferent nerve fibres) and impossible to ascertain which receptors are involved: the injection of drugs which stimulate endings is valuable for pilot experiments the reports of which are confined only to the laboratory notebook. Most of the value of these three methods has been, not to elucidate which receptors in which heart chambers were involved in a reflex phenomenon, but to describe the possible range of effects which *might* evolve from a proper analytical study of this topic. In this regard it does seem, for instance, that stimulating the receptors discharging into ventricular C fibres, results in a bradycardia and hypotension (see review by Thorén, 1979a). Most of the comment on these means of initiating reflexes will be found in Chapter 7 where effects on the peripheral vascular system are discussed.

However, some of the experiments have involved changes in heart rate. Oberg & Thorén (1973) described experiments in which they examined compound action potentials and conduction velocities in cardiac vagal nerves; particularly they observed three fibre populations in two dogs and two in a third. They were able to divide the fibres examined into two groups; one which was fast conducting was stimulated by low intensity stimuli (4 V, 0.01–0.02 ms duration) and claimed to be a 'low threshold' myelinated group; a second group claimed to be a slow conducting 'higher threshold' non-myelinated group were activated by a higher intensity stimulus (4 V, 1–2 ms duration). Oberg & Thorén (1973) gave mean conduction velocities for the few experiments with no expression of range of results or statistical tolerance limits or even a statistical demonstration that the two groups were different in any respect. They also admit that 'It should be realised, however, that exact figures for conduction velocities are difficult to establish with the present set-up because of the relatively short distance between stimulating and recording electrodes.' However, it may be assumed that, as they claim, one of the groups ('low threshold') would consist mainly of myelinated fibres and the other non-myelinated, probably with an adequacy to justify pilot experiments involving stimulation of the nerves and observation of effects. Thus using these techniques Oberg & White (1970a) and Oberg & Thorén (1973) could claim that stimulation of myelinated fibres in the vagal cardiac nerves resulted in only slight increases in heart rate with the carotid arteries not occluded, which were greater when the carotid arteries were occluded. With a higher intensity of stimulation, presumably affecting both myelinated and non-myelinated fibres, it was found (Oberg & White, 1970a; Oberg & Thorén, 1973) that there was a decrease in heart rate whether the carotid arteries were occluded or not. A similar bradycardia (and hypotension) had been reported 20 years before this by Neil & Zotterman (1950) who found that the reflex effects were elicitable only if the electrical stimulation of the cardiac vagal branches were sufficiently powerful to excite the small fibres of the Aδ or C fibre type.

It is not possible to estimate where the stimulated afferent fibres originate, i.e. where the receptors are or even whether they are in the lungs or in the heart. Recordings of impulse activity in afferent fibres of the caudal cardiac nerve (Donoghue, Fox & Kidd, unpublished observation) have shown that it contains nerve fibres originating in mechanoreceptors in the lung as well as the heart. Activity in afferent fibres from the lungs had also previously been noticed in small branches of the vagus from the heart found behind the pulmonary artery (Dawes & Widdicombe, 1953) and by Oberg & Thorén (1973) who reported 'Occasionally, one or a few lung inflation receptor afferents can also be identified (Thorén, unpublished data)', in the 'right cardiac nerve'. In this regard it is interesting that Neil reports (Heymans & Neil, 1958; p. 211) that stimulation of the most obvious 'cardiovagal' branch on the right in the cat resulted in bradycardia, hypotension and tachypnoea. Over the course of an hour or so the respiratory response to stimulation disappeared suggesting that the afferent fibres causing this response were different from those causing the circulatory responses. By gross dissection the nerve appeared to originate in the vein but, as pointed out, there is no proof it did not, partly at least, have its site of origin in the lung.

Similar criticisms can be levelled at experiments in which the 'sympathetic' afferent nerve fibres were stimulated and small increases in heart rate obtained. Though in some experiments the heart rate was unaffected (e.g. Peterson & Brown, 1971) or not commented upon (e.g. Purtock, Colditz, Seagard, Igler, Zuperku & Kampine, 1977), in others (e.g. Malliani, Parks, Tuckett & Brown, 1973) there was a tachycardia when the 'sympathetic' afferents were activated by stimulating branches of the ansae subclaviae in an afferent direction. But again, the origin of the receptors involved could not even be estimated. Least of all, there is no indication of whether atrial receptors are involved or not.

Cooling the vagi to block tonic activity (e.g. Oberg & White, 1970a; Mancia, Donald & Shepherd, 1973) has not only provided evidence that some pressor effects are mediated by the vagi, but also that an increase in heart rate is observed, indicating that afferent, or possible efferent fibres, were involved before cooling. Differential cooling affecting tonic activity has provided little evidence of differential effects as opposed to its use during discrete stimulation of atrial receptors (see Chapter 6). Anodal block is said to be a more selective way to block myelinated afferent fibres (e.g. Mendell & Wall, 1964; Thorén, 1979a). However, there is dispute as to its effectiveness in discriminating between different populations of nerve fibres and it has even been shown that stimulation of non-myelinated fibres occurs (e.g. Hopp et al., 1980; see also Chapter 7). Such a block has been of little or no use in investigating reflex changes in heart rate resulting from possible stimulation of atrial receptors. Blocking vagal nerves during hypoxia which caused bradycardia in cats (Thorén, 1973) and guessing where the receptors involved might be, seems a singularly unproductive way of investigating the function of cardiac receptors.

A third blunderbuss technique for the supposed investigation of atrial receptors is the use of drugs, injecting them into various parts of the circulation and observing the responses. Mostly this technique has been used to investigate the Bezold–Jarisch reflex, the reponse of which consists of bradycardia, hypotension and

Stimulation by methods not involving distension

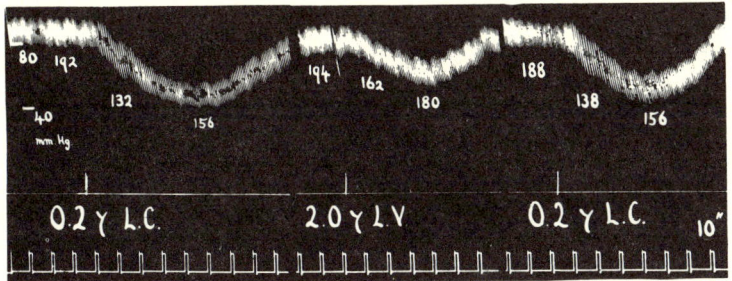

Fig. 5.4. Dog 5.8 kg. Pentobarbital. Blood pressure recorded by a membrane manometer from femoral artery, heart rate from ECG in beats·min^{-1} indicated by figures below pressure tracing. Injection of 0.2 μg veratridine into the main left coronary artery (LC) causes a greater fall of blood pressure and heart rate than 2.0 μg in the cavity of the left ventricle (LV). Time in 10 s intervals. (From Dawes, 1947.)

apnoea; the first two components, bradycardia and hypotension, are now thought to emanate from receptors in the heart, mainly the left ventricle, discharging into non-myelinated fibres in the vagi (e.g. see Thorén, 1979a; Donald & Shepherd, 1978; Hainsworth et al., 1979; Chapter 7). The best use of this technique was made by Dawes (1947). Dawes, in a beautiful study of the Bezold–Jarisch reflex, (Dawes, 1947; Dawes & Comroe, 1954) by selectively injecting small doses of veratridine at various points in the heart and central circulation, concluded at that time 30 years ago, that the main site of receptors involved was in the left ventricle (e.g. Fig. 5.4); the prediction was subsequently confirmed (see Chapter 7). But again, using this technique has not advanced the story of atrial receptors.

6 REFLEX EFFECTS ON THE HEART, II: DISCRETE STIMULATION OF ATRIAL RECEPTORS

In Chapters 4 and 5 it is concluded that, of the reported techniques claimed to stimulate atrial receptors, the one using small balloons with the left lung tied off at the root (first described by Ledsome & Linden, 1964b), is preferable. Also from Chapter 5, which chronologically presents the reports of the attempts to stimulate portions of the atria, it is apparent that the investigations by the Leeds group predominantly argue that if care is taken discretely to distend (Chapter 4) only those areas of the atria known histologically (Chapter 2) and electrophysiologically (Chapter 3) to contain atrial receptors then consistent responses are obtained. Others argue differently but appear possibly to be stimulating receptors other than atrial receptors. The arguments for and against the propositions put forward by the Leeds group are now presented.

In summary we suggest there is evidence to show that stimulation of atrial receptors results in a reflex increase in heart rate, the afferent nerves of which are in the vagi and the efferent nerves solely in the sympathetic nerves. Stimulation of the atrial receptors results in an increase in activity in the sympathetic nerves to the sinu-atrial node though not to cardiac muscle (no positive inotropic effect) and a decrease in activity in nerves to the kidney, there being also an increase in urine flow partly a result of the lower activity in nerves but mainly as a result of a blood-borne agent (the effects on the kidney are described in Chapter 10).

Evidence for an increase in heart rate

In Leeds the responses to stimulation of atrial receptors have been investigated in various preparations in the anaesthetised dog: by distending small balloons inserted into the three left pulmonary vein–atrial junctions, into two pulmonary vein–atrial

Evidence for an increase in heart rate

junctions and the left atrial appendage, into one or both atrial appendages, distending a left atrial pouch containing the atrial receptors and by distending a balloon at the superior vena caval–right atrial junctions. The results of all these investigations are displayed in Table 6.1 and are discussed below.

Ledsome & Linden (1962, 1964b) distended the small balloons in the pulmonary vein–atrial junctions (see Chapter 4 for details of methods) and observed an increase in heart rate in every experiment; in 78 distensions in 24 dogs there was an average increase in heart rate of 24 beats·min^{-1} (range 2–89). One of the best examples from their investigations is shown in Fig. 6.1; the increases in heart rate were calculated by subtracting the mean of the heart rate recorded in the control periods, before and 3 min after distension, from the heart rate during distension, giving an increase in this experiment of 77 beats·min^{-1}. No change in mean arterial blood pressure was observed and the change in pulse pressure, pulmonary artery pressure and the small falls in left atrial pressure and right atrial pressure are assumed to result from the increase in heart rate caused by the stimulation of left atrial receptors. It was shown by sectioning and cooling the vagi and by sectioning the ansae subclaviae or blocking the effects of sympathetic nerves with drugs, that the afferent nerve of the reflex was in the vagi and the efferent solely in the sympathetic nerves to the heart (see later for detailed evidence).

In experiments since then and following the discovery of atrial receptors in the appendages (Floyd et al., 1972; Chapter 2) another small balloon was placed in the left atrial appendage in addition to one in the upper pulmonary vein and one in the middle pulmonary vein; distension of these balloons again caused an increase in heart rate (Kappagoda, Linden & Mary, 1975) and an example from this work is shown in Fig. 6.2. Here it can be seen that the heart rate before distension of the balloons was 94 beats·min^{-1}, during distension was 162 beats·min^{-1}, and 3 min after distension was 116 beats·min^{-1}, giving a mean increase in heart rate of 57 beats·min^{-1}. Ten distensions of three balloons in five dogs resulted in a mean increase in heart rate of 35 beats·min^{-1} in these animals with a range of initial heart rates from 48 beats·min^{-1} to 133 beats·min^{-1}. The same afferent and efferent nerves were shown to be involved.

Table 6.1. *Distension of various parts of the vein/atrial regions in the dog*

Site of distension	No. of dogs	No. of distensions	Increase in heart rate (beats·min^{-1}) mean (range)	Initial heart rate (beats·min^{-1}) mean (range)	References
A Leeds group					
1 *Left atrium*					
(a) Left upper pulmonary vein–atrial junction	4	8	13 (7–22)	—	Kappagoda, Linden & Saunders (1972)
(b) Two junctions: left upper and middle pulmonary vein–atrial junctions	6	24	11	89 (48–133)	Kappagoda, Linden & Mary (1975)
	6	12	22	89 (48–133)	Kappagoda, Linden & Mary (1975)
	11	27	25 (8–54)	100 (56–139)	Kappagoda, Linden, Scott & Snow (1975)
(c) Three junctions – upper, middle and lower,	24	78	24 (2–89)	91 (36–168)	Ledsome & Linden (1964b)
	10	30	35 (5–68)	127 (61–193)	Carswell et al. (1970)
	10	20	18 (4–43)	110 (75–210)	Ledsome & Hainsworth (1970)
	12	37	21 (6–90)	148 (107–217)	Furnival et al. (1971)
	5	31	25 (8–48)	97 (65–134)	Harry et al. (1971)
	9	24	17 (5–41)		Kappagoda, Linden & Snow (to be published)
upper, middle + appendage	5	10	35	89 (48–133)	Kappagoda, Linden & Mary (1975)
	9	50	27 (9–60)	92 (39–118)	Kappagoda, Linden & Sivananthan (1979)
	21	21	23 (5–53)	100 (51–165)	Linden et al. (1979)

(d) Two junctions: right upper and middle vein–junction	43	78	22 (3–89)	123 (64–213)	Karim et al. (1972)
	3	8	31 (15–53)		Kappagoda, Linden & Snow (to be published)
II *Right atrium*					
Superior vena cava–atrial junction	16	65	18 (5–73)	133 (60–202)	Kappagoda, Linden & Snow (1972a)
III *Atrial appendages*					
Left	9	38	20 (7–61)	120 (61–185)	Kappagoda, Linden & Saunders (1972)
Right	3	7	12 (3–20)	126 (82–158)	Kappagoda, Linden & Saunders (1972)
Left and right	14	50	22 (7–59)	109 (64–162)	Kappagoda, Linden & Saunders (1972)
IV *Left atrial pouch*	10	33	10 (3–27)	137 (88–239)	Ledsome & Linden (1967)
B Other group					
Three left pulmonary vein–atrial junctions					
(a) Intact brain	32	109	18		Albrook, Bennion & Ledsome (1972)
	5	15	26 (5–76)	141 (103–168)	Burkhart & Ledsome (1974)
	7	21	19 (4–37)	141 (49–242)	Burkhart & Ledsome (1978)
(b) Decerebrate	5	15	16 (2–27)	107 (58–196)	Burkhart & Ledsome (1974)

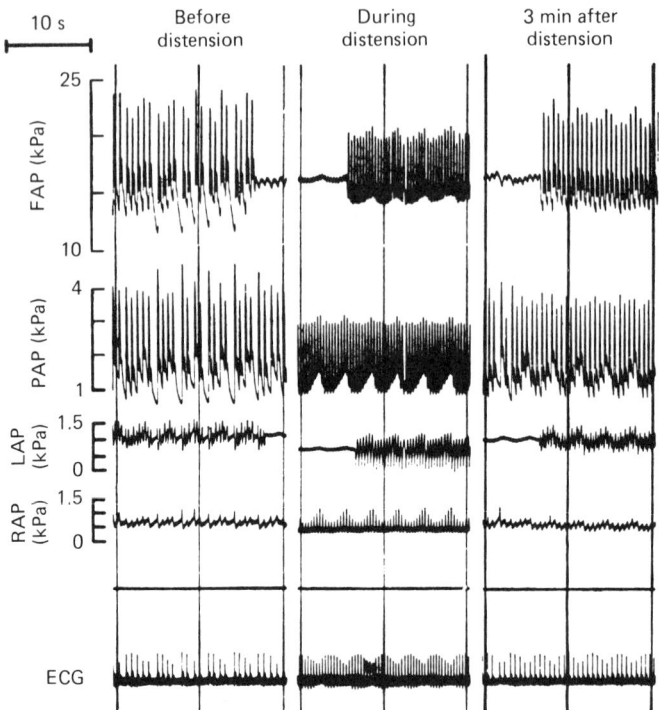

Fig. 6.1. Effects of stimulation of left atrial receptors on the heart rate of one dog, illustrating, not the best, but one of the better responses. Records from above downwards: femoral arterial pressure (FAP); pulmonary arterial pressure (PAP); left atrial pressure (LAP); right atrial pressure (RAP); datum line; and the electrocardiogram (ECG). The three panels show records before, during, and at 3 min after distension of the balloons. The change in heart rate from 80 to 170 to 105 beats·min^{-1} gave an increase of 77 beats·min^{-1} by averaging the heart rates before and after distension and subtracting the result from the heart rate during distension. (From Ledsome & Linden, 1964b.)

In 14 more anaesthetised dogs small latex balloons tied to stiff nylon catheters were introduced either into the left atrial appendage alone or into both atrial appendages. The balloons were placed in the tips of the appendages and tied in position and the nylon catheters were clamped so as to hold the balloons out of the atrial cavity and away from other tissue, particularly the ventricles. It was possible then to distend the balloons with up to 3 cm^3 of saline without obstruction to flow through the

Evidence for an increase in heart rate

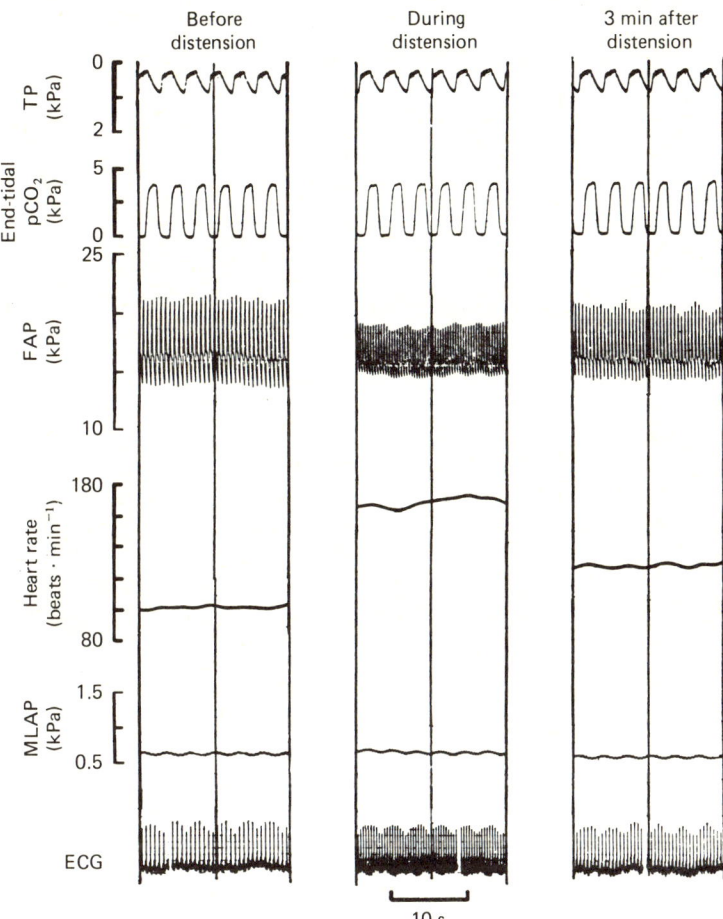

Fig. 6.2. Effect of stretching the left upper and middle pulmonary vein–atrial junctions and the left atrial appendage (three balloons). From above downwards, tracheal pressure (TP); end-tidal pCO_2; femoral arterial pressure (FAP); heart rate; mean left atrial pressure (MLAP); and the electrocardiogram (ECG). Records obtained immediately before distension of the balloons (heart rate, 94 beats·min^{-1}), during distension (heart rate 162 beats·min^{-1}) and 3 min after distension (heart rate 116 beats·min^{-1}). Mean increase in heart rate 57 beats·min^{-1}. (From Kappagoda, Linden & Mary, 1975.)

atrium or altering the atrial pressure (Kappagoda, Linden & Saunders, 1972). Thirty-eight distensions of the left atrial appendage alone, seven distensions of the right atrial appendage alone, and 50 distensions of both atrial appendages simultaneously were performed in the 14 dogs. An increase in heart rate was observed during each period of distension. For the distension of a balloon in the left atrial appendage the heart rate before distension was 119.8 beats·min^{-1} (mean; range 61–185), during distension was 140.0 beats·min^{-1} (mean; range 72–218) and 3 min after distension was 123.1 beats·min^{-1} (mean; range 60–183); the mean increase in heart rate being 20 beats·min^{-1} (mean; range 7–61). For distensions of the right atrial appendage the mean increase in heart rate was 12 beats·min^{-1} (mean; range 3–20) and for right and left together the increase was 22 beats·min^{-1} (mean; range 7–59). There was no correlation between the increases in heart rate and small changes in mean arterial pressure. There was also no correlation between the increase in heart rate and the changes in mean left and mean right atrial pressure. Sympathetic blockade and cooling of the vagi allowed the same conclusion as above, that the efferent pathway of the reflex was solely in the sympathetic nerves to the heart and the afferent pathway was at least partially in the vagal nerves. In order to determine the receptors involved in this reflex the effect of crushing the base of both atrial appendages on the response was studied in six dogs. After the control responses were observed clamps were placed across the bases of the appendages and left *in situ* for 10 min. The response to stretch of the atrial appendage was abolished in each animal. In four of these animals the left upper pulmonary vein–atrial junction was also stretched by distending small balloons in the manner of Ledsome & Linden (1964b) both before and after crushing the bases of the appendages. In all four animals the characteristic response of an increase in heart rate was present on both occasions indicating the integrity of the pathway mediating a reflex increase in heart rate following stimulation of left atrial receptors at the vein–atrial junctions. From these experiments it is possible to conclude that distension of balloons in the appendages was stimulating receptors in the atrial appendage and not stretching those in the upper pulmonary vein–atrial junctions.

Evidence for an increase in heart rate

In another series of experiments (Ledsome & Linden, 1967) an isolated pouch of the left atrium was constructed by placing a specially made clamp across the left atrium in anaesthetised dogs; the pouch was then distended by means of pulsatile changes in pressure. It was shown that the same reflex response of an increase in heart rate could be elicited and the same afferent and efferent nerves were involved. High pressures of the order of about 5–7 kPa were necessary to elicit a moderate increase in heart rate of 10.3 beats·min^{-1} (mean; range 3–27) (Ledsome & Linden, 1967); high pressures, similar to these, of the order of 2.5–5 kPa were required by Kidd *et al.* (1966, 1978) to cause a moderate increase in action potentials from atrial receptors (up to about 10 spikes·s^{-1}) at similar rates of pulsation (see Fig. 4.8). By evoking the Law of Laplace (see Chapters 3 and 4), it was suggested that the tension in the wall of the pouch and therefore the stretch of receptors would be much less even though the pressure in the lumen was higher, since the pouch had a radius of curvature about four times smaller than that of the whole atrium. This investigation served to provide more circumstantial evidence for the hypothesis that the atrial receptors were involved in this reflex response. No bradycardia was observed during any of these investigations.

Also in Table 6.1 can be seen the results of stimulating the receptors in the right atrium. A special cannula was created (see Chapter 4) that could be inserted into the external jugular vein of anaesthetised dogs to enable the superior vena caval–right atrial junction to be distended without blocking the venous return or changing the pressure in the right atrium. Distension of the terminal balloon to stimulate the right atrial receptors always resulted in an increase in heart rate (Kappagoda, Linden & Snow, 1972*a*). An example of a typical response is shown in Fig. 7.4. In 65 distensions in 16 dogs there was an increase in heart rate of 18 beats·min^{-1} (mean; range 5–73); these increases in heart rate were observed to occur from an initial control heart rate of 133 beats·min^{-1} (mean; range 60–202). There was no relationship between the small changes in arterial pressure or the superior vena caval pressure and the changes in heart rate. By cooling each vagus in turn the afferent pathway of the reflex was again shown to be in the vagi. Cooling the nerve to 6 °C (thermode temperature 5 °C) blocks conduction in myelinated nerve fibres of the size attached to atrial receptors, and reduced this response of an increase in heart rate; the response of an increase in heart rate when a vagal nerve was cooled was less than the response either before cooling or after rewarming the nerve. From these results it was possible to conclude that the afferent pathway of this reflex was at least partly in the vagi. The efferent pathway of this reflex was also shown to be in the sympathetic nerves; crushing both ansae subclaviae or blocking the action of sympathetic nerves with drugs, completely abolished the response of an increase in heart rate. No bradycardia was observed after sympathetic blockade; it may be significant that in the three dogs in which the right ansa alone was sectioned the response was completely abolished, though more experiments will obviously have to be completed before any definite conclusions could be made. There was no evidence to conflict with the hypothesis that the response to stimulation of right atrial receptors was the same as stimulation of left atrial receptors and that the afferent and efferent pathways were in the vagal and sympathetic nerves respectively.

It can be seen from Table 6.1 that if we lump together the responses to distension of one, two or three areas of the atria in the investigations completed in Leeds and reported above, together with the two investigations reported from Vancouver using the same stimulus (Albrook *et al.*, 1972; Burkhart & Ledsome, 1974), we find that during 23 investigations reported in 14 publications, 811 distensions of discrete areas of the atria in 251 dogs resulted in an increase in heart rate, the mean of the mean increases being 19 beats·min^{-1} (range of mean 10–35).

Nevalainen *et al.* (1980) studied the effect on heart rate of distending a balloon positioned at the left upper pulmonary vein–atrial junction in anaesthetised and unanaesthetised dogs. They showed that significant increases in heart rate occurred during distension of the balloon in the unanaesthetised dog, and in dogs anaesthetised with chloralose but not in dogs anaesthetised with pentobarbital. The increases in heart rate persisted throughout the duration of the distension of the balloon (8 min). Although it is likely that the increase in heart rate was caused by stimulation of atrial receptors, the report of Nevalainen *et al.* (1980) does not establish that the atrial receptors were involved in the response of increases in heart rate. Small dogs were used

(8–10 kg) and it could be argued that distension of the balloon might have caused obstruction to blood flow and reduction in blood pressure; the left atrial pressure and the arterial blood pressure were not measured and the volume used to distend the balloon was not given. Furthermore it is impossible meaningfully to compare the magnitude of the increase in heart rate between the two types of anaesthesia and in the unanaesthetised state. No information is given on the level of anaesthesia, the acid–base status and the variability of the heart rate during distension in the unanaesthetised state.

During the many investigations from Leeds reported above, it has been suggested that the anatomical pathway responsible for the reflex increase in heart rate during distension of the small balloons in the left and right atrio–venous junctions and appendages consisted of the following: an afferent pathway comprising Paintal-type atrial receptors discharging into myelinated fibres in the vagal nerves and efferent pathway solely in the sympathetic nerves. Several reviews (i.e. Paintal, 1973a; Shepherd, 1973) insisting that other pathways are involved and the observations that C fibres may be stimulated by distension of the left atrium (Thorén, 1979a) and that 'sympathetic' afferent fibres show increased activity with the stimulus caused by distension of small balloons (Holton, 1977), make it pertinent to present the evidence for our conclusion in more detail, as follows.

Afferent pathway of reflex

Section or cooling of the vagi in the chest and neck has always reduced or abolished the response. By sectioning or cooling the vagal nerves at various levels within the chest and neck, so as to block the nerve impulses from the atrial receptors, it was shown (Ledsome & Linden, 1964b) that the response to distension of pulmonary vein–atrial junctions was first reduced and then abolished. Sectioning the vagal nerves at the level of the right lung root and at the level of the upper border of the aorta on the left eliminated afferent nerves emanating from atrial receptors and abolished the responses. The fact that the control heart rate was unchanged and that the carotid sinus reflexes were intact was shown by occluding the carotid arteries, allowed the conclusion that the efferent vagal nerves had not been sectioned.

Table 6.2. *Vagal afferent pathway: increase in heart rate* ($beats \cdot min^{-1}$)

	Control			Section or cooling the vagi in:					
				Chest			Right vagus		
	No. dogs	No. dist.	Increase in heart rate ($beats \cdot min^{-1}$) mean (range)	No. dogs	No. dist.	Increase in heart rate ($beats \cdot min^{-1}$) mean (range)	No. dogs	No. dist.	Increase in heart rate ($beats \cdot min^{-1}$) mean (range)
a. Leeds group									
I *Left atrium*									
(a) Three junctions:	6	6	36 (13–77)	2	2	2.5 (2–3)	—	—	—
upper, middle and	10	30	35 (5–68)	—	—	—	—	—	—
lower pulmonary	3	6	29	—	—	—	—	—	—
vein/atrial	7	45	27 (9–60)	—	—	—	—	—	—
II *Right atrium*	6	20	21 (7–41)	—	—	—	5	6	6 (0–13)
III *Atrial appendages*									
Left	1	2	32 (22–43)	—	—	—	1	1	4
Left and right	4	18	31 (9–59)	—	—	—	4	6	3.5 (0–10)
IV *Left atrial pouch*	3	3	10 (0–11)	3	3	1 (0–3)	—	—	—

Vagal section or cooling

Results from the several investigations discussed in the previous section are collected together in Table 6.2 which shows the results of sectioning or cooling the vagal nerves to a temperature adequate to block the activity in myelinated nerves of the size connected to atrial receptors (conduction velocities of 10–$35 \; m \cdot s^{-1}$) in each of the previously reported investigations. The responses to distension of the three left pulmonary vein-atrial junctions, the superior caval–right atrial junction, the atrial appendages and a pouch of left atrium are shown before and after the sectioning or cooling of one or both vagi in the chest or in the neck. All the results are further summarised in Table 6.3 where it can be seen that in 16 dogs during four separate investigations, 25 distensions of the left atrial balloons following sectioning or cooling of both vagi in the chest or neck resulted in the response of only 0.7 $beats \cdot min^{-1}$ (average of the means of the four investigations; range 0–2); a control response to distension before the sectioning or cooling of the vagi was 32 $beats \cdot min^{-1}$ (average; range 25–36). That it is essential to cool or section both vagi is apparent from the results of the electrophysiological studies (e.g. Coleridge *et al.*, 1957; Coleridge *et al.*, 1964*b*). It could be concluded from these investigations that receptors in the right atrium and those in the

Left vagus			Both vagi			
No. dogs	No. dist.	Increase in heart rate (beats·min⁻¹) mean (range)	No. dogs	No. dist.	Increase in heart rate (beats·min⁻¹) mean (range)	References
4	4	2.5 (0–10)	1	1	0	Ledsome & Linden (1964b)
—	—	—	5	5	0	Carswell et al. (1970)
—	—	—	3	6	2	Ledsome & Hainsworth (1970)
—	—	—	7	13	1 (0–3)	Kappagoda, Linden & Sivananthan (1979)
4	4	11 (0–21)	—	—	—	Kappagoda, Linden & Snow (1972)
—	—	—	—	—	—	Kappagoda, Linden & Saunders (1972)
3	3	32 (15–53)	—	—	—	Kappagoda, Linden & Saunders (1972)
—	—	—	—	—	—	Ledsome & Linden (1967)

pulmonary veins on the right side of the left atrium mainly discharged into fibres in the right vagus, and also that receptors in the left side of the left atrium discharged mainly into fibres in the left vagus (e.g. see Fig. 4.1). But there was still a large number of receptors with fibres in the opposite vagus.

Electrophysiological evidence

As has been referred to earlier and in Chapters 3 and 4, Kidd et al. (1966, 1978) using two different preparations, small balloons in the pulmonary vein–atrial junctions and a pouch created from part of the left atrium containing the atrial receptors, recorded action potentials in slips of nerve dissected from the left vagus in the neck. It was concluded that both methods of distension of parts of the atrium result in excitation of atrial receptors (Chapter 4).

The receptors were located in the regions which had previously been delineated on both histological and electrophysiological grounds as the area in which left atrial receptors with myelinated vagal afferent fibres are to be expected (Coleridge et al., 1957; Coleridge et al., 1964b; Chapters 2, 3 and 4). Patterns of discharge before distension or the application of the clamp were characteristic of those for myelinated fibres attached to type B

Table 6.3. *Afferent and efferent pathway: summary of published results*

Drug or intervention	Increase in heart rate (beats·min^{-1}) average of mean values		No. of investigations	No. of publications	Total no. of	
	Control average (range of means)	After drug or intervention average (range of means)			Distensions	Dogs
Section of vagi in						
chest	23 (10 and 36)	2 (1–25)	2	2	5	5
neck						
Right	28 (21–32)	4 (3.5–6)	3	2	19	10
Left	29 (21–36)	15 (2.5–32)	3	3	15	11
Both	32 (27–36)	0.7 (0–2)	4	3	25	16
Sympathetic blockade						
Section of ansae subclaviae	25 (16–31)	4.5 (0–16)	5	4	20	18
Propranolol (0.5 mg·kg^{-1})	23 (11–60)	3.8 (0–9.8)	10	7	55	41
Bretylium tosylate (10 mg·kg^{-1})	21 (11–35)	0.6 (0–2)	9	7	100	54

Afferent pathway of reflex

and intermediate receptors (Paintal, 1972, 1973a). The number of impulses and the pattern of discharge during distension of the balloons were similar to and were also characteristic of those observed from atrial receptors with vagal myelinated fibres during infusion and expansion of blood volume.

Other evidence for the involvement of these receptors in the heart rate reflex response derives from the consideration of the mean and pulsatile pressures within the pouch with the resultant impulse frequencies and differences in threshold observed between the pouch and the reconstituted whole left atrium (see Chapter 4).

From a study of action potentials the observations are compatible with the previous studies in which reflex alterations in heart rate were observed. No evidence so far conflicts with the hypothesis that the most likely receptors to be involved in the reflex increase in heart rate are the Paintal-type atrial receptors attached to vagal myelinated fibres.

Grading the stimulus

It was suggested (Paintal, 1973a) that this reflex mechanism might be a 'trigger' response such that once the threshold to the receptors was reached the response mounted so rapidly that in effect this reflex could not contribute very much to the physiological control of the circulation. Because of this possibility it was thought necessary to grade the stimulus and attempt to get a 'dose–response' curve. However, in the earlier experiments it was not possible to obtain a correlation between the magnitude of stretch thought to be imposed and the increase in heart rate. As detailed in Chapter 4 attempts to show the 'stretching force' imposed on the vein–atrial junctions suggested that with larger volumes in the balloons less 'stretching force' could be imposed; it was possible that the balloons moved in relation to the atrial wall (see Chapter 4).

However, this problem was solved by grading the stimulus to the receptors in another way. Once it had been found that the distension of the atrial appendages with small balloons caused a reflex increase in heart rate (Kappagoda, Linden & Saunders, 1972a, b) and that each atrial appendage contained about ten atrial receptors in the dog, it was possible to stimulate successively

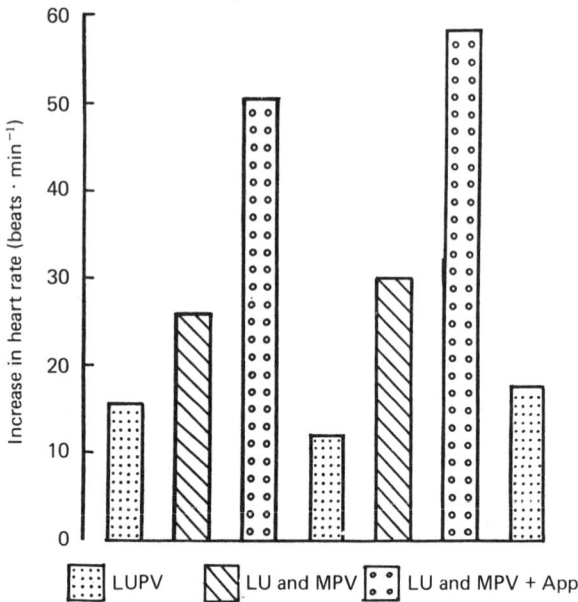

Fig. 6.3. Gradation of the responses to distension of the balloons: LUPV, distension of the balloon in left upper pulmonary vein alone; LU and MPV, distension of the two balloons in left upper and middle pulmonary veins respectively; LU and MPV + App, distension of the three balloons in the left upper and middle pulmonary veins and in the left atrial appendage respectively. The responses are expressed as increases in heart rate (beats·min^{-1}). (From Kappagoda, Linden & Mary, 1975.)

different areas of receptors and therefore successively greater numbers of receptors; distensions of the balloons first at one atrio–venous junction, secondly at two atrio–venous junctions, and thirdly at two atrio–venous junctions together with the distension of the left atrial appendage, were completed (Kappagoda, Linden & Mary, 1975). The pulmonary vein–atrial junctions were each distended with 1 cm^3 of warm saline and the atrial appendage with 2 cm^3. An example from one dog is shown in Fig. 6.3. In six dogs 24 distensions of a single pulmonary vein–atrial junction resulted in an increase in heart rate 10.8 beats·min^{-1} (mean; range 6–18); 12 distensions of the two pulmonary vein–atrial junctions, an increase in heart rate of 22.2 beats·min^{-1} (mean; range 12–37); and by distending the appendage in addition (i.e. 10 distensions of three balloons simultaneously) an increase in 35.2 beats·min^{-1} (mean; range 22–57) was observed. Single balloon distensions were obtained both before and after the multiple balloon distensions. The difference between any two of the groups of results was statistically significant. Thus when the stimulus to the atrial receptors is graded by successively recruiting groups of atrial receptors the response of an increase in heart rate is also graded (Kappagoda, Linden & Mary, 1975), giving evidence of spatial summation within the central nervous system. The area stimulated by these balloons is small compared to the total area in which atrial receptors are to be found, e.g. the right atrial receptors, atrial receptors on the right side of the left atrium and an unknown number on the left side of the left atrium would not be stimulated in this series of experiments.

Recently Greenwood & Kappagoda (1980) have used an 'expanding' spherical wire cage on a stainless steel cannula to distend the superior caval–right atrial junction and obtain an increase in heart rate. Although they have not specifically identified the receptors stimulated by this technique it is probable that Paintal-type right atrial receptors were affected (see Chapter 5); the heart rate increases were blocked by bretylium tosylate. It is likely therefore that the 'summation' of the increases in the heart rate observed in their experiments resulting from simultaneous stretching of right (metal cage) and left (small balloons) atrio–venous junctions, originated as a summation of effect of stimulating right and left Paintal-type atrial receptors. Such a response allows the conclusion that the right and left atrial receptors act as one group in a possible control system regulating heart rate. It is probable that if all the atrial receptors could be simultaneously stimulated a very much larger increase in heart rate would result allowing the suggestion that the reflex may be of considerable importance in regulation of the circulation. However, it may be concluded again, from this series of experiments, that the most likely receptors to be stimulated by the distension of small balloons at the pulmonary vein–atrial junctions are the atrial receptors which discharge into myelinated fibres in the vagal nerves.

Reflex effects on the heart, II

Differential cooling of the vagi

Yet a further series of experiments positively correlated the vagal myelinated fibres attached to the atrial receptors with the response of an increase in heart rate and eliminated C fibres from any association. This step was thought to be necessary because it had been reported during several investigations (e.g. Sleight & Widdicombe, 1965; Coleridge et al., 1973; Thorén, 1976a; Thames, 1979 and see Chapters 2 and 3) that there were also receptors in the atrium which discharge into C fibres (conduction velocity less than 2.5 m·s^{-1}) in the vagal nerves. Thorén (1976a) has shown an increase in C fibre discharge of up to 20 impulses·s^{-1} when pressures were raised in the atria up to 3–4 kPa. Thus it was probable that the distension of the balloons was also exciting these receptors and it is possible that the C fibres could be involved in the heart rate-reflex response. Therefore in three groups of experiments in this investigation, the responses of an increase in action potentials in myelinated fibres, in C fibres and the increase in heart rate during stimulation of the atrial receptors were examined whilst progressively cooling the vagi in the neck (Kappagoda, Linden & Sivananthan, 1979). First, various cooling thermodes were examined and one finally constructed 2.5 cm wide which when cooled, resulted in the temperature in the centre of the nerve (at mid-thermode, 1.25 cm along the cooled segment of the nerve) being at the same temperature as the surface of the thermode (at mid-thermode) – a detailed description of the 2.5 cm wide thermode is reported by Linden, Mary & Weatherill (1981). Because cooling was relatively slow this relationship remained the same (difference < 0.1 °C) during cooling. However, at least one minute was allowed at each temperature before records were taken.

From previous experiments it was known that atrial receptors discharged during the control period at a mean frequency of 30–40 impulses·s^{-1} and that on distension of a small balloon in the pulmonary vein–atrial junction with 1 cm^3 warm saline this discharge increased to a frequency of 80–120 impulses·s^{-1}. It was also known that these fibres had a conduction velocity in our experiments of the order of 10–35 m·s^{-1}. Also from several reports published by Paintal, (Paintal, 1963a, 1965a, b, 1966) it

Afferent pathway of reflex

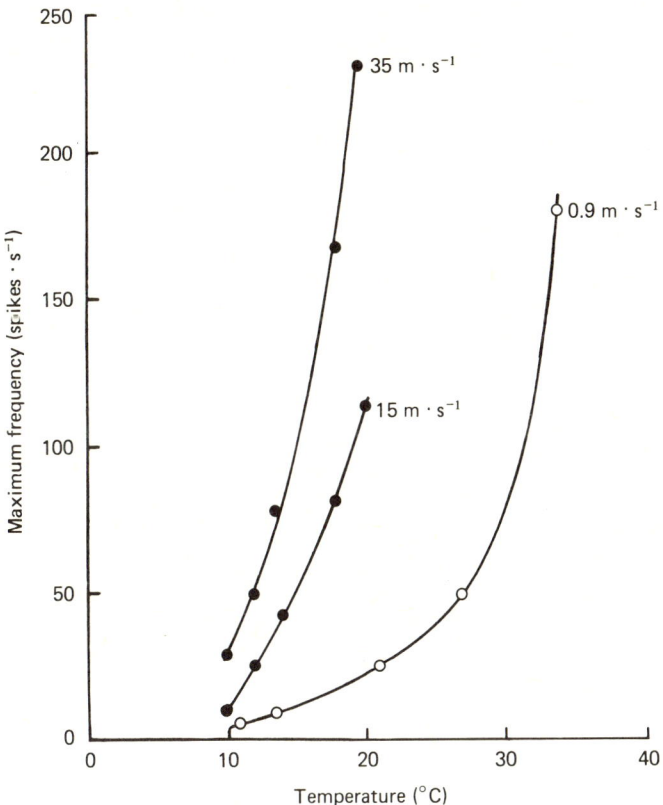

Fig. 6.4. Maximum frequency of impulses conducted by myelinated fibres with conduction velocities of 35 m·s^{-1} and 15 m·s^{-1} (from Paintal, 1972); and of a C fibre of conduction velocity 0.9 m·s^{-1} (from Franz & Iggo, 1968). Ordinate: impulses in nerve fibres, spikes·s^{-1}; abscissa: temperature of nerve on cooling thermode. (From Linden, 1979.)

could be suggested that differential cooling might selectively block the activity of atrial receptors discharging into myelinated fibres as opposed to others, particularly receptors discharging into non-myelinated (C) fibres. That a cooling temperature of about 10–12 °C might be critical in this regard could be concluded by comparing Paintal's (1966) results obtained from myelinated fibres with those of Franz & Iggo (1968) in a non-myelinated fibre. A diagram published by Paintal (1966) shows that the maximum frequency of impulses which a myeli-

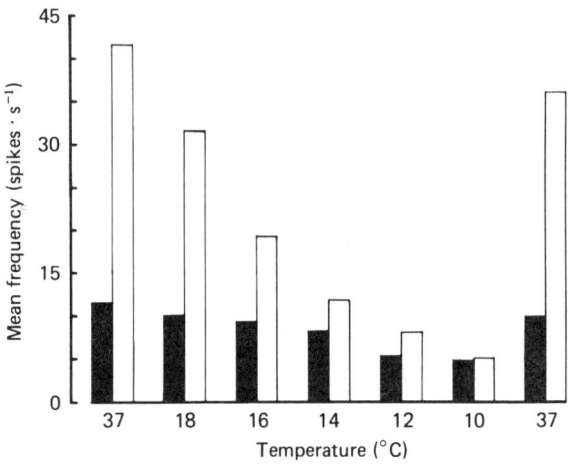

Fig. 6.5. The effect of cooling the vagus on the response in a type B atrial receptor to distension of a balloon at a pulmonary vein–atrial junction. The results of one experiment are shown in the form of a histogram. Ordinate, mean frequency of discharge (spikes·s^{-1}); abscissa, temperature of vagus (°C). The black columns represent the average frequency during the two control periods and the white columns represent the frequency during the period of distension. The difference between the test and control was minimal when the vagus was cooled to 10 °C. (From Kappagoda, Linden & Sivananthan, 1979.)

nated nerve fibre can conduct depends on the temperature and the conduction velocity, i.e. in any one fibre the effect of cooling is frequency dependent. Part of Paintal's figure is shown redrawn in Fig. 6.4; the results of cooling two myelinated fibres, one with a conduction velocity of 35 m·s^{-1}, one with 15 m·s^{-1}, are shown. As the nerve is cooled the maximum frequency at which impulses can pass through the cold block is indicated by each curve. For instance, at 16 °C it can be seen that a frequency of 120 impulses·s^{-1} would just get through the cold block in a fibre conducting at 35 m·s^{-1}, and at 12 °C a frequency of 30 impulses·s^{-1} would just not pass the block in a fibre conducting at 15 m·s^{-1}. The first hypothesis to be tested was that the increases in numbers of action potentials brought about by distending the balloons in the pulmonary vein–atrial junctions would be gradually blocked as the vagi were cooled; the results of one experiment in one dog are shown in Fig. 6.5 and the

Afferent pathway of reflex

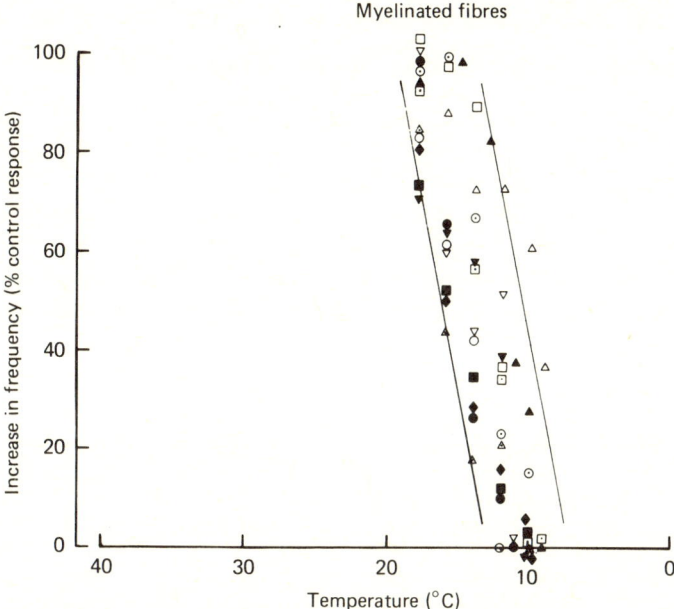

Fig. 6.6. Response of the increase in action potentials in myelinated vagal fibres resulting from distension of balloons in pulmonary vein–atrial junctions, to cooling of the vagus in 2 °C steps. Each point represents the response of the increase in action potentials (mean frequency), at each temperature of the vagus, expressed as a percentage of the response with the vagus at 36–37 °C. Each symbol represents the response in one nerve fibre. Twelve fibres with conduction velocities ranging from 9 to 37.5 m·s^{-1} were examined in eight dogs. The responses at 36–37 °C were all rated 100% responses and are not shown in the diagram. The two continuous lines are drawn by eye to enclose all the responses to cooling and are the same as in Fig. 6.8. (From Kappagoda, Linden & Sivananthan, 1979.)

results of the examination of 12 fibres in eight dogs are shown in Fig. 6.6.

As seen in Fig. 6.5 the response in the myelinated fibre was first obtained with the vagus at a temperature of approximately 37 °C (first control response). The vagus was cooled in 2 °C decrements and the distension repeated at each temperature. The process was continued until a response (i.e. an increase in mean frequency above the control value at that temperature) was no longer elicited. The vagus was then rewarmed to 37 °C and the second control response obtained. It was found that the response in this myelinated fibre to distension of the balloon (expressed as an increase in mean frequency above the control value) was 30.2 spikes·s^{-1} at 37 °C, 10.3 spikes·s^{-1} at 16 °C and 0.3 spikes·s^{-1} at 10 °C. On rewarming the vagus at 37 °C the increase was 25.1 spikes·s^{-1}. Twelve such fibres were examined in this way in eight dogs; the response was abolished over a range of 12–8 °C. In order to compare the data from all the dogs, the response at a particular temperature was expressed as a percentage of the average of the two control responses obtained at 37 °C. The results from all these fibres are summarised and shown in Fig. 6.6. The oblique lines include the majority of the data; they are the same lines as shown in Fig. 6.8, where they are drawn by eye to include all the data. Thus it is concluded that the response of atrial receptors, which discharge into myelinated vagal afferent fibres, to distension of the balloons, is slightly attenuated (approximately 30% reduction) when the vagus is cooled to 16 °C and is considerably reduced (approximately 70% reduction) at 12 °C. It is abolished when the vagus is cooled to approximately 10 °C. It could be concluded from this evidence that the myelinated fibres involved were attached to atrial receptors and therefore atrial receptors were being stimulated by the distension of the small balloons.

In the next group of experiments the effect of the same graded cold blockade of both cervical vagi on the increase in heart rate obtained in response to distension of balloons at the vein–atrial junctions and the atrial appendage, was studied. The response to distension of the balloons was first obtained with the vagi at approximately 37 °C (first warm control response). The vagi were then cooled to a temperature between 18 °C and 8 °C, and the response was repeated. Finally, the vagi were rewarmed and a second warm control response elicited. In this way the response to distension of balloons at three or four different temperatures was examined in each animal down to the temperature at which it was abolished. In each instance the 'cool' response was preceded and followed by a 'warm' one. The results from one experiment are shown in Fig. 6.7 which shows the entire experiment in diagrammatic form. It can be seen that when the vagi were cooled to 10 °C no increase in heart rate was observed on distension of the balloons. The initial control heart rate at this stage was greater than that observed in the test

Afferent pathway of reflex

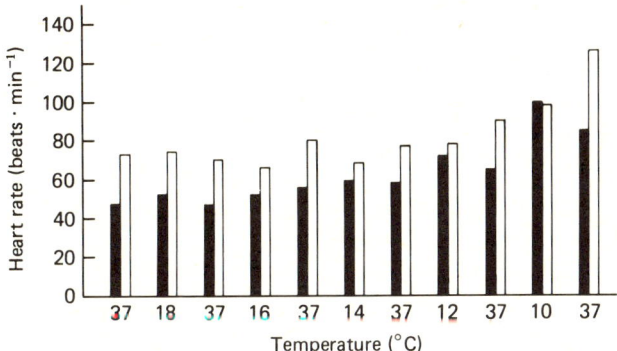

Fig. 6.7. The effect of cooling both cervical vagi on the increase in heart rate resulting from distension of the balloons at the left pulmonary vein–atrial junctions. The results of one experiment are shown in the form of a histogram. Ordinate, heart rate (beats·min^{-1}); abscissa, temperature of vagus (°C). The black columns represent the average heart rate during the two control periods (beats·min^{-1}) and the white columns represent the heart rate during the period of distension. The response of an increase in heart rate is abolished at 10 °C. (From Kappagoda, Linden & Sivananthan, 1979.)

periods in the early stages of the experiment. However, when the vagi were warmed for the last time the control heart rate was similar to that observed when the vagi were cooled to 10 °C. On this occasion the heart rate increased by 41 beats·min^{-1} when the balloon was distended. Experiments similar to this one were completed with the vagi cooled to various temperatures in nine dogs. In these animals a total of 50 responses were obtained at 36–37 °C. The mean increase in heart rate was 27.3 beats·min^{-1} (range 9–60). In order to compare the results in one dog with those obtained in another, in each dog the responses at any one temperature were expressed as a percentage of the average of all the warm control responses in that animal. These results are summarised in Fig. 6.8; the oblique lines are drawn by eye to include all the data. From these results it is concluded that the response of an increase in heart rate was slightly reduced (approximately 20% reduction) at 16 °C and greatly diminished at 12 °C (approximately 70% reduction). It was abolished between 8 and 12 °C.

There is a general similarity in the effect of cooling the vagi on the heart rate response to that of cooling the vagi on the increase in action potentials in myelinated fibres discharging as

Reflex effects on the heart

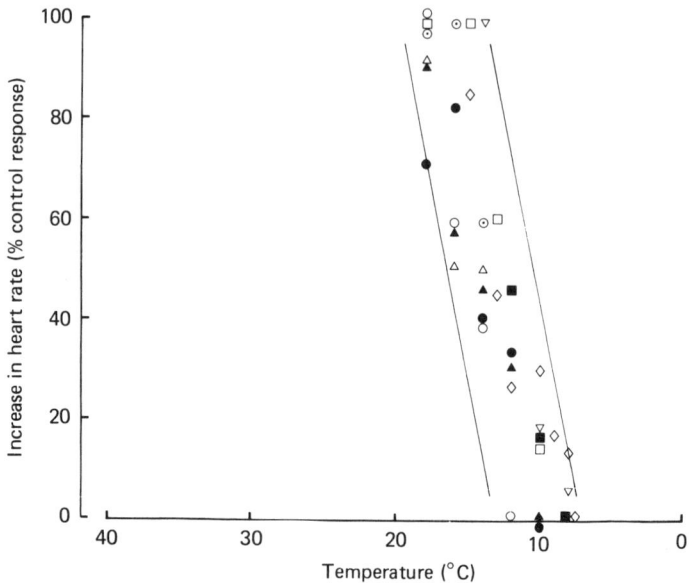

Fig. 6.8. Response of the increase in heart rate resulting from distension of balloons in the pulmonary vein–atrial junctions, to cooling of the vagi in steps to 8 °C. Each point represents the response of the increase in heart rate at each temperature of the vagi expressed as a percentage of the control responses obtained with the vagi at 36–37 °C; the control responses were obtained before and after the cooled response. Each symbol represents the results from one dog. The responses at 36–37 °C were all rated 100 % responses and are not shown in the diagram. The continuous lines are drawn by eye to enclose all the responses to cooling and are the same as those in Fig. 6.6. (From Kappagoda, Linden & Sivananthan, 1979.)

a result of stimulating atrial receptors; parallel lines drawn on Fig. 6.8 enclose all the responses to an increase in heart rate to cooling of the vagi and the same lines drawn on the previous figures (Fig. 6.6) enclose all but three responses of increases in action potentials on cooling. Thus it may be concluded that the effects of cooling the vagal nerves in a stepwise fashion are the same on both the response of an increase in action potentials to distension of the balloons and the response of an increase in heart rate to distension of the balloons. It is therefore concluded, following this positive correlation, that Paintal-type atrial receptors and the myelinated fibres in the vagus are involved in the afferent pathway of this reflex.

Afferent pathway of reflex

The next series of experiments eliminated the C fibres as being even partly responsible. There is only one report (Franz & Iggo, 1968) of a C fibre, the impulse traffic in which was examined whilst cooling; this response has been plotted alongside those of Paintal in Fig. 6.4. The C fibre had a conduction velocity of 0.9 m·s^{-1} and it can be seen that a frequency of about 20 impulses·s^{-1} (a frequency observed by Thorén (1976a) to be conducted in C fibres when the pressure in the atrium was raised) would just not get through the cold block at 16 °C – well above the blocking temperature of our reflex response; the usual discharge in C fibres of less than 5 impulses·s^{-1} would still be passing through the cold block even at 12 and 10 °C. This investigation therefore examined C fibres which increased their discharge during distension of the small balloons in the vein–atrial junctions and subsequently the temperature of the vagal nerves was decreased in 2 degree steps. The first control response was elicited with the vagi at approximately 37 °C. The effect on the response of cooling the vagus was calculated in the same manner as for myelinated fibres being cooled, as above. The vagi were cooled and the distension was repeated at each stage, until the response was abolished (i.e. there was no increase in mean frequency over the control values). The vagus was then rewarmed and a second warm control response was elicited.

Fig. 6.9 illustrates the responses obtained in two fibres. It shows a fibre (conduction velocity 1.2 m·s^{-1}) which had an initial spontaneous discharge of 10.7 spikes·s^{-1}. This discharge increased to 30 spikes·s^{-1} during distension of the balloons and returned to 8.3 spikes·s^{-1} during the final control period. When the vagus was cooled to 17 °C, the control discharge was 5.3 spikes·s^{-1} and increased to 6.1 spikes·s^{-1} during distension of the balloon and returned to 5.0 spikes·s^{-1}. On rewarming the vagus the response attained its previous magnitude (initial control 10.2 spikes·s^{-1}; test 27.0 spikes·s^{-1}; final control 7.7 spikes·s^{-1}). In contrast Fig. 6.10 shows a fibre (conduction velocity 1.5 m·s^{-1}) which had no spontaneous activity. It increased to 7.4 spikes·s^{-1} during balloon distension and ceased to discharge during the final control period. This response was still present (3.7 spikes·s^{-1}) when the vagi were cooled to 6 °C.

In order to compare the data from different investigations, the response in a particular fibre at a given temperature was

Reflex effects on the heart

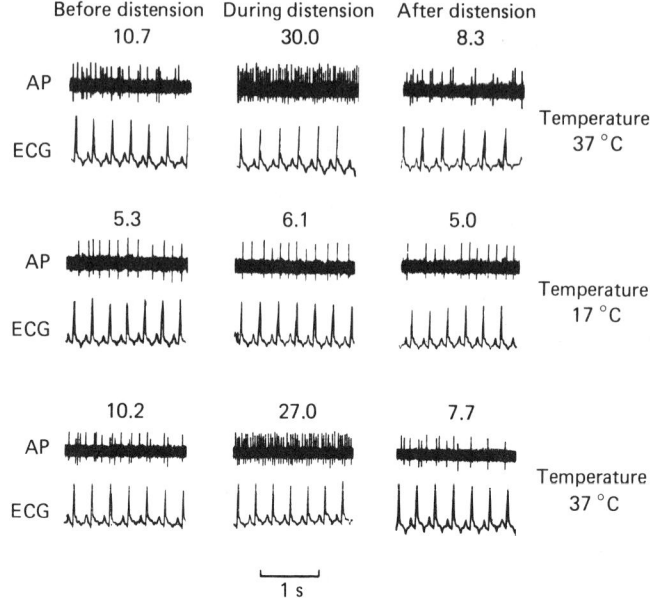

Fig. 6.9. The effect of cooling the cervical vagus on the response in a non-myelinated fibre to distension of a balloon at the left pulmonary vein–atrial junction. Fibre had a frequency of approximately 10 spikes·s^{-1} during the control period and a conduction velocity of 1.2 m·s^{-1}. The figure shows portions of experimental records taken with the vagus at 37 (initial control response), 17 and 37 °C (final control response). Each record shows the action potentials (AP) and the electrocardiogram (ECG). The number above each tracing is the mean frequency (spikes·s^{-1}). It is seen that the response was virtually abolished by cooling the vagus to 17 °C. (From Kappagoda, Linden & Sivananthan, 1979.)

expressed as a percentage of the average of the warm responses as for the myelinated fibres above. These results are summarised in Fig. 6.11. It was found that graded cold blockade did not affect the response in non-myelinated fibres in the same quantitative manner as it did in the myelinated fibres. The response was attenuated over a much wider range of temperature. It seems there is little similarity between the response in C fibres to progressive cooling and that of the heart rate response. The same two continuous lines drawn on Figs. 6.6 and 6.8 that enclosed the results of the previous two investigations have been

Afferent pathway of reflex

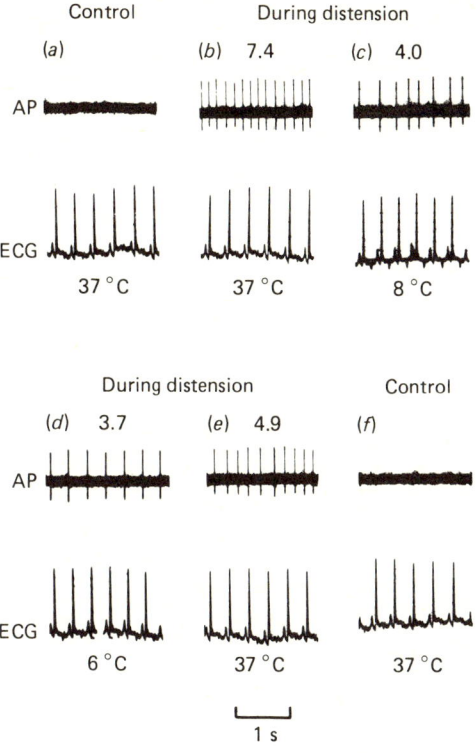

Fig. 6.10. The effect of cooling the cervical vagus on the response in a non-myelinated fibre to distension of a balloon at a left pulmonary vein–atrial junction. The fibre was inactive during *all* the control periods and had a conduction velocity of 1.5 m·s^{-1}. The figure shows portions of experimental records taken with the vagus at 37, 8 and 6 °C. Each record shows the action potentials (AP) and the electrocardiogram (ECG). The number above each tracing of spike potentials is the mean frequency calculated over 1 min. Since this fibre was inactive during the control periods only two control records at 37 °C are shown ((*a*) and (*f*)). (*b*), (*c*), (*d*) and (*e*) are portions of records taken during periods of distension (i.e. test records). It is seen that the response was not abolished even when the vagus was cooled to 6 °C. There were small cyclical changes in heart rate in this animal. There was no response in changes in heart rate to distension of the balloons, presumably because of the extensive dissection of the vagus nerve. (From Kappagoda, Linden & Sivananthan, 1979.)

Reflex effects on the heart

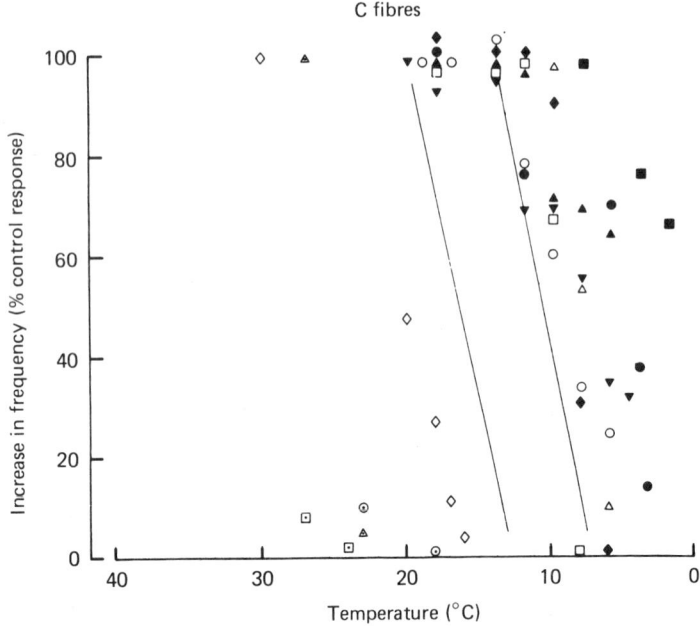

Fig. 6.11. Response of the increase in action potentials in non-myelinated fibres (i.e. C fibres) resulting from distension of balloons in the pulmonary vein–atrial junctions, to cooling of the vagus in 2 °C steps. Each point represents the response of the increase in action potentials (mean frequency) at each temperature of the vagus, expressed as a percentage of the response with the vagus at 36–37 °C. Each symbol represents the responses in one nerve fibre. Twelve fibres with conduction velocities $< 2 \text{ m} \cdot \text{s}^{-1}$ were obtained in 22 dogs. The responses at 36–37 °C were all rated 100% responses and are not shown in the diagram. The continuous lines are the same as those in Figs. 6.6 and 6.8. Note that nearly all the responses to cooling lie outside these lines. (From Kappagoda, Linden & Sivananthan, 1979.)

drawn on Fig. 6.11; it is obvious that these two lines enclose hardly any of the responses of C fibres to cooling.

There was a large range of response in receptors attached to C fibres in that the discharge in the control period was 3.2 spikes·s^{-1} (mean; range 0–11.8) and this discharge rose to 13.9 spikes·s^{-1} (mean; range 1.3–33.6) during distension of the balloons with the vagi warm. However, considering the data presented in Fig. 6.11 it is possible to infer that there are two

Afferent pathway of reflex

populations in this group of non-myelinated fibres. Of the twelve fibres examined, eight had a relatively low frequency of 0.72 spikes·s^{-1} (mean; range 0–1.8) during the control period, which increased to 6.5 spikes·s^{-1} (mean; range 1.3–12.5) during stimulation. These fibres were blocked at a lower temperature than the myelinated fibres. The other four fibres had a frequency during the control period of 7.9 spikes·s^{-1} (mean; range 0.1–11.8) and increased to 28.5 spikes·s^{-1} (mean; range 23.1–33.6) during stimulation; these fibres were blocked at a higher temperature than the myelinated fibres. There was no difference between the conduction velocities of this group of four fibres and the group of eight fibres showing a lower frequency of discharge on distension of the balloons. At both 16 °C and 12 °C the response of the high-frequency group are fully blocked whilst less than 5% of the response of the low-frequency group are blocked at 12 °C. Thus there is no relationship between the response of the C fibres and the response of the increase in heart rate to cooling the vagi. It is probable that the rates of discharge in the four fibres which are higher than those usually observed in C fibres are a result of the artificial presence of the balloons causing abnormal local increases in tension – and even greater increases in tension during distension of the balloons, which would account for the higher discharge rates. What was being examined in these experiments was the *effect* of the distension of the balloons at the vein–atrial junctions, i.e. the difference between the frequency of spikes observed during the control period and that observed during the distension. Under these conditions the reflex response of action potentials in myelinated fibres and increases in heart rate positively correlated whereas it must be concluded it is highly unlikely that the C fibres are concerned in the reflex response of an increase in heart rate to stimulation of receptors by the small balloon.

Non-vagal pathway

This investigation also helps to resolve two other aspects of the reflex. In previous investigations the afferent path of the reflex has been investigated by cooling the cervical vagi to 5 °C (e.g. Ledsome & Linden, 1964a; Kappagoda, Linden & Saunders,

1972a, b). This procedure has been criticised on the grounds that such cooling affects the animal to a degree which renders it unable to respond to the stimulus (Malliani et al., 1973); for instance cooling the vagi to 5 °C resulted in a control heart rate which on occasion exceeded that obtained during the period of stimulation when the vagi were warm. Recently it has also been demonstrated that distension of the balloons at the vein–atrial junctions causes an increased discharge in 'sympathetic' afferent fibres (Holton, 1977; Holton, Kidd & Koley, to be published). The technique of cooling the vagi to 5 °C did not permit the conclusion that the vagi were the sole afferent path of this reflex increase in heart rate. However, in the present study it has been shown that by graded cooling of the cervical vagi the response of an increase in heart rate could be attenuated at a considerably higher temperature (12–10 °C) than that at which a significant increase in the control heart rate occurred (Kappagoda, Linden & Sivananthan, 1979). Also the abolition of the reflex increase in heart rate by cooling the vagi to 10–12 °C indicated that this reflex response was unlikely to be related to the 'sympathetic' afferent fibres originating from the atrial wall.

In conclusion it seems from these items of evidence that the atrial receptors which have been stimulated by small balloons in the vein–atrial junctions and which are causing the reflex increase in heart rate are the Paintal-type atrial receptors which are attached to myelinated fibres of a conduction velocity of the order of $10-35 \text{ m} \cdot \text{s}^{-1}$. It seems that this afferent pathway is in the vagal nerves.

Efferent pathway of the reflex

Blockade of sympathetic nerves

Because the response of an increase in heart rate took 30 s to 5 min to decay following the removal of distension of the balloons, it was considered that the efferent limb of the reflex could be in the sympathetic nerves to the heart. Thus, as pointed out in the discussion of the reports already presented, section of the right and left ansae subclaviae (which contain all the sympathetic efferent nerves to the heart in the dog) and the use of sympathetic blocking drugs (propranolol; bretylium tosylate),

Table 6.4. *Sympathetic efferent pathway: increase in heart rate (beats·min⁻¹)*

	Control			Blockade of sympathetic nerves									
				Section of ansae subclaviae			Propranolol (0.5 mg·kg⁻¹)*			Bretylium tosylate (10 mg·kg⁻¹)			
	No. dogs	No. dist.	Increase in heart rate (beats·min⁻¹) mean (range)	No. dogs	No. dist.	Increase in heart rate (beats·min⁻¹) mean (range)	No. dogs	No. dist.	Increase in heart rate (beats·min⁻¹) mean (range)	No. dogs	No. dist.	Increase in heart rate (beats·min⁻¹) mean (range)	References
a. Leeds group													
I *Left atrium*													
(a) Two pulmonary vein/ atrial junctions	11	27	25 (8–54)	—	—	—	10	22	9.8 (0.5–22)	3	3	2 (0–7)	Kappagoda, Linden, Scott & Snow (1975)
	5	5	31 (17–53)	4	4	5 (0–16)	2	2	14 (12 and 16)	—	—	—	Ledsome & Linden (1964b)
(b) Three pulmonary vein/ atrial junctions	2	2	60 (38 and 81)	—	—	—	6	6	3	3	3	0	Carswell et al. (1970)
	3	6	19	—	—	—	3	3	0	5	5	1 (0–3)	Ledsome & Hainsworth (1970)
	12	37	21 (6–90)	6	6	0	—	—	—	—	—	—	Furnival et al. (1971)
Two pulmonary veins + appendage	5	10	35	—	—	—	—	—	—	—	—	—	Kappagoda, Linden & Mary (1975)
(c) Two junctions – right upper and middle pulmonary vein/atrial	43	78	22 (3–89)	[Section and/or propranolol]			5	7 (4.5–10)	34	77	2 (0–6)	Karim et al. (1972)
	3	8	31 (15–53)	2	4	16.5 (12 and 21)	3			2	5	0.8 (0–25)	Kappagoda, Linden & Snow (to be published)
II *Right atrium*	9	9	16 (9–30)	3	3	0	4	4	0 (0–1)	2	2	0	Kappagoda, Linden & Snow (1972a)
III *Atrial appendages*													
Left } 8 dogs	4	4	14 (9–24)	—	—	—	4	3	1.5 (0–6)	1	1	0	Kappagoda, Linden & Saunders (1972)
Right }	3	3	16 (11–20)	—	—	—	3	3	0	—	—	—	Kappagoda, Linden & Saunders (1972)
Left and right	6	6	24 (17–38)	3	3	1 (0–3)	4	4	1.5 (0–6)	1	1	0	Kappagoda, Linden & Saunders (1972)
IV *Left atrial pouch*	5	5	11 (5–20)	—	—	—	2	2	1 (0–2)	3	3	0	Ledsome & Linden (1967)

* In the case of Kappagoda, Linden, Scott & Snow (1975), atenolol was administered instead.

showed that the efferent limb of the reflex was solely in the efferent sympathetic nerves to the heart. Some of the investigations carried out in Leeds have been extracted and are shown in Table 6.4 where the effect of blockade of sympathetic nerves on the increase in heart rate is shown. Results are again summarised in Table 6.3 where it can be seen that in five different investigations there were 20 distensions of the balloons in 18 dogs following section of both ansae subclaviae; the control increase in heart rate was 25 beats·min^{-1} (average of means; range 16–31) and that following section of the ansae subclaviae the response was reduced to 4.5 beats·min^{-1} (average of means; range 0–16). In 41 dogs, 55 distensions of the balloon in 10 separate investigations resulted in a control increase in heart rate of 23 beats·min^{-1} (average of means; range 11–60) which, after adrenoreceptor blocking drugs (propranolol or atenolol) had been administered to the animal, was reduced to 3.8 beats·min^{-1} (average of means; range 0–9.8). Explanation of this residual response lies in the fact that these drugs are competitive antagonists and the release of noradrenaline in sufficient concentration even in the presence of blocking drugs still has an effect (e.g. Ledsome et al., 1965). The administration of bretylium tosylate (10 mg·kg^{-1}) abolishes all remaining increases in heart rate; bretylium tosylate blocks the action of all efferent sympathetic nerves without affecting central connections of cardiac reflexes or efferent vagal nerves (Ledsome & Linden, 1964a). In 54 dogs, 100 distensions of the small balloons in nine separate investigations caused an increase in heart rate of 21 beats·min^{-1} (average of the means; range 11–35) in the control period before the administration of bretylium tosylate, and 0.6 beats·min^{-1} (average of the means; range 0–2) after bretylium tosylate.

Electrophysiological evidence

Karim, Kidd, Malpus & Penna (1972) distended each of the two upper right pulmonary vein–atrial junctions in a similar manner to that of Ledsome & Linden (1964b). The stellate ganglion and ansa subclavia were exposed by removing the third rib and a small segment of the internal thoracic vein. Recordings were made using conventional techniques until 'few fibre' prepara-

Efferent pathway of reflex

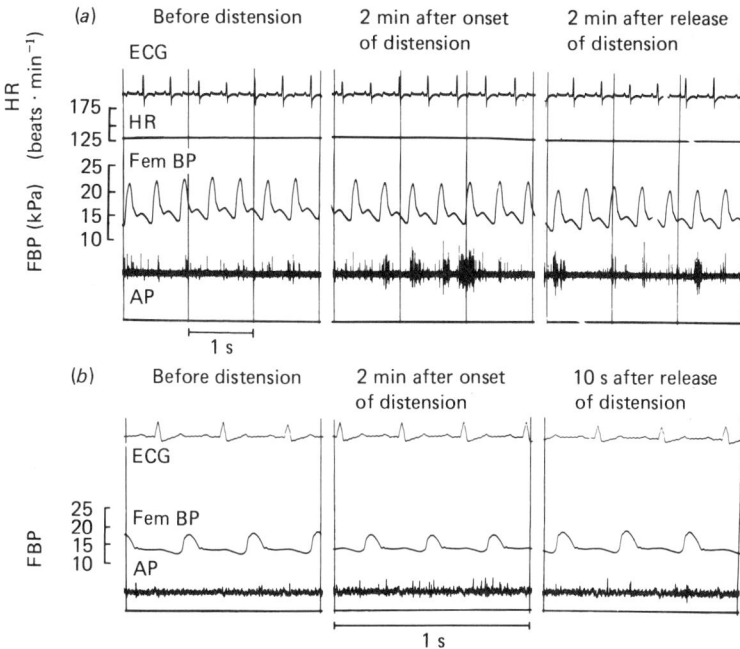

Fig. 6.12. Records of electrocardiogram (ECG); heart rate (HR); femoral blood pressure (FBP) and action potentials (AP), from two strands (a) and (b) from the right inferior cardiac sympathetic nerves. Action potentials of both strands increased significantly during balloon distension without any changes in FBP and HR. (From Karim et al., 1972.)

tions of the sympathetic efferent fibres were obtained. In each dog a reflex increase in heart rate to distension of the balloons was elicited about half an hour after the operative procedure had been completed. In 43 dogs, 78 distensions of the pulmonary vein–atrial junctions resulted in a mean increase in heart rate of 22 beats·min^{-1} (range 3–89). To prevent any possible alteration in the number of action potentials (impulses·s^{-1}) which might occur simply as a result of the change in the heart rate, this reflex increase in heart rate was abolished or reduced to less than 6 beats·min^{-1} either by tying the right ansa subclavia or by blocking the sympathetic effect with drugs. A typical response of a cardiac sympathetic strand (multi-fibre preparation) to distension of the balloon without any change in mean systemic

159

Table 6.5. *The effect of distension of the pulmonary vein–atrial junctions on the impulse activity of the inferior cardiac sympathetic efferent nerves before and after cooling (5 °C) or section of the vagal nerves in the neck*

		Percentage change in impulse activity			
Dog no.	Strand no.	Control distension	After vagal cooling	After vagal rewarming	After vagal section
11	1	+22.6	—	—	0
13	1	+21.3	—	—	0
15	1	+19.6	0	+18.5	0
16	1	+19.0	—	—	0
17	1	+47.2	—	—	0
18	1	+36.7	−8.4	+22.4	—
18	2	+34.5	0*	+17.0	0
20	1	+63.6	+13.0	+40.3	0
21	1	+20.0	−12.7*	+19.0	—
21	1	+19.0	0	+25.5	—

— procedure was not adopted; 0 indicates no change; * only right vagus nerve was cooled. (From Karim *et al.*, 1972.)

arterial blood pressure and heart rate is shown in Fig. 6.12. (Fig. 6.12(*a*) shows the response in a multi-fibre preparation and Fig. 6.12(*b*) a similar response in a 'few fibre' cardiac sympathetic strand). The mean impulse frequency increased significantly during distension in both strands. In 14 dogs, 27 distensions of the right pulmonary vein–atrial junctions resulted in an increase in frequency of impulses in each of 15 'few fibre' strands of the inferior cardiac branch of the right stellate ganglion. When the impulse frequency obtained during distension was compared with the frequency during two control periods the mean increase was 28% (range 7–64%). The response of nine strands to distension of the balloon was abolished when both vagal nerves were either cooled to 5 °C or sectioned in the neck as shown in Table 6.5. The spontaneous activity of the strands did not significantly change after cooling or section of the vagal nerves; the mean values of the activity of these strands before and after vagal cooling or section were 23.9 impulses·s^{-1} (s.e. ±4.9) and 25.1 impulses·s^{-1} (s.e. ±5.2) respectively. It is interesting to

Efferent pathway of reflex

note that in this investigation it was observed that renal sympathetic efferent nerve activity decreased at the same time as the cardiac sympathetic nerve activity increased (see Chapter 10; Fig. 10.4) whilst there were no changes in activity in other peripheral nerves (see Chapter 7).

The vagal efferent component

In spite of the claims to the contrary there is little evidence to support the assertion (Albrook et al., 1972; Burkhart & Ledsome, 1974; Ledsome, 1979) that there is a vagal component to this reflex. The findings of Hakumäki (1970, 1972) that, during an infusion to elicit the Bainbridge reflex in dogs, there was a withdrawal of activity in efferent vagal nerves to the heart as well as an increase in activity in sympathetic nerves, can be explained by the fact that many receptors, both within the heart and outside would be being stimulated (see Chapter 4).

Similar criticism can be levelled at the work of Chapman & Mittmann (1975) and Chapman, Mittmann, Prickett & Richmond (1978) who examined activity in single cardiac efferent fibres of the vagus whilst distending a balloon in the left atrium to obstruct the mitral orifice and thus flow through the atrium. Not surprisingly they obtained changes in activity in efferent vagal nerves but it is not possible to accept that such an experiment establishes the involvement of the atrial receptors in this response. Distension of the atrium in this manner would stimulate various types of receptors (see Chapter 4) and also lead to effects secondary to the fall in cardiac output. No evidence was given by them that atrial receptors were involved. The work of Kollai et al. (1978) claims that stretch of the right and left atria of anaesthetised dogs results in either an increase or a decrease in heart rate. Stretch of the right atrium was claimed to increase the activity in both vagal and sympathetic efferent fibres claimed to be innervating the heart. Stretch of the left atrium produced biphasic changes in cardiac sympathetic efferent fibres. It is never possible to be certain that efferent fibres examined like this are in fact innervating the heart as they may have been passing over it. But a much greater criticism of this work making it difficult to treat as a serious attempt to elicit responses specifically from atrial receptors, is the fact that the stimulus was inadequate (see Chapter 5 for criticism). But Burkhart & Ledsome (1974) used a discrete stimulus similar to that used in Leeds and claimed that the efferent vagal nerves were involved. Burkhart & Ledsome (1974) using small balloons, although always obtaining responses of an increase in heart rate, claim that part of this increase results from a reduction in vagal tone. Although they are showing only very small increases in heart rate attributable to a vagal component it is important to point out that there are explanations for their results other than stimulation of atrial receptors. It may be noteworthy that in the investigations of Burkhart & Ledsome (1974) smaller animals were used and these were in the prone position; it is possible that such a small size and such a position allowed the balloons to take up relatively more volume of the left atrium and provide obstruction to flow through it. Again, there was no measurement of left atrial pressure throughout the investigation and it is not possible to conclude whether or not there was evidence of obstruction of flow of blood through the atrium (see Chapter 4). Burkhart & Ledsome (1974) investigated the reflex essentially in two preparations, one which was decerebrate and the second which had a high spinal section and in which the blood pressure was maintained by an infusion of noradrenaline. An important criticism of this paper stems from their records in which they examine three preparations in each of the two groups. The first group of the animals were decerebrate. A small increase in heart rate (6 beats·min^{-1}) was observed in these animals after giving bretylium tosylate and propranolol. This increase in heart rate was not obtained following vagal section. However, after cervical vagotomy in these animals it is noticed that even with the small balloons, distension caused a fall in blood pressure (of up to 3 kPa) which must have resulted from an obstruction in the left atrium. It may therefore be concluded that the obstruction was also present before cervical vagotomy, possibly causing a fall in output, change in arterial baroreceptor stimulation and a subsequent vagally induced increase in heart rate. Therefore, the increase in heart rate is vagally induced but not attributable to stimulation of atrial receptors.

In the second group, following cervical vagotomy after high spinal section, there were even greater falls in blood pressure (up to 8 kPa) when the balloons were distended. Thus, using the same argument it is easier to explain the now greater increases in heart rate observed during distension of the balloons and after high spinal section but before cervical vagotomy. Ledsome (1979) persists in his claim that there is a vagal efferent limb to the reflex saying 'The suggestion of Kappagoda, Linden, Scott & Snow (1975) that these changes were secondary to circulatory obstruction and a decrease in arterial baroreceptor stimulation is unacceptable as in these experiments arterial pressure increased during distension of the pulmonary vein–atrial junction (Burkhart & Ledsome, 1974, Fig. 3).' It is difficult to conclude from this figure that stimulation of baroreceptors was not changed: noradrenaline was being infused continuously throughout the experiment; the standard errors are so great there is probably no significant rise in blood pressure even of the 0.3 or 0.4 kPa indicated; it is not evident that there was a normal distribution of the results, e.g. their Fig. 5; there may have been great changes in pulse pressure allowing much less baroreceptor stimulation; some contribution to the small increase (? statistical) in *mean* blood pressure could have been caused secondary to the increase in heart rate – this latter point could have been checked by pacing the heart. It seems unlikely therefore, from all the argument, that the observed vagal responses are mediated through atrial receptors.

In this regard evidence from Leeds, part of which is based on the distension of small balloons in the pulmonary vein–atrial junctions before and after giving bretylium tosylate (10 mg·kg^{-1}) appears pertinent. There is evidence that this drug blocks the effect of stimulation of sympathetic nerves to the heart and yet allows free access of afferent nerves to the efferent vagal nerves to the sinu-atrial node (Ledsome & Linden, 1964a). Evidence for the statement that distension of small balloons in the pulmonary vein–atrial junctions does not cause an increase in heart rate (or any change in heart rate) following administration of bretylium tosylate has been obtained many times in this laboratory, the first occasion being by Ledsome & Linden (1964b).

In view of this controversy Kappagoda, Linden, Scott & Snow (1975) made a careful study of this reflex, blocking the sympathetic action with a β-adrenoreceptor blocking drug (atenolol; ICI Ltd) which could be used at ten times the dose at which propranolol could be used before getting secondary depressive reactions and yet the drug itself was almost equipotent with propranolol; and also, again, carefully using bretylium tosylate to block the effects of activity in sympathetic nerves to the heart. Care was taken to set up the preparation so that there was no possibility at all of the heart 'sitting on' the pulmonary vein balloons and therefore allowing some obstruction of the left atrium upon distension; during distension of the balloons observation of the records of atrial and systemic arterial pressure allowed judgements to be made on this issue (see Chapter 4). It was necessary to carry out these experiments under carefully controlled conditions and important to establish definite criteria by which results could be accepted for analysis. After an initial control period of at least 2 min the balloons were distended slowly (each over a period of 30 s) and the distensions were maintained for a period of 2–3 min. The blood pressure in the femoral artery, both atria, the pressure in the trachea, the end-tidal pCO_2, the ECG and the analogue output from the cardiotachometer were continuously recorded throughout the entire period. Further experimental records were obtained during a final control period of 3–8 min after the release of the distension. Experiments in which distension of the balloons was associated with a decrease in mean arterial pressure greater than 0.25 kPa or increases in mean left atrial pressure greater than 0.1 kPa as compared with the values obtained during the initial period, were not accepted for analysis. Further, the above techniques, when recording experimental data, also allowed the documentation of any transient changes in blood pressure which could follow distension of the balloon. Twenty-seven distensions of the upper pulmonary vein–left atrial junction were performed in 11 dogs and an increase in heart rate was observed during each distension. The increase in heart rate was 24.8 beats·min^{-1} (mean; range 8–54; S.E. of mean ± 3.1). There were no significant changes in arterial pressure or atrial pressure during these manoeuvres. Eight dogs were then given atenolol followed by bretylium tosylate and the remaining three dogs were given bretylium tosylate alone. In 20 distensions in eight dogs after the injection of atenolol the calculated increase in heart rate was 9.8 beats·min^{-1} (mean; range 0.5–21.5; S.E. of the mean ± 1.8). The magnitude of the increase in heart rate was significantly less during distensions performed after administration of the drug than those performed before. In 22 distensions in 10 dogs after the injection of bretylium tosylate the calculated increase in heart rate was 2.3 beats·min^{-1} (mean; range -2 to $+8$; S.E. of the mean ± 0.8). At the end of these experiments the carotid arteries were occluded and a tachycardia was observed at the beginning of each occlusion. A bradycardia was immediately associated with the release of the occlusion in each instance. From this evidence the explanation of the increase in heart rate following atenolol is that even with these high blocking doses the concentration of noradrenaline at the site of action following release from sympathetic nerves is so great that it overcomes the antagonism of the competitive adrenoreceptor blocking drug. Such a conclusion is supported by the work of Ledsome et al. (1965) who stimulated sympathetic nerves to the heart before and after the injection of propranolol when only 75 % response to maximal stimulation of nerves was obtainable with the usual blocking dose (0.5 mg·kg^{-1}). There was also great variation to blockade of stimulation, e.g. even 3 mg·kg^{-1} propranolol (about six times the effective dose in anaesthetised dogs) only abolished 70 % of the maximal response to stimulation of sympathetic nerves in one dog. Also, Donald, Ferguson & Milburn (1968) in racing greyhounds observed heart rates of 192 beats·min^{-1} after 2 mg·kg^{-1} propranolol in an animal watching the others race as well as of 300 beats·min^{-1} in the racing animals after blockade – any heart rate over about 140 beats·min^{-1} *must* occur as a result of the effect of catecholamine. This same β-blockade reduced almost completely the increase in heart rate observed in response to the infusion of isoprenaline. It may be suggested that most of the above evidence shows only that maximal or near maximal effects are partially blocked; and that small reflex sympathetic increases in heart rate, of say 20–40 beats·min^{-1}, would be totally blocked. Without evidence such a conclusion would be dangerous; such a complete block would have to be demonstrated (by what means?) on each and every occasion before any residual increase in heart rate could be attributed to less activity in efferent vagal nerves. This evidence and this argument suggest it is not possible completely to block the effects of activity in sympathetic nerves with β-receptor antagonists and particularly it is not possible to block reflex effects.

It was concluded that there was really no justification for using β-receptor antagonists alone to define the efferent reflex pathways in sympathetic nerves. Therefore bretylium tosylate was used in addition to atenolol to block sympathetic nerves to the heart. This drug was selected because it produces specific blockade of sympathetic nerves to the heart (Boura & Green, 1959; Ledsome & Linden, 1964a) without affecting changes in heart rate mediated through vagal efferent nerves (Ledsome & Linden, 1964a) or the release of adrenaline from the adrenal medulla (Boura & Green, 1959). After demonstrating that bretylium tosylate blocked the effect on the heart rate of maximal stimulation of the ansae subclaviae, Ledsome & Linden (1964a) also showed that reflexes mediated through the vagi to the heart were left intact. The increase in heart rate produced by occlusion of the common carotid arteries was the same or greater after injection of bretylium tosylate (10 mg·kg^{-1}) compared with the control values. Results similar to these were obtained in an investigation of Kappagoda, Linden, Scott & Snow (1975). The reflex increase in heart rate produced by inflation of the lungs, known to act only through the vagal efferent pathway, was unchanged after injection of bretylium tosylate (Ledsome & Linden, 1964a). Thus there is indisputable evidence that after injection of bretylium tosylate, reflexes mediated by vagal efferent nerves remain intact. It is unlikely that bretylium tosylate affects central nervous activity; after the administration of bretylium tosylate Karim et al. (1972) observed changes in activity in efferent sympathetic nerves in response to stimulation of left atrial receptors showing that vagal afferent nerves carrying impulses from left atrial receptors still had access to sympathetic efferent nerves, particularly cardiac nerves but also renal nerves. The suggestion that bretylium tosylate may have a direct action on the heart has been contradicted by evidence that the administration of bretylium tosylate in dogs causes a reduction in heart rate, resulting not only from a decrease in sympathetic activity but also from an increase in vagal activity; evidence for the latter statement is provided by the fact that the control heart rates were in the order of 55 beats·min^{-1}, about 65–69 beats·min^{-1} lower than the heart rates reported in dogs in similar condition acutely denervated (e.g. Harry, Kappagoda, Linden & Snow, 1973). In addition, it is known that section of the vagi after bretylium tosylate results in a vast increase in heart rate (e.g. Fig. 5, Ledsome & Linden, 1964a; 60 beats·min^{-1} before section of the vagi and 192 beats·min^{-1} after). In fact this preparation provides an ideal background for the demonstration to students of reflexes involving increases in heart rate possibly mediated by vagal nerves. In spite of these conditions distension of the balloons resulted in a mean increase in heart rate of only 2 beats·min^{-1}; small increases of the order of magnitude that were observed in three out of five dogs in which the efferent sympathetic nerves were maximally electrically stimulated after bretylium tosylate (Ledsome & Linden, 1964a). These findings all suggest that there is no evidence for the existence of a vagal efferent component in this reflex.

No bradycardia

Another controversy which arises in spite of the evidence produced above that stimulation of atrial receptors always results in an increase in heart rate requires illumination; in spite of this evidence it is widely believed that the heart rate response to stimulation of atrial receptors is dependent on the initial heart rate (e.g. Coleridge & Coleridge, 1972; Paintal, 1973a; Shepherd, 1973). Paintal in a recent review (1973a) concludes, 'Thus it can provisionally be concluded that stimulation of left atrial type B receptors of the dog causes either a reflex tachycardia or bradycardia, depending on the initial heart rate and the reflex fall in blood pressure under most experimental conditions.' However, a critical examination of the literature quoted by Paintal (1973a) in support of these two conclusions does not warrant such a statement. The claim that there is a reflex fall in blood pressure under most experimental conditions is refuted in Chapter 7.

There are several reasons for adhering to the original conclusion that the reflex which is evoked by stimulating the Paintal-type atrial receptors involves only a sympathetic efferent pathway and in no way involves vagal efferent nerves. That this reflex does not involve vagal efferent nerves causing an *increase* in heart rate has been expounded above. The following argument suggests that the view that there may be an increase or a *decrease* in heart rate is erroneous. First, in all experiments in this laboratory there has never been a decrease in heart rate and all the evidence has pointed to a single sympathetic efferent pathway responsible for the observed increase in heart rate (see Tables 6.1–6.4). Some of the 'evidence' for the bi-phasic response has been provided by Shepherd and co-workers in two reports (Edis & Shepherd, 1969; Edis *et al.*, 1970). These authors claim to have observed, during stimulation of atrial receptors, a reflex reduction in blood pressure and a bradycardia or tachycardia, depending on the initial heart rate. At low heart rate a tachycardia was recorded and at high heart rate a bradycardia was recorded. No change in heart rate was observed with initial heart rates of the order of 140–150 beats·min^{-1}. However, the technique for stimulation of atrial receptors did not satisfy at least two primary criteria, i.e. localisation of the stimulus and the ability of the stimulus to stimulate the receptors under investigation. These criteria had been satisfied during the original investigation of Ledsome & Linden (1964b) where small balloons each about 2 mm long were distended in the vein–atrial junctions (see Chapter 4); the same technique had been shown to be capable of stimulating atrial receptors as shown by Kidd *et al.* (1966, 1978; see Chapter 3), although such an investigation would not exclude the possibility that the receptors discharging into C fibres might also be stimulated but unrecognised. That the C fibres are not involved in this reflex of an increase in heart rate has been shown previously in this chapter.

In the preliminary communication of Edis & Shepherd (1969) three balloons each having a volume of 3–4 cm^3 were distended at the pulmonary vein–atrial junctions. Injections of such large volumes would undoubtedly have obstructed the flow of blood through the left atrium which has a volume of less than 20 cm^3. In a subsequent paper Edis *et al.* (1970) described much smaller injections of saline (0.25–2 cm^3) into balloons which were 1.5 cm in length. The balloons used by Ledsome & Linden (1964b) and subsequently by Kidd *et al.* (1966, 1978) were much smaller (approximately 2 mm long) and when distended with 1 cm^3 of warm saline acquired a spherical shape of diameter about 0.8 cm. Whilst one cannot be certain of the shape acquired by a balloon 1.5 cm in length when distended with 0.2–2 cm^3 of saline (Edis *et al.*, 1970), it is unlikely that it will assume a spherical shape or stretch the vein–atrial junctions in a discrete

Efferent pathway of reflex

circumscribed manner. Indeed there was no evidence to suggest that the stimulus was capable of stimulating left atrial receptors. The evidence presented in their paper (Edis *et al.*, 1970) does, however, support the alternative hypothesis that some of the effects noticed were attributable either to obstruction to flow or to stimulation of other cardiovascular receptors. For instance, distension of the balloons with 2 cm^3 of saline was invariably accompanied by a measurable, significant diminution in cardiac output. In the presence of such changes it is clearly not possible to eliminate the secondary effects nor to attribute either the changes in heart rate or the changes in blood pressure to stimulation of left atrial receptors alone.

Edis *et al.* (1970) claimed that the changes in heart rate observed from stretching the left pulmonary vein–atrial junctions were reflexly induced. They attempted to elucidate the efferent pathway involved by the use of atropine and propranolol. Intravenous administration of propranolol did not prevent the *increase* in heart rate and the administration of intravenous atropine sulphate did not prevent a *decrease* in heart rate evoked by distension of the balloons.

These two results taken individually do not provide any evidence of reflex involvement in the response. In addition, if a reflex was involved it was not the reflex increase in heart rate attributable to stimulation of atrial receptors, in which the efferent nerves are solely in the sympathetic nervous system, since (in the investigation of Edis *et al.*, 1970) propranolol did not reduce the response of an increase in heart rate. It has been suggested by Furnival, Linden & Snow (1971) that at least one conclusion could be that there is no evidence of nervous involvement in their response at all.

Pelletier & Shepherd (1973) and Shepherd (1973) have pointed out that there were differences between their experiments and those from Leeds; they draw no conclusions from these differences. It is therefore important to consider the stated differences and the implications as follows. Shepherd (1973) pointed out that both aortic nerves were sectioned and carotid sinuses were vascularly isolated so that no influence from aortic or carotid baroreceptors would be observed. Thus no secondary effects should result from stimulation of these baroreceptors. In this respect it is worth pointing out that in our laboratory with the carotid sinuses perfused at various constant pressures Carswell, Hainsworth & Ledsome (1970a) distended balloons at the left pulmonary vein–atrial junctions and always obtained a reflex increase in heart rate. In all other experiments carried out in our laboratory without controlled pressures in the sino-aortic areas, distension of the balloons in the left pulmonary vein–atrial junctions and at the junction of the superior vena cava and the right atrium and in both atrial appendages have always resulted in tachycardia. During 811 distensions in 251 dogs there was always an increase in heart rate. The initial heart rates varied between 36 and 239 beats·min^{-1} (see Table 6.1); there should be little if any effective stimulation of baroreceptors at the high heart rates. There is a distinct possibility that other receptors could be responsible for the bradycardia and hypotension observed by Shepherd and others; as pointed out above, stimulation of small areas of the large pulmonary veins at the hilum of the lungs and over the whole of the left atrium have caused discharges of action potentials into slips of vagal nerves with conduction velocities slower than those attributable to atrial receptors and it is concluded that these fibres come within the C fibre range (conduction velocity less than 2.5 m·s^{-1}). Shepherd comments that he used larger balloons, therefore it is possible that these larger balloons of Edis et al. (1970) could have stimulated C fibre endings. Predicting the effects of increased activity in these C fibres from known responses to stimulation of other similar fibres emanating from the ventricle (e.g. Sleight, 1979), would suggest that the C fibres from the atrium could be responsible for any bradycardia and hypotension observed from stretching atrial muscle. However, though there is at the moment no evidence of such a cause and effect relationship, a recent investigation (Kappagoda, Linden & Sivananthan, 1979; see Chapter 3) has shown that the transient fall in blood pressure seen in about a third of the distensions with small balloons is caused by an increased activity in non-myelinated fibres (C fibres). It may be that with a greater stimulus to the receptors an increased activity in these C fibres could effect also a decrease in heart rate (cf. activation of ventricular receptors and C fibres, Chapter 3). Another possible explanation of Shepherd's results is that other receptors, remote

Summary

from the immediate area of distension, were involved; as pointed out above, there was evidence of an obstruction to flow through the atria in Shepherd's experiments.

Though there is little discussion of the function of myelinated afferent vagal fibres in relation to heart rate, it does seem that Donald & Shepherd (1978, p. 452) in their review now accept that only a reflex tachycardia is evoked by stimulating Paintal-type atrial receptors.

No positive inotropic response

In a further investigation involving the stimulation of left atrial receptors, Furnival et al. (1971) inserted the small balloons into the left pulmonary vein–left atrial junctions and showed again that distension of these balloons caused a reflex increase in heart rate with the efferent pathway solely in the sympathetic nerves. In expectation of a concomitant positive inotropic response the effect of stimulation of the left atrial receptors on the inotropic state of the left ventricle was studied using a known sensitive index of inotropic changes, i.e. the maximal rate of rise of pressure in the left ventricle (dP/dt_{max}) which had previously been shown to be an adequate index under the circumstances of this investigation (Furnival, Linden & Snow, 1970). Though stimulation of left atrial receptors resulted in an increase in heart rate of up to 90 beats·min^{-1} there were no significant concomitant changes in dP/dt_{max}. It was concluded that activity in this discrete efferent pathway does not include an inotropic effect on the left ventricle, and therefore the reflex involved only those sympathetic nerves which innervate the sinu-atrial node.

Summary

From the evidence it is apparent that, as has previously been stated, the most likely receptors to be stimulated by the small balloons at the pulmonary vein–atrial junctions are the Paintal-type atrial receptors (Paintal type B and intermediate; Kappagoda et al., 1976, 1977b) which cause only an increase in heart rate. The afferent limb of the reflex is solely in myelinated nerve fibres in the vagi and the efferent solely in sympathetic nerves.

Reflex effects on the heart

There is no concomitant positive inotropic response. The most reasonable explanation of the bradycardia and hypotension observed by others is that some other receptors in the vicinity are involved, e.g. those attached to C fibres or receptors remote from the area stimulated.

7 ATRIAL RECEPTORS: THE SYSTEMIC AND PULMONARY CIRCULATIONS

Atrial receptors are but one group out of many groups of receptors within the chest which, on stimulation, evoke responses in the systemic and pulmonary circulations. Before discussing the reports of investigations claiming to involve atrial receptors in such reflex responses it is necessary briefly to describe reflexes emanating from receptors known to be present within the chest. With knowledge of the background of the functions of these other receptors, the function of atrial receptors can then be properly judged.

Receptors within the chest

Investigations to determine the receptors, situated within the chest, which could be involved in reflex changes in the systemic circulation have been reported for more than 100 years. The techniques used have been similar to those described in Chapter 5 when responses of changes in heart rate were examined. Thus the injection of drugs, mechanical distension, infusion, perfusion and localised distension of the chambers of the heart and circulation, blocking possible tonic effects in the vagal nerves and stimulating compound nerves near the heart have all been used to demonstrate effects on arterial blood pressure. In the quest to examine changes in vasomotor control most of these techniques suffer from the same disadvantages as enumerated in Chapter 5, as well as difficulties in assessing active constriction or dilatation of the vessels. However, using these techniques reflex vasodilatation and constriction have been claimed to result from stimulation of receptors in the heart, pulmonary artery and aorta, and in the lungs.

Atrial receptors: systemic and pulmonary circulations

Cardiac receptors

In a search for receptors within the chest which could cause vasodilatation much of the work has involved a study of the Bezold–Jarisch reflex, a reflex resulting in apnoea, bradycardia and hypotension. Reflexes resulting in bradycardia have been discussed in Chapter 5 and here it is intended to refer mainly to changes in systemic arterial pressure.

In 1867 Bezold & Hirt observed that intravenous injections of veratrum resulted in a reduction in blood pressure and heart rate, as well as apnoea. These responses were abolished by cutting the vagi and hence were thought to be reflex in nature. Jarisch and his co-workers (e.g. Jarisch & Henze, 1937; Jarisch & Richter, 1939; Jarisch & Zotterman, 1948) confirmed these results and since that time these responses have been known as the Bezold–Jarisch reflex. These early experiments have been repeated by several groups of investigators with a view to ascertaining, first, the organ from which the afferent impulses for this phenomenon originated and secondly, the identity of the receptors within that organ. It is not possible to review the extensive literature on this topic but references should be made to the recent reviews (e.g. Paintal, 1973b; Donald & Shepherd, 1978; Hainsworth et al., 1979; Thorén, 1979a).

The technique for using chemical substances by application or injection, in an attempt to stimulate receptors in the heart and lungs, was refined in an excellent investigation by Dawes (1947) who found that this response could be elicited by the injection of small doses of veratridine into the various cavities of the heart, great vessels and coronary arteries of cats and dogs. However, the greatest reflex fall in blood pressure and the heart rate was observed when the injections were made to the area of supply of the circumflex and anterior descending coronary arteries, suggesting that receptors in the ventricles were involved. Small responses were also elicited by the injection of the drug into the lungs; but Dawes (1947) indicated that the most likely site for the receptors of the Bezold–Jarisch reflex was the left ventricle. Later Dawes & Comroe (1954) suggested the reflex be called the coronary chemoreflex.

Subsequently, when techniques for recording action potentials in the afferent nerves from the heart became available, Coleridge

Receptors within the chest

et al. (1964*b*) and Sleight & Widdicombe (1965) were able to demonstrate in the dog that injection of veratridine into the coronary arteries activated the receptors in the ventricles which discharged into the vagi (see Chapter 3 for an account of the electrophysiology). They concluded that these receptors were responsible for the Bezold–Jarisch reflex. It appears likely that ventricular receptors do, at least in part, mediate the Bezold–Jarisch reflex though the precise identity of the type of receptor remains in doubt, particularly because veratridine is a nonspecific stimulus to the cardiac receptors (e.g. Neil & Joels, 1961; Brown, 1964; Thorén, 1979*a*).

In parallel with these pharmacological investigations, there were several attempts mechanically to stimulate receptors in the heart so as to elicit the Bezold–Jarisch reflex. Daly & Verney (1927) observed that increasing the pressure in the left side of the heart while keeping the aortic pressure constant resulted in a bradycardia (see Chapter 5). This result was confirmed in 1959 by Aviado & Schmidt, who observed that increasing the pressure in a vascularly isolated left atrium resulted in no reflex responses, but when the left ventricle was included in the perfusion circuit bradycardia and hypotension were obtained. They were unable to perfuse the left ventricle alone. In an earlier publication Aviado and his colleagues studied the effect of increasing the pressure in a vascularly isolated right atrium which also resulted in a bradycardia and hypotension (Aviado *et al.*, 1951).

Since then numerous studies have been completed involving vagal afferent fibres with receptors claimed to be in the heart, the increased activity in which has been claimed to cause changes in the peripheral circulation (e.g. Oberg & Thorén, 1972*a*; Thorén, 1972; Donald & Shepherd, 1978; Hainsworth, Kidd & Linden, 1979). Methods claimed to stimulate ventricular receptors and evoke circulatory responses have included such techniques as the injection of drugs (e.g. Sleight, 1964; Bergel & Makin, 1967; Sleight, Lall & Muers, 1969; Abrahamsson & Thorén, 1972; Oberg & Thorén, 1972*a*; Feigl, 1975); haemorrhage (e.g. Oberg & White, 1970*b*; Pelletier, Edis & Shepherd, 1971; Oberg & Thorén, 1972*b*); occlusion of the coronary arteries and cardiac infarction (e.g. Kolatat, Ascanio, Tallarida & Oppenheimer, 1967; Thorén, 1972, 1976*b*); occlusion of coronary sinus (Muers & Sleight, 1972*a,b*); stimulating com-

Atrial receptors: systemic and pulmonary circulations

pound (afferent) nerves (e.g. Oberg & White, 1970a; Abrahamsson & Thorén, 1972; Oberg & Thorén, 1973); vagal blockade or section (e.g. Guazzi, Libretti & Zanchetti, 1962; Pillsbury, Guazzi & Freis, 1969; Oberg & White, 1970a; Mancia, Donald & Shepherd, 1973; Thorén, Donald & Shepherd, 1976; Thorén, Shepherd & Donald, 1977; probably mechanical distension (e.g. Ross *et al.*, 1961; Zoller, Mark, Abboud, Schmid & Heistad, 1972). All claims included a response of a fall in blood pressure, many a bradycardia.

Therefore from these pharmacological and physiological investigations the general view to emerge was that stimulation of receptors in the heart and large vessels resulted in a decrease in peripheral resistance. But without fail not one of these investigations provided evidence that ventricular receptors were involved – none had attempted to show, or suggested, that atrial receptors were involved.

'Cardiopulmonary' receptors

It is pertinent here to comment on the term 'cardiopulmonary' receptors, a term which is now being used in reports of some investigations claiming to demonstrate reflex responses (e.g. Guazzi *et al.*, 1962; Mancia, Donald & Shepherd, 1973; Mancia, Romero & Shepherd, 1975; Mancia, Shepherd & Donald, 1976; Thorén *et al.*, 1977; Jarecki, Thorén & Donald, 1978; Takeshita, Mark, Eckberg & Abboud, 1979). 'Cardiopulmonary' receptors are said to have been responsible for responses which are elicited by a stimulus before, but not after vagal section. Thus the warning on vagal section given in Chapter 4, to take care, is not heeded. As is explained earlier in this chapter there are many reflexes emanating from receptors in the chest. Therefore the term 'cardiopulmonary' receptors covers very many receptors within the thorax, discharging into myelinated and nonmyelinated fibres, originating in heart (ventricles and atria), lungs, vessels, bronchi, pleura, interstitial tissue and passing into the central nervous system through all routes including afferent nerves in the vagi and sympathetic rami. Various receptors when stimulated cause various responses, tachycardia and bradycardia through the vagi and/or 'sympathetic' afferent nerves (with and without positive inotropic effects), increases and decreases in blood pressure (transient and sustained), diametrically opposite effects on some blood vessels and not others, effects on sodium excretion, renin and urine flow, respiration, etc. (see Chapters 2–10 for references). It is time the term was abandoned and experiments designed to chase this 'Holy Grail' were not even considered.

Pulmonary artery receptors

Receptors on the walls of the pulmonary artery of cats and dogs have been described by Swan & Whitteridge (1956), Bianconi & Green (1959), Coleridge & Kidd (1960) and Coleridge, Kidd & Sharp (1961), and a relationship to pulmonary artery pressure as the stimulus has been described (Coleridge & Kidd, 1961). Attempts to elucidate reflex responses from the receptors in the pulmonary artery by this group have shown that perfusion at lower pressures (less than 8 kPa) resulted in hypotension whilst perfusion at higher pressures (greater than 10.5 kPa) produced hypertension (Coleridge & Kidd, 1963), though all these pressures are relatively high; stimulating drugs (capsaicin) caused a hypotension, some of which was attributable to receptors in the pulmonary artery (Coleridge, Coleridge & Kidd, 1964a). Hyman (1968) has claimed that non-occlusive distension of the pulmonary arteries in lightly anaesthetised dogs causes pulmonary vasoconstriction; but it is likely that the technique has other effects than solely the stimulation of receptors in the pulmonary artery.

Recently, after commenting that recent reviews (e.g. Korner, 1971; Paintal, 1973a) considered that previous attempts to examine reflexes during distension of the pulmonary arteries had led to equivocal results, Ledsome & Kan (1977) proceeded to demonstrate that stimulating 'receptors lying in or close to the walls of the pulmonary artery' causes a reflex (vagal afferent fibres) peripheral constriction. An interesting finding was that a decrease in temperature of the perfusate in their isolated pouch of the pulmonary artery caused a fall in systemic vascular resistance.

Thus various reflex effects on the peripheral circulation are obtainable from this site depending on the means of stimulation.

Atrial receptors: systemic and pulmonary circulations

Aortic baroreceptors and chemoreceptors

A milestone in the study of the function of receptors in the heart and circulation was the publication of a review by Heymans & Neil (1958). They pointed out then, and it is still accepted, that stimulation of baroreceptors in the carotid sinus and aortic arch by increasing the systemic blood pressure causes hypotension and bradycardia. The aortic arch has been difficult to examine but recently (e.g. Hainsworth, Ledsome & Carswell, 1971; Pelletier, Clement & Shepherd, 1972) it has been confirmed that, though threshold and sensitivity of the receptors in the aortic arch are different from those in the carotid sinus, the reflex effects on the heart rate and peripheral resistance of stimulating the receptors are directionally the same.

Heymans & Neil (1958) also reviewed the function of chemoreceptors known to exist in the aortic and carotid bodies. The problem discussed at that time of whether stimulation of chemoreceptors in the carotid body resulted in a bradycardia or tachycardia was finally resolved by Daly & Scott (1958). They used several techniques to eliminate other relevant variables and showed that stimulation of chemoreceptors and allowing secondary changes in respiration to occur resulted in a tachycardia; stimulating chemoreceptors in the carotid body, without secondary reflexes being involved, caused a bradycardia. This difference allowed the explanation that reflexes from the lung, resulting from changes in respiration caused by the stimulation of chemoreceptors, were causing the tachycardia (see next section), but emphasised that stimulation of chemoreceptors in the carotid body caused a bradycardia. Comroe & Mortimer (1964) inserted coils of tubing between the cut ends of both carotid arteries to delay the arrival of blood to the carotid bodies. Injections of chemicals, which stimulated the chemoreceptors, into the aortic arch resulted in an early tachycardia (attributed to aortic chemoreceptors) followed by a bradycardia (attributed to carotid chemoreceptors). These results have been confirmed and extended recently: stimulation of chemoreceptors in carotid bodies, isolated from circulation, resulted in bradycardia and a negative inotropic response (Hainsworth, Karim & Sofola, 1979); whereas stimulating aortic chemoreceptors in an isolated pouch of the aorta caused

Receptors within the chest

a tachycardia and a positive inotropic response, i.e. opposite effects (Karim, Hainsworth, Sofola & Wood, 1980).

It is accepted (e.g. Heymans & Neil, 1958; Daly & Scott, 1962; Daly, Hazzledine & Howe, 1965; Hainsworth & Karim, 1973) that stimulation of aortic or carotid chemoreceptors causes a peripheral vasoconstriction, which has to be dissociated in some investigations from hypoxic effects on the central nervous system (e.g. Hainsworth & Karim, 1973).

Receptors in the lungs

Reflexes from the lungs, with effects on peripheral resistance, have been examined for many years. Widdicombe (1973), in a review, classifies lung afferent fibres as emanating from pulmonary stretch receptors stimulated by normal degrees of inflation; irritant receptors, stimulated by greater degrees of inflation, inhalation of irritants, congestion, oedema, etc.; J-receptors, which are juxta pulmonary capillary receptors and stimulated by chemicals, especially phenyl diguanide, injected into the pulmonary circulation. Stimulation of these receptors reflexly affects the circulation primarily, and also secondarily, to invoked respiratory changes.

For example, inflation of the lungs has been reported to cause tachycardia or bradycardia, a negative inotropic response in ventricular muscle and systemic vasodilatation (e.g. Anrep, Pascual & Rossier, 1936; Daly & Scott, 1958; Daly & Hazzledine, 1963; Ledsome & Linden, 1964a; Daly, Hazzledine & Ungar, 1967; Daly & Robinson, 1968; Fillenz, 1969; Glick, Wechsler & Epstein, 1969; Hayashi, 1969). Recently Hainsworth (1974) has gone some way to explaining many of the conflicting results by attention to the methodology showing that: (1) reflex tachycardia was observed from inflation of normally perfused lungs with 1–2 kPa pressure; (2) the reflex bradycardia usually occurred during (a) inflation of normally perfused lungs with a pressure of 3–4 kPa pressure, (b) inflation with 2 kPa pressure immediately following hyperinflation, and (c) inflation with 1–4 kPa in an artificially perfused lung. Vascular resistance increased during inflation at lower pressures and sometimes decreased at higher inflation pressures. More recently Greenwood, Hainsworth, Karim, Morrison & Sofola (1980) have shown that lung inflation,

Atrial receptors: systemic and pulmonary circulations

under conditions which result in the response of a tachycardia, does not change the inotropic state of the heart, whereas the response of bradycardia is accompanied by a negative inotropic change. The mechanisms of these responses were not investigated and are unknown, but the results emphasise a variability of response dependent on experimental method.

Summary

This brief description of reflex effects of tachycardia and bradycardia, vasoconstriction and vasodilatation occurring in response to stimulation of receptors in the chest near, both physically and haemodynamically, to the atria, emphasises the difficulty in claiming a particular response to emanate from the atrial receptors unless meticulous care has been taken to eliminate the above possible explanations.

Atrial receptors and the systemic circulation

When examining the role of atrial receptors in this quest it is important to realise that, as discussed in Chapters 2 and 3, there are three types of receptor ending to be considered: (1) unencapsulated end-organs discharging into vagal myelinated fibres, (2) receptors discharging into vagal non-myelinated fibres, and (3) receptors discharging into 'sympathetic' afferent fibres. Reports claiming to show reflexes in which these three groups of receptors are involved will be discussed here.

Atrial receptors discharging into myelinated vagal fibres

Left atrial receptors. Stretching the pulmonary vein–atrial junctions has been extensively employed as a technique for stimulating left atrial receptors which discharge into the vagal myelinated and non-myelinated afferent fibres and also the receptor endings which discharge into sympathetic afferent nerves (Chapters 3 and 6). Using a 'selective' cold block of the vagus, it is possible to link reflex responses to either one or other of the vagal afferent fibres (see Chapter 6). Conversely abolition of a reflex response by interfering with the vagi alone would render the participation of sympathetic afferent fibres unlikely.

The systemic circulation

Thus, it can be concluded that under specific conditions, stretching the pulmonary vein–atrial junctions remains a valid technique for investigating reflex effects on the peripheral circulation mediated by the complex unencapsulated nerve endings discharging into myelinated fibres in the vagi (see Chapter 6).

Carswell *et al.* (1970*a*) investigated the peripheral circulation using a hind limb perfused at constant flow, during distension of balloons positioned at the pulmonary vein–atrial junctions in anaesthetised dogs. In the first series of experiments, the carotid sinus pressure was uncontrolled and they observed that stretching the vein–atrial junctions resulted in a reflex increase in heart rate and a small but statistically significant fall in the perfusion pressure of the hind limb. Since these manoeuvres were accompanied by changes in systemic pulse pressure (with no significant changes in mean pressure) a further series of experiments were performed in which the pressures in both carotid sinuses were controlled over a wide range. They observed no significant decrease in limb perfusion pressure during distension of the balloons at either low or high carotid pressure (Fig. 7.1). In fact at the higher carotid pressure there was an increase in mean pressure. The authors' interpretation of these findings was that 'it cannot therefore be concluded that the small decrease in perfusion pressure observed in the steady state in the first group of experiments represents direct reflex response to stimulation of left atrial receptors'. In addition, they also claimed that the fact that the changes in vascular resistance were small could not have been due to damage to vasomotor nerves to the limb because large changes in vascular resistance occurred immediately following changing the pressure in the carotid arteries either by changing the carotid perfusion pressure or by occluding the common carotid arteries. In the former experiments the carotid arteries were perfused at various pressures so that the control vascular resistance in the limb varied over a wide range; thus the absence of a reproducible vasomotor response on distension of the pulmonary vein–atrial junctions in these experiments could not be explained by the limb vessels being already in a state of maximal dilatation or maximal constriction. In a later investigation, Mason & Ledsome (1974) repeated the experiments described above and arrived at substantially the

Atrial receptors: systemic and pulmonary circulations

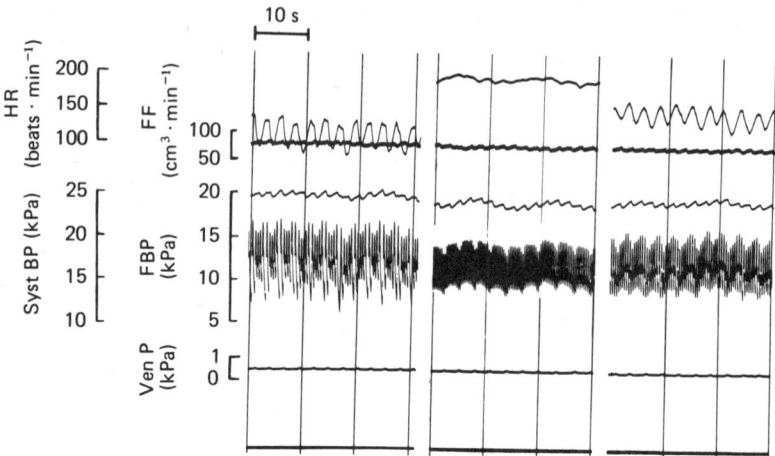

Fig. 7.1. Effects of distension of the pulmonary vein–atrial junctions in a dog in which a large increase in heart rate occurred. Dog 13 kg. Femoral artery perfusion, aorta not occluded. From above downwards heart rate, femoral perfusion flow, femoral perfusion pressure, systemic arterial pressure (recorded in the right femoral artery) and venous pressure. HR, heart rate (beats·min^{-1}); FF, femoral perfusion flow (cm^3·min^{-1}); FBP, femoral perfusion pressure (kPa); Syst BP, systemic arterial pressure (kPa); Ven P, venous pressure (kPa). First panel recorded immediately before distension of the pulmonary vein–atrial junctions; second panel, after 2 min of distension; third panel, 2 min after release of distension. (From Carswell et al., 1970a.)

same conclusions regarding the effect of stimulating left atrial receptors on the vascular resistance of the hind limb.

The effect of the stimulation of atrial receptors on vascular resistance in the kidney has a particular relevance to urine flow and sodium excretion, and evidence pertaining to that topic is examined in Chapter 9. Essentially the conclusion is that distension of the left atrium could exert an influence reflexly on the renal circulation but the precise identification of the receptors involved must await further experiments.

The effect of stimulating left atrial receptors on the peripheral veins of dogs has been studied (Snow, Kappagoda & Linden, 1978, unpublished) using the isovolumic limb and spleen preparation as described by Webb-Peploe & Shepherd (1968) and Webb-Peploe (1969). It was found that distension of the vein–atrial junctions resulted in an increase in heart rate and no significant changes in the venous tone in the hind limb, fore limb and spleen. It was also observed that in each animal carotid occlusion resulted in an increase in venous tone in these regions under investigation.

These findings on the resistance and capacitance vessels of the systemic circulation are supported by another investigation involving stimulation of left atrial receptors. Karim *et al.* (1972) found that distension of the pulmonary vein–atrial junctions in the dog resulted in no significant change in the activity in lumbar and splenic sympathetic nerves (Figs. 7.2 and 7.3), a finding which contrasted with the effect on the renal nerves (see Chapter 10).

Right atrial receptors. Several investigations claim to have demonstrated that the vasoconstrictor tone of the arteries in the limbs is affected by the receptors in the right heart and pulmonary circulation. In 1951 Aviado *et al.* demonstrated that perfusion of a vascularly isolated right atrium resulted in a bradycardia and hypotension. There have been several investigations in recent years which have attempted to confirm these findings in man (Roddie, Shepherd & Whelan, 1957; Brown, Goei, Greenfield & Plessaras, 1966; Ardill, Bannister, Fentem & Greenfield, 1967; Zoller *et al.*, 1972; Johnson, Rowell, Neiderberger & Elsman, 1974).

Roddie *et al.* (1957) studied the effect of changes in posture on the vasoconstrictor tone in human skeletal muscle. They observed that passively raising the legs of recumbent human subjects resulted in reflex dilatation of blood vessels in skeletal muscles. This procedure was accompanied by an increase in central venous pressure. Brown *et al.* (1966), Ardill *et al.* (1967), Zoller *et al.* (1972), and Johnson *et al.* (1974) used procedures which diminished central venous pressure. This reduction was achieved by subjecting the lower half of the body to negative pressure which results in pooling of blood in the lower extremities (see Brown *et al.*, 1966). As a consequence, all the above workers were thus able to demonstrate a concomitant reduction in blood flow to the limbs, i.e. the opposite of the response demonstrated previously by Roddie *et al.* (1957). From the results of these experiments it was suggested that receptors in the low pressure

Atrial receptors: systemic and pulmonary circulations

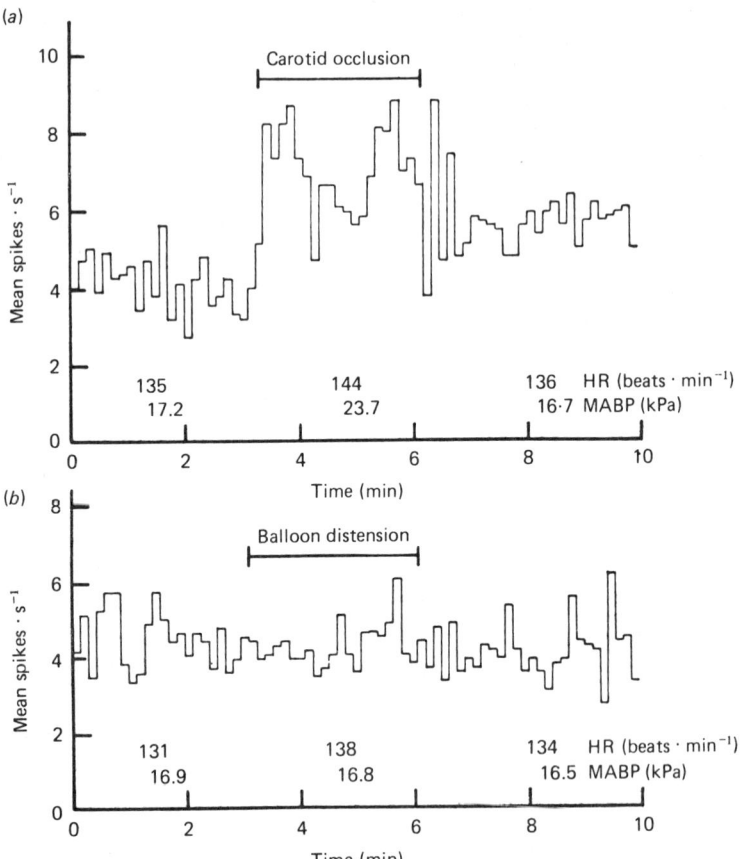

Fig. 7.2. Continuous records of mean frequency (spikes·s^{-1}) of a lumbar sympathetic nerve strand showing a significant response to carotid occlusion (a), and no response to balloon distension (b). HR, heart rate; MABP, mean arterial blood pressure. (From Karim et al., 1972.)

areas exerted an influence on the tone of the peripheral blood vessels. There are, however, certain difficulties in the interpretation of the results of these experiments; many of the receptors discussed at the beginning of this chapter would have been involved. It is clear from the data published by Brown et al. (1966) and Ardill et al. (1967) that significant changes in cardiac output and blood pressure occurred during the period

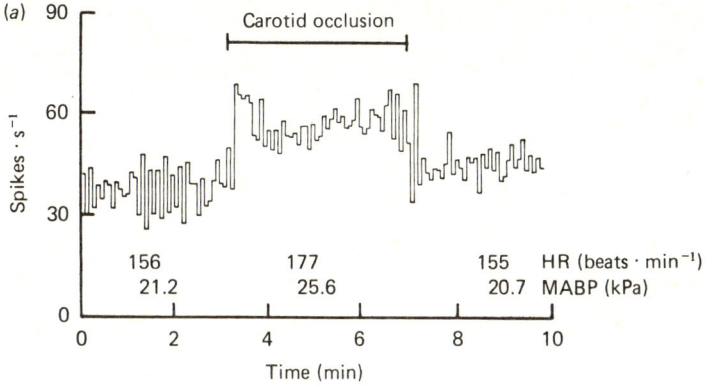

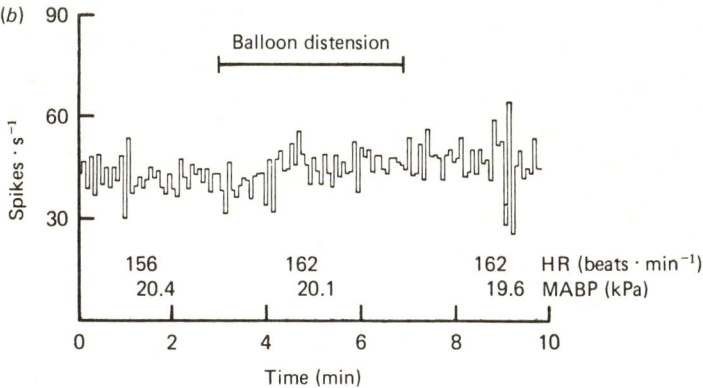

Fig. 7.3. Continuous records of mean fequency (spikes·s^{-1}) of a splenic sympathetic efferent nerve strand showing a significant response to carotid occlusion (a), and no response to balloon distension (b). HR, heart rate; MABP, mean arterial blood pressure. (From Karim et al., 1972.)

of negative pressure, which could account for the changes in blood flow to the limb. In the experiments of Zoller et al. (1972) and Johnson et al. (1974) no significant changes in blood pressure were observed. From these observations it was concluded that the baroreceptors were not involved in the reflex and that the change in peripheral blood flow was the result of activation of a discrete reflex from the low pressure areas of the circulation. However, it is not possible to conclude that there were no changes in baroreceptor activity because there was no discernible change in blood pressure; following changes in cardiac output (venous return had decreased) the baroreceptors would have changed their discharge and reflex adjustments would have taken place. The authors are not justified in their conclusion that receptors in the low-pressure area were involved.

However, receptors in the right atrium could be affected during both the above investigations; subjecting the lower body to a negative pressure of -1 to -2 kPa resulted in a fall of mean right atrial pressure of 0.5 kPa. It is possible that this change in central venous pressure could affect the complex unencapsulated nerve endings in the right atrium (Kappagoda, Linden & Snow, 1972a, b; Chapter 3) but probably not receptors discharging into the sympathetic afferents (see Chapter 3). However, it must be concluded that the role of these receptors attached to sympathetic afferent fibres in the regulation of the resistance vessels is unknown.

Indirect evidence argues against these receptors influencing the tone of capacitance vessels. In the investigations described by Kappagoda, Linden & Snow (1972a, b) distension of a balloon in the superior vena caval–right atrial junction resulted in stimulation of the complex unencapsulated endings and also a reflex increase in heart rate. In these experiments (see Chapters 4 and 6; Fig. 7.4), the whole of the blood flow in the superior vena cava was transferred to the femoral vein by means of a pump. The output of the pump was not altered during either the test period or the control periods before and after the test period. Thus the venous return from the superior vena cava was constant throughout any one experiment. Under these circumstances any change in venous tone would be reflected as a change in pressure in the superior vena cava. Such an observation was not made during these experiments, thus providing strong circumstantial evidence that the stimulus did not affect the venous tone.

In summary, it is concluded that the complex unencapsulated nerve endings in the left atrium do not exert a significant influence either on the capacitance vessels or on the resistance vessels of the systemic circulation. The evidence concerning the complex unencapsulated nerve endings in the right atrium is less

The systemic circulation

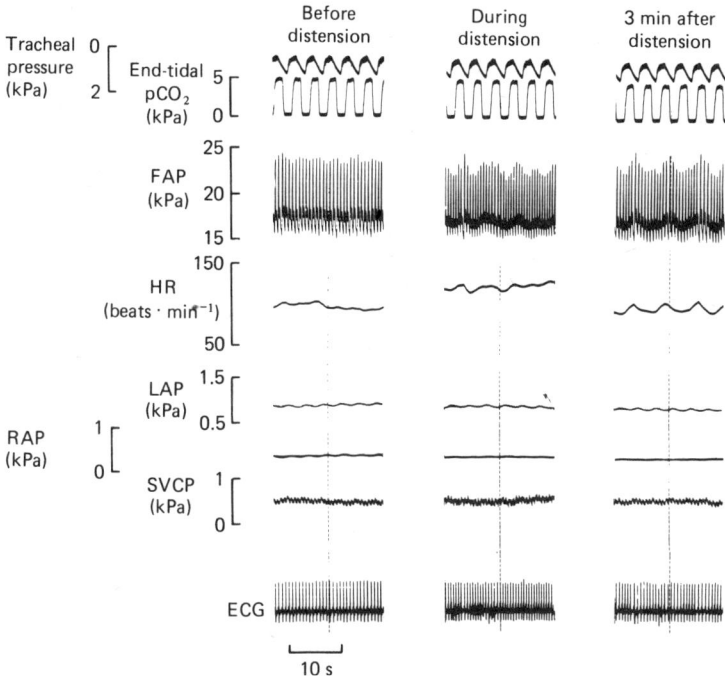

Fig. 7.4. Effects of stretching the junction between the superior vena cava and the right atrium. From above downwards, tracheal pressure, end-tidal pCO_2, femoral arterial pressure (FAP), heart rate (HR), left (LAP) and right (RAP) atrial pressures, superior vena caval pressure (SVCP) and the electrocardiogram (ECG). Records obtained immediately before distension of balloon A (heart rate 97 beats·min^{-1}), during the distension (heart rate 126 beats·min^{-1}) and three min after removal of the distension (heart rate 106 beats·min^{-1}). Mean increase in heart rate 25 beats·min^{-1}. (From Kappagoda, Linden & Snow, 1972a.)

complete but it is likely that they also do not influence the peripheral vessels.

Receptors discharging into non-myelinated vagal fibres

The second group of vagal afferent fibres which has been investigated in recent years consists of the non-myelinated vagal fibres which carry impulses from atrial receptors (see Chapter 3).

Atrial receptors: systemic and pulmonary circulations

Several attempts have been made in the last ten years to elucidate the mechanisms in which these non-myelinated fibres are involved. Oberg & White (1970a) observed in anaesthetised dogs with denervated aortic baroreceptors, that cooling the cervical vagi to 0 °C resulted in an increase in systemic blood pressure which is accompanied by vasoconstriction in skeletal muscle, intestine and kidney. From these findings the authors concluded that certain vagal afferent fibres exerted a tonic restraint on the vasomotor centre.

In an effort to locate the source of these tonically inhibitory nerves, Oberg & Thorén (1973) investigated the effect of stimulating the right caudal cardiac nerve in the cat. This nerve is believed to carry the bulk of the afferent nerves from the heart which are destined for the vagus. By studying the evoked compound action potentials, these authors claimed that this nerve contained two main types of fibres – namely a low-threshold myelinated group and a high-threshold non-myelinated group (see Chapter 5). Stimulation of the nerve at a strength sufficient to activate the myelinated fibres alone resulted in a small increase in heart rate and vasoconstriction in renal and muscle vessels. Cooling the cervical vagi to 0 °C resulted in abolition of the response indicating that sympathetic afferent fibres were not involved in the response. Since the cooling was carried out in a single step, it is not possible to conclude that the responses were mediated solely by myelinated nerves (see Chapters 3 and 6) particularly when the frequencies of stimulation applied to the nerves were as stated (60–80 Hz).

On the other hand, when the nerve was stimulated to activate the high-threshold non-myelinated group, there was a marked bradycardia, a fall in blood pressure and vasodilatation. These results were used to strengthen the earlier claim that the non-myelinated vagal fibres exerted a tonic inhibitory effect on the vasomotor tone. However, the basic criticism that the precise organ of origin of the fibres stimulated was unknown, remains unanswered.

It is also relevant at this stage to consider the experiments of Edis *et al.* (1970) who studied the effect of distending balloons positioned at the pulmonary vein–atrial junctions (see Chapter 5 for criticism of this work in relation to changes in heart rate). Although the stimulus was nominally similar to that applied by

Carswell *et al.* (1970*a*), the effect on the systemic vascular resistance was different in that a relatively more sustained fall was observed. The balloons used by the former were considerably larger than those by Carswell *et al.* (1970*a*) and it is conceivable that the responses evoked by them were a result of activation of receptors other than those discharging into myelinated fibres. Such an interpretation of these results appears justified on the basis of the work of Lloyd who demonstrated that increasing pressure in the left atrium (Lloyd, 1972), and the left pulmonary vein–atrial system in particular (Lloyd, 1975), produced a fall in systemic resistance. Although the stimulus in the former investigation was not limited to the atrium, the effect was abolished by vagotomy. Lloyd (1975) also observed a transient fall in systemic vascular resistance in response to an abrupt change in left atrial pressure; when a square wave stimulus was applied there was an immediate reduction in resistance followed by a recovery towards the control state. Recently Lloyd & Friedman (1977) whilst confirming that distension of the left atrium and pulmonary veins resulted in a transient fall in systemic resistance also showed that this fall in resistance involves vessels in the skin, skeletal muscle, kidney and the large intestine. There are obvious similarities between this effect and the transient fall in blood pressure noted during the distension of balloons positioned at the pulmonary vein–atrial junctions (see later in this chapter).

Continuing to investigate the nature of the receptors stimulated, Shepherd and his colleagues used another technique to examine the non-myelinated afferent fibres in the vagus, involving the cooling of the cervical vagus (Thorén, Mancia & Shepherd, 1975). The study was conducted in anaesthetised rabbits. The aortic and carotid sinus nerves were first cut and then the cervical vagi were cooled to 12, 8, 6 and 0 °C. They observed that progressive cooling of the vagi resulted in an increase in aortic blood pressure and the effect was maximal at 0 °C (Fig. 7.5). They also investigated the effect of graded cooling of the vagi on the spontaneous activity of myelinated fibres in the aortic nerve (i.e. baroreceptor) and in the vagus (i.e. pulmonary stretch receptor). It was found that spontaneous activity was minimal at 8 °C and abolished at 6 °C. Thus cooling from 6 to 0 °C resulted in no further change in myelinated fibres

Atrial receptors: systemic and pulmonary circulations

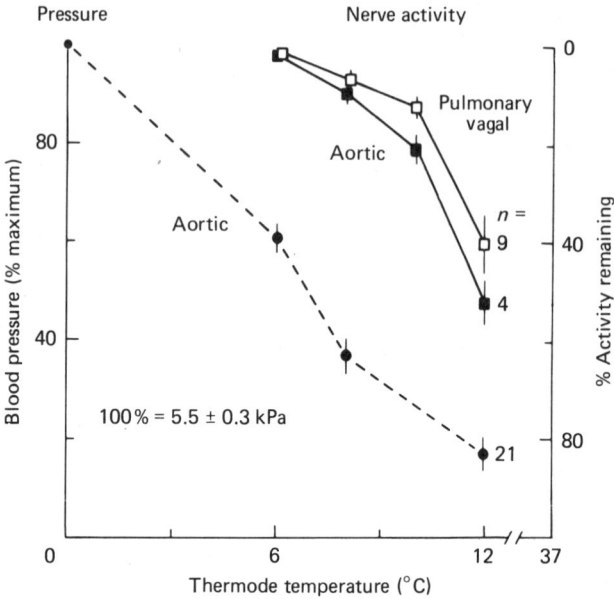

Fig. 7.5. Mean (±S.E.) increases in aortic blood pressure (●) obtained by cooling of vagal nerves to 12, 8, 6 and 0 °C and for changes in nerve activity in vagal afferent fibres from lungs (pulmonary stretch receptors) (□) and aortic baroreceptor afferents (■) during cooling of vagal and aortic nerves to 12, 10, 8, 6 and 0 °C. Changes in the nerve traffic are calculated as traffic remaining (%), with nerve activity at 37 °C as 100%. (From Thorén et al., 1975.)

but nevertheless resulted in a further increase in aortic blood pressure. This effect was attributed, probably correctly, to the removal of the activity in non-myelinated nerves in the vagi which the authors claimed originated from the 'cardiopulmonary' region.

Mancia & Donald (1975) then performed a complex series of experiments on anaesthetised dogs subjected to denervation of both the carotid and aortic baroreceptors. The vagi were cut at the level of the diaphragm and the activity of vagal fibres originating in the chest was interrupted by cooling the vagi in the neck. By the incorporation of several extracorporeal perfusion circuits, the authors proceeded to remove the whole heart, ventricles alone, the lungs alone and both the heart and

The systemic circulation

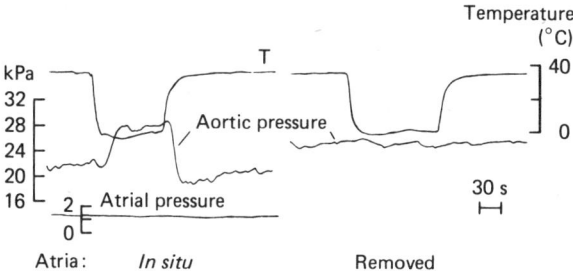

Fig. 7.6. Left: increase in aortic blood pressure during vagal block with only the atria *in situ* (ventricles removed). Right: absence of the increase after removal of the atria. Original tracings from a dog with its carotid sinuses denervated, its aortic nerves cut, its vagi divided at the diaphragm, and its lungs removed. The temperature record (T) was obtained from a thermistor at the surface of one vagus. (From Mancia & Donald, 1975.)

lungs from the chest in various groups of animals. It was found that in each condition, except the last, cooling the vagi to 0 °C resulted in an increase in blood pressure indicating that non-myelinated fibres from the lung, atria and ventricles exerted a 'tonic' inhibitory effect on vasomotor activity. An example of this effect in a dog in which only the atria were *in situ* is shown in Fig. 7.6. It is clear that the increase in blood pressure observed on cooling the vagi was abolished after removal of the atria. In those dogs with only the atria *in situ*, injection of veratridine (0.5 $\mu g \cdot kg^{-1}$ in 0.5 cm^3 of saline) into the artery to the sinus node resulted in a fall in blood pressure. Thus, though these were heroic experiments, the conclusion that activity in the non-myelinated fibres emanating from the atria contributes to the tonic inhibitory effect on the 'vasomotor centre' in the dog is inescapable. It has also been shown (see earlier in this chapter) that the Bezold–Jarisch effect, as defined in response to injections of veratridine, can originate from the atria and not solely from the ventricles.

Mancia, Shepherd & Donald (1975), using techniques similar to the above, showed that interruption of the afferent non-myelinated fibres in the cervical vagus also resulted in diminution of blood flow in the hind limb and the kidney. It is possible that fibres originating in the atria contributed to this phenomenon. Such a conclusion could also be drawn from the investigation

Atrial receptors: systemic and pulmonary circulations

of Kahl, Flint & Szidon (1974) where increasing or decreasing left atrial pressure was associated with a fall or rise in renal vasomotor tone, respectively. Though this is a complex situation, atrial receptors could have been involved in this reflex response (see below).

Discrete stimulation of atrial receptors. It is necessary now to re-examine the effect of distension of small balloons at the pulmonary vein–atrial junctions. Stretch of the pulmonary vein–atrial junctions with the small balloons stimulates atrial receptors which transmit impulses in myelinated vagal fibres (Kidd *et al.*, 1966; Kappagoda, Linden & Sivananthan, 1979; Chapters 3 and 6) and recently it has also been shown that such a stimulus is capable of causing an increased activity in non-myelinated vagal afferent fibres originating in the atria (Kappagoda, Linden & Sivananthan, 1979; Chapter 6). However, on repeating the stimulus after cooling the cervical vagi to 8–12 °C, it was found that the *increase* in impulse traffic in the myelinated fibres was no longer observed when the small balloons were distended. In addition at this temperature the response of an increase in heart rate was also abolished (Kappagoda, Linden & Sivananthan, 1979; Chapter 6).

However, Carswell *et al.* (1970a) did not observe any changes in peripheral resistance during stimulation of atrial receptors using the same technique of distension of small balloons at the pulmonary vein–atrial junctions. There is, however, one other aspect of the response of the systemic resistance vessels to stretching of the vein–atrial junctions. In the experiments which were performed to demonstrate a reflex increase in heart rate it was found that in some experiments distension of the balloons was accompanied by a transient decrease in blood pressure which lasted 10–15 s (Fig. 7.7). In the initial publication by Carswell *et al.* (1970a) it was observed in one-third of the dogs. In subsequent publications (see Burkhart & Ledsome, 1977) it has been claimed that it is a much more frequent observation.

In the hands of the Leeds group, in recent years, this observation is relatively rare and is seen in approximately 5–10 % dogs. Even when it is observed, it can be eliminated by adjusting the rate of injection of saline into the balloon (Kappagoda, Linden & Sivananthan, 1979). In the example shown by Carswell

The systemic circulation

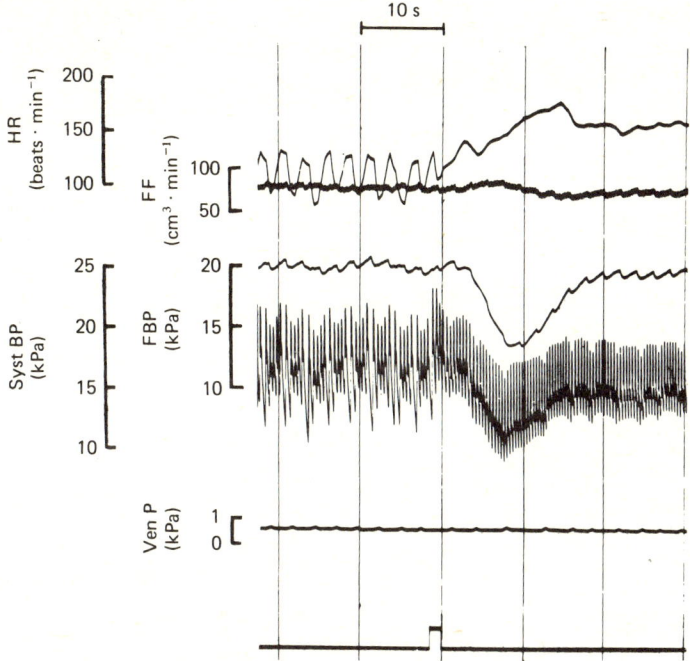

Fig. 7.7. Changes occurring immediately following distension of the pulmonary vein–atrial junctions at signal. Dog 13 kg. Femoral artery perfusion, aorta not occluded. From the above downwards heart rate, femoral perfusion flow, femoral perfusion pressure, systemic arterial pressure (recorded in the right femoral artery), venous pressure and signal marker. HR, heart rate (beats·min^{-1}); FF, femoral perfusion flow (cm^3·min^{-1}); FBP, femoral perfusion pressure (kPa); Syst BP, systemic arterial pressure (kPa); Ven P, venous pressure (kPa). (From Carswell *et al.*, 1970*a*.)

et al. (1970*a*) it is clear that each inflation was completed in 1–2 s (Fig. 7.7). The technique now adopted in Leeds is slightly different in that the injections into each balloon are completed in 5–10 s and this difference could account for the relative rarity of the observations (Fig. 7.8). Nevertheless, the question which remains is whether the response is an effect originating in the complex unencapsulated nerve endings.

For reasons described in Chapter 6, any response to stimulation of the complex unencapsulated nerve endings should be

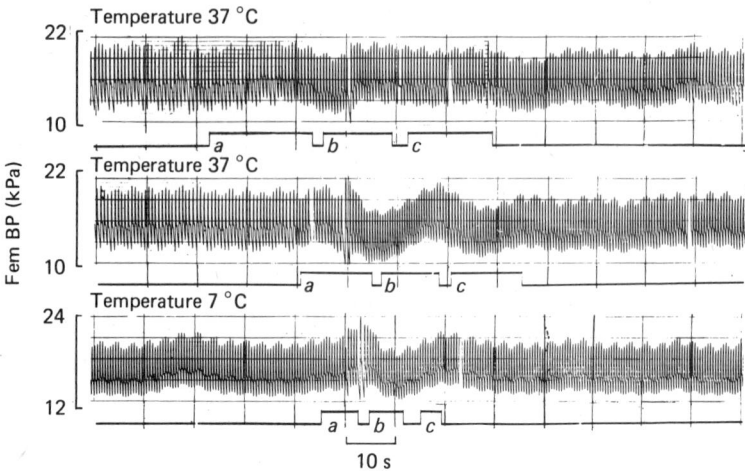

Fig. 7.8. The effect of distension of the balloons at the pulmonary vein–atrial junctions on the systemic blood pressure. Each record shows the femoral blood pressure (Fem BP) and the event marker. (a) Distension of the left superior pulmonary vein–atrial junction; (b) distension of the left middle pulmonary vein–atrial junction; and (c) distension of the left lower pulmonary vein–atrial junction. The length of the 'event' indicates the time taken to distend the respective balloons. Upper record: vagi at 37 °C. Slow distension of the balloons producing a small transient reduction in blood pressure. Middle record: vagi at 37 °C. Rapid distension of the balloons producing a relatively greater transient reduction in blood pressure. Bottom record: vagi at 7 °C. Rapid distension of the balloons producing a transient reduction in blood pressure. The magnitude of this response is similar to that in the middle record. (From Kappagoda, Linden & Sivananthan, 1979.)

diminished by cooling the vagi towards 12 °C and abolished between 12 and 8 °C. In an attempt to investigate the mechanisms of this transient phenomenon on blood pressure, the vagi were cooled in stages in several dogs in which the response was observed (Kappagoda, Linden & Sivananthan, 1979). At each temperature the stimulation was repeated. It was found that the response was virtually unaffected by cooling to 8 °C (Fig. 7.8) and was still present at 5 °C. This finding taken together with its dependence on the rate of injection into the balloon suggests strongly that this transient effect on systemic arterial pressure is a phenomenon mediated by receptors other than the complex unencapsulated endings, probably receptors discharging into

The systemic circulation

the non-myelinated fibres in the vagi. The transient and ephemeral nature of the response is entirely consistent with the behaviour of atrial receptor endings which discharge into C fibres (see Chapters 3 and 6).

Koizumi, Ishikawa, Nishino & Brooks (1975), using balloons, weights and threads attached to various parts of the atria, examined reflex responses, also observing transient responses. They obtained both increases and decreases in heart rate and attributed some of their results to changes in arterial blood pressure and venous return. During distension of balloons at the pulmonary vein–atrial junctions they observed early bradycardia followed by an increase in heart rate; though such an effect could be a result of haemodynamic changes secondary to the bizarre stimuli, a possible explanation is that the early response is a transient response which is caused by increased activity in non-myelinated fibres in the vagus as explained above and by Kappagoda, Linden & Sivananthan (1979) (also see Chapter 6).

Afferent fibres in sympathetic rami

The electrophysiology of atrial receptors discharging into nerve fibres in the sympathetic rami has been described in Chapter 3. The evidence linking these receptors and afferent nerves with reflex changes in the peripheral blood vessels is reviewed below.

Before discussing the investigations which have a particular relevance to atrial receptors it is important briefly to consider some of the numerous reports claiming responses from stimulation of receptors in the ventricles or elsewhere in the chest, and discharging through afferent fibres in the sympathetic rami. Reviews of this topic may be found in Donald & Shepherd (1978) and Hainsworth, Kidd & Linden (1979).

Many general experiments using fairly blunderbuss techniques have shown that stimulation of 'sympathetic' afferent fibres causes changes in peripheral vessels. For instance, recently Purtock *et al.* (1977) have stimulated the sympathetic rami (which include T 1–3), after section distal to the spinal cord, and observed either constriction or dilatation of the renal vessels depending on the frequency of stimulation. Such experiments are typical of a large series of experiments studying responses of changes in heart rate (e.g. Malliani *et al.*, 1973; see Chapter

5), changes in myocardial contractility (e.g. Malliani, Peterson, Bishop & Brown, 1972), increases in blood pressure (e.g. Peterson & Brown, 1971) and changes in activity in renal nerves (e.g. Weaver, 1977; Weaver et al., 1979). Alternatively experiments involving 'sympathetic' afferent fibres have been completed where the heart, large vessels or parts of them have been 'stimulated' and action potentials in the sympathetic nerves or reflex responses have been examined; increased coronary artery pressure, myocardial ischaemia and coronary occlusion evoked a reflex change (Brown, 1967; Milliani, Schwartz & Zanchetti, 1969; Brown & Malliani, 1971; Uchida & Murao, 1974b); increases in arterial blood pressure were shown, in spinal vagotomised cats, to cause an increased discharge in efferent sympathetic nerves (Malliani, Pagani, Recordati & Schwartz, 1971); reflex effects on arterial blood pressure and very small changes in heart rate and myocardial 'contractility' have been demonstrated by stretching a part of the wall of the thoracic aorta (Lioy et al., 1974); the application of chemicals including dripping solutions containing potassium ions on to the supposed receptor sites on the left ventricle has also caused the activity in the 'sympathetic' afferent fibres to increase (Uchida & Murao, 1974a; Reimann & Weaver, 1980).

A closer look at one or two of the reports will illustrate the difficulties in elucidating reflex mechanisms involving 'sympathetic' afferent fibres but great credit must be given to Brown, Malliani, Uchida and their groups for bringing this important problem to the fore. In an attempt to elucidate the reflex effect of stimulating the receptors which discharge into these sympathetic nerves, Peterson & Brown (1971) studied the effect of stimulating the inferior cardiac and pericoronary nerves in the cat (Fig. 7.9). They found that stimulation of the inferior cardiac nerve resulted in an increase in blood pressure but no change in heart rate. This response was present after cervical vagotomy. It was abolished by cutting the thoracic sympathetic trunk below the third ramus, the vertebral nerve and the first three rami communicantes. It was also abolished by cutting the central connections of the stellate ganglia. Sectioning the spinal cord at the C_1 level did not abolish the response though it was diminished in magnitude. Finally they found that sympathetic blockade with phenoxybenzamine resulted in the abolition of the

The systemic circulation

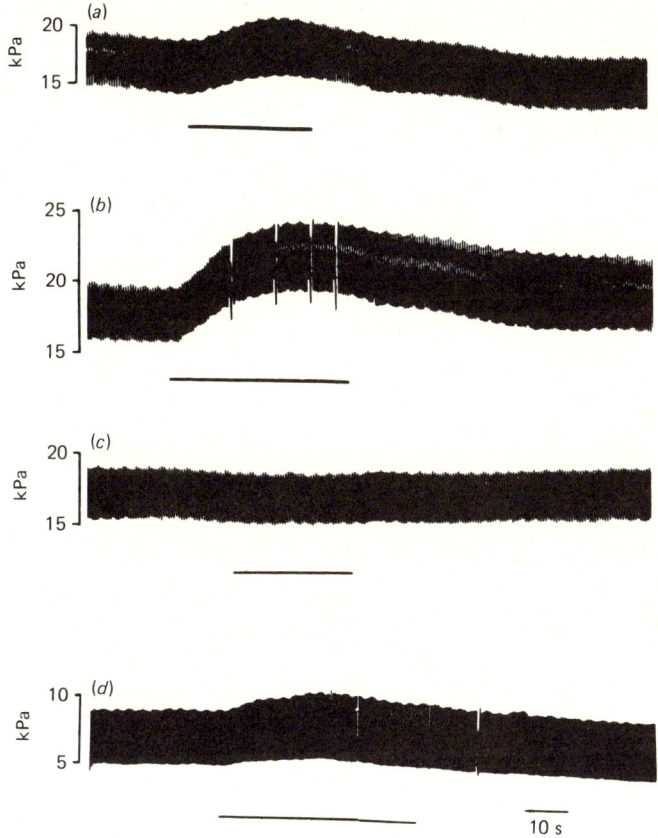

Fig. 7.9. Blood pressure responses to stimulation of the central end of the cut inferior cardiac nerve. (*a*) Response with all other nerves intact; 2.5 V, 15 stimuli·s^{-1}, 5 ms duration. (*b*) Response after bilateral cervical vagotomy; 2.5 V, 15 stimuli·s^{-1}, 5 ms duration. (*c*) Response after section of all central sympathetic connections from the stellate ganglion; 10 V, 15 stimuli·s^{-1}, 5 ms duration. (*d*) Response after bilateral cervical vagotomy in a spinal animal; 5 V, 15 stimuli·s^{-1}, 5 ms duration. (From Peterson & Brown, 1971.)

response, thus indicating that the rise in blood pressure resulted from sympathetic vasoconstriction. These results led the authors to the conclusion that the response was a reflex mediated by afferent fibres in the upper thoracic rami communicantes. The efferent pathway was in the sympathetic outflow to the blood vessels and the central connections were at least partially in the spinal cord.

Peterson & Brown (1971) also showed that the inferior cardiac nerve contained both myelinated and non-myelinated fibres. The stimulus parameters used in the experiments quoted above were such that they would have activated both types of fibres. However, they attempted to differentiate between the effects of increased activity in these two groups of fibres by using different stimuli. Stimuli with a strength of 10 V and duration of 0.05 ms when applied to the inferior cardiac nerve activated the myelinated fibres alone and resulted in a small increase in blood pressure while stimuli of a strength of 10 V and 0.1 ms activated the non-myelinated fibres as well and resulted in a much greater increase in pressure.

In order to define the origin of these fibres Peterson & Brown (1971) studied the effect of stimulating the pericoronary nerve. The authors showed that after cutting both vagi this procedure resulted in an increase in blood pressure. However, with the vagi intact a bradycardia and hypotension were seen in the majority of animals – a finding which was attributed to the existence of vagal non-myelinated afferent fibres emanating from the heart. The implication in this claim is that these fibres have traversed the pericoronary nerve and then leave it to join the cardiac vagal branches and continue into the central nervous system. Sectioning the stellate ganglia and the third and fourth rami abolished the response of an increase in pressure. Once again the response was abolished by the administration of phenoxybenzamine and was preserved (though diminished) by sectioning the cord at C_1. Stimulation of the pericoronary nerve at voltages which were supramaximal only to myelinated fibres resulted in a small increase in blood pressure. When the strength was increased to exceed the threshold for non-myelinated fibres a large rise in blood pressure was observed. Furthermore, stimulation of the pericoronary nerve only evoked a component from non-myelinated fibres in the compound action potentials recorded from the inferior cardiac nerve. No myelinated component was evident in it and this apparent anomaly was attributed to technical difficulties. However, these findings clearly demonstrated a continuity of nerve fibres between the pericoronary nerve and the inferior cardiac nerve.

The systemic circulation

Taken collectively, one possible explanation for their findings was that stimulation of fibres originating in the heart, and traversing in turn the pericoronary nerve, the inferior cardiac nerve and the upper cervical sympathetic rami, resulted in an increase in blood pressure which was at least in part a spinal reflex. One cannot, however, conclude with certainty that these fibres do originate from the atria (cf. Uchida, 1979) or that the non-myelinated fibres in pericoronary nerves are, in fact, afferent fibres.

In subsequent years this response has been intensively investigated by Malliani and his colleagues (see Malliani, 1979, for review). The essential conclusions of these investigations are given below. Repeating the above experiment but using a different anaesthetic Malliani et al. (1973) were able to demonstrate an increase in heart rate in cats in addition to the increase in blood pressure. This response was also shown to be a reflex which had a pathway similar to that shown by Peterson & Brown (1971). Using electrophysiological techniques, Schwartz et al. (1973) showed that stimulation of the inferior cardiac nerve and the pericoronary nerve also resulted in reduction in activity in vagal efferent fibres and an increase in sympathetic efferent fibres. These changes appeared to be unaffected by mid-collicular decerebration.

Malliani et al. (1972) have shown that the stimulation of the inferior cardiac nerve also resulted in an increase in ventricular 'contractility' – a finding which is again compatible with the electrophysiological findings described above. In addition, Pagani, Schwartz, Bishop & Malliani (1975) have shown that stimulation of cardiac nerves also appears to affect the dimension of the thoracic aorta.

Recently Weaver (1977) has investigated the effects of stimulating afferent nerves to the sympathetic chain (a nerve to the stellate ganglion) and of large infusions, in the anaesthetised cat with the carotid sinus nerves and vagi sectioned. On stimulating the afferent nerves it was found that there was first an excitatory and then an inhibitory effect on the activity in efferent nerves to the kidney; later (Weaver et al., 1979) these different effects were attributed to different groups of afferent nerves. Activity in efferent nerves to the kidney decreased during the infusions. The blood pressure rose or fell and to some extent the variation was related to the frequency and strength of the stimulus. It was concluded that receptors discharging into 'sympathetic' afferent fibres and having their site of origin in the 'cardiopulmonary' area could affect the activity in nerves to the kidney. It is probably valid to draw this limited conclusion from such blunderbuss techniques, but what receptors are involved and whether the effects are primary or are secondary to the changes in blood pressure cannot be discerned.

Summary

These experimental results clearly indicate the existence of reflex mechanisms emanating from the heart which exert an influence on the sympathetic and vagal outflow. The sympathetic afferent component of the reflex is at least partially mediated through spinal centres. There is, however, no direct evidence to link the afferent nerves with the atrial receptors demonstrated by Uchida & Murao (1974c) and Kostreva et al. (1975) but in view of their multifocal origin such a situation seems probable. That many of these fibres have a multifocal origin was discovered many years ago (Holmes & Torrence, 1959) and recently extensively re-examined by Coleridge, Coleridge, Dangel, Kidd, Luck & Sleight (1973) (see Chapter 3). Such multifocal origins of many of these fibres suggest that the receptors discharging into them will not subserve discrete responses involved in the particular control of any circulatory parameter.

Atrial receptors and the pulmonary circulation

Compared with the effects on the systemic circulation, there has been relatively little interest in the reflex effects of stimulating atrial receptors on the pulmonary circulation. No encouragement can be obtained from the observation that effects on respiration are not part of the reflex response. Ledsome & Hainsworth (1970) showed that stimulating left atrial receptors, presumably discharging into myelinated fibres in the vagi, had no effect on the respiration. No significant changes in respiratory rate or tidal volume were recorded although they were consistently able to demonstrate the reflex increase in heart rate. Such a mechanism affecting respiration had previously been reported by Daly, Ludany, Todd & Verney (1937) and Aviado *et al.* (1951) who suggested that distension of the pulmonary veins and stimulation of pulmonary venous receptors caused a reflex tachypnoea. It is therefore considered unlikely that stimulation of these unencapsulated left atrial receptors makes any significant contribution to the hyperpnoea of muscular exercise.

Also no change, in response to the same discrete stimulus, was observed in the pulmonary circulation. Distension of the left pulmonary vein–atrial junctions in anaesthetised dogs (Ledsome & Linden, 1964b) did not result in any significant changes in mean pressure in the pulmonary artery even though the procedure resulted in a reflex increase in heart rate. Using the same stimulus as Ledsome & Linden (1964b) Furnival, Linden & Snow (unpublished) examined the effect of distending the pulmonary vein–atrial junctions on the 'tone' in pulmonary veins. The preparation devised by Snow (1973) involved a right heart bypass and perfusion of the right lung. Stimulation of left atrial receptors by distending the left upper pulmonary vein–atrial junction was without effect on the resistance to flow in the pulmonary veins, although an increase in heart rate was observed. The 'viability' of the preparation and validity of this technique was established by demonstrating a reflex constriction of the pulmonary veins in response to occlusion of the carotid arteries. Thus it was concluded that increased activity in left atrial receptors did not effect either veno-constriction or veno-dilatation.

In contrast to these studies, Lloyd & Schneider (1969) studied the effect of distending the left heart and the pulmonary veins on vascular tone. They found that at a constant rate of blood flow through the lungs the form of the relationship between the 'pulmonary venous' pressure and the pulmonary artery pressure was described by a sigmoid curve. Left ventricular pressure was measured but 'The data were obtained with pump-perfused dogs so arranged that the left atrium and ventricle served as extensions of the pulmonary venous system.' For left ventricular pressures less than 2.7 kPa the slope of the curve was less than unity, and for pressures exceeding 3.6 kPa the slope was unity. Between left ventricular pressures of 2.7 and 3.6 kPa the slope was greater than unity. This sigmoid shape of the curve was altered by ganglionic blockade but not by vagotomy. Subse-

Atrial receptors: systemic and pulmonary circulations

quently Lloyd & Schneider (1970) showed that sectioning the stellate ganglia also altered the shape of the curve, thus indicating the basic reflex nature of the response. The authors suggested that the receptors involved in this response may be the ones which discharge into the sympathetic afferent fibres (cf. Malliani, 1979), though such a proposition remains highly speculative.

In another study, Hyman & Sanchez (1969) inserted a balloon into a single pulmonary vein under radiographic control, in lightly anaesthetised dogs with intact chests. They obtained increases in pulmonary arterial and venous pressures in response to distension of the balloon. They concluded that there was reflex constriction of pulmonary vessels because little change was observed in dogs subjected to vagotomy and atropine. However, the rises in pulmonary venous and arterial pressures were the same, suggesting a back-pressure effect even with the small change in atrial pressure, though the effects observed in the perfused section probably did not have this cause. The small changes in atrial pressure and systemic arterial pressure with and without vagal blockade (completed in a different group of dogs) suggest that the very large balloons (4–5 cm^3) were causing some obstruction. The hazards in using vagotomy as a means of demonstrating reflexes have already been commented on in Chapter 4. Also if one accepts that there was a reflex response there is no indication in this report as to which receptors were involved; in very lightly anaesthetised animals, such as these, the question of stimulating pain fibres arises. A reasonable conclusion from this group of experiments is that there may have been an effect which was not entirely mechanical.

Thus, in summary, it appears that there is little evidence to suggest that the complex unencapsulated atrial receptors exert any influence on the pulmonary circulation, though such a role for the other atrial receptors cannot be excluded, as the hypothesis has not been tested.

8 CENTRAL CONNECTIONS OF ATRIAL RECEPTORS

General background

Before examining the evidence of the sites of termination of afferent fibres attached to atrial receptors, it is necessary briefly to discuss the evidence contributing to the knowledge of the possible termination of afferent fibres from the circulation in the chest. Numerous investigations involving a variety of techniques, have provided evidence that cardiovascular afferent fibres which run in the vagal nerves, enter the medulla and terminate in, or close to, the nucleus of the tractus solitarius near to the obex (for reviews see Kirchheim, 1976; Kidd, 1979, 1980) but there is considerable overlap in this area.

Anatomical and histological evidence has clearly defined the nucleus of the tractus solitarius as the major site of termination for afferent fibres (see Kidd, 1979). For example, Cottle (1964) determined the distribution of degenerating fibre terminals following division of small groups of the vagal nerve rootlets and concluded that the vagal afferent fibres were distributed in the intermediate, caudal and commissural regions of the nucleus of the tractus solitarius. The afferent nerves from cardiac receptors must be assumed to terminate within this distribution to the dorso-medial and ventro-lateral areas of the nucleus tractus solitarius although it should be remembered that the divided rootlets also contain afferent fibres from other origins within the afferent vagal distribution.

Electrical stimulation of the cervical vagal nerves evoked 'slow wave' activity with latencies appropriate to action potentials in myelinated afferent fibres, from the intermediate and commissural section of the nucleus tractus solitarius, the nucleus intercalatus and the dorsal motor nucleus of the vagus in the medial brain stem; more laterally, responses were also evoked from the region of the nucleus ambiguus (Lam & Tyler, 1952; Harrison & Bruesch, 1954; Anderson & Berry, 1956; Hellner & Baumgarten, 1961; Porter, 1963). Other studies to determine the distribution of the non-myelinated fibres, which constitute the majority of the afferent fibres within the cervical vagal nerves, indicate a similar distribution within the brain stem of the anaesthetised cat and dog (Lam & Tyler, 1952; Fussey, Kidd & Whitwam, 1973). However, the cervical vagal nerves contain afferent fibres from areas other than the heart, and more recently in Leeds, Kidd and his group (Kidd, 1980) have restricted the origins of afferent fibres excited, by stimulating the central end of the right vagal cardiac nerve in the anaesthetised cat (Donoghue, Fox, Kidd & Koley, 1977, 1980). The latencies of the 'slow wave' and 'multi-unit' activity evoked by such stimulation fell into two major categories, early and late. Short latency responses, 4–50 ms, had afferent fibres with conduction velocities of 3–37 m·s^{-1}. These responses were mainly distributed in the medial and lateral areas of the nucleus of the tractus solitarius, the lateral edge of the area postrema and the dorsal motor vagal nucleus; more laterally, evoked responses were found in the region of the nucleus ambiguus. Long latency responses, 60–250 ms were associated with afferent fibres having conduction velocities of 0.6–2.5 m·s^{-1} distributed in the medial and lateral part of the nucleus of the tractus solitarius, the area postrema, the dorsal motor nucleus of the vagus and the parahypoglossal area.

Although such responses are initially useful in defining projections of cardiac vagal afferent fibres, they are difficult to interpret. In such recordings it is difficult to separate presynaptic and postsynaptic components and to distinguish afferent and efferent contributions. Therefore Kidd and his group (Kidd, 1980), using metal microelectrodes, recorded activity extracellularly from single neurones which were excited with long latencies appropriate to afferent vagal C fibres; the conduction velocities in the afferent fibres were measured. Using various criteria (Kidd, 1980), they were able to show that 34 neurones were excited synaptically and 17 were excited non-synaptically, but they were unable to distinguish whether the latter group were afferent or efferent in nature. These neurones were in the medial part of the nucleus of the tractus solitarius and in the dorsal motor nucleus of the vagus.

General background

In these experiments, the intensity of the electrical stimulus to the right vagal cardiac nerve was such that both myelinated and non-myelinated fibres were excited. Thus, responses were obtained from neurones driven synaptically by the non-myelinated fibres to determine whether the same neurone was also activated by myelinated fibres within this nerve. In no case was it possible to demonstrate an early evoked response, although frequently early compound evoked waves from other neurones were present. Thus, although more subtle tests for sub-threshold convergence effects have not yet been applied, Kidd (1980) suggests that the evidence at present favours a working hypothesis that the non-myelinated afferent fibres terminate in an area of the brain stem which is coextensive with the area of termination of the myelinated fibres of the right vagal cardiac nerve and that the two afferent inputs are separate; individual neurones activated by the non-myelinated afferents from the heart do not appear to receive a convergent influence from myelinated fibres from the same region.

Clearly further studies are required, but the possibility that the two types of afferent fibres – myelinated and non-myelinated – may have separate brain stem connections is of great interest in view of the recent evidence postulating that 'cardiopulmonary' vagal non-myelinated fibres may have a tonic role in the control of the peripheral vasculature (Thorén *et al.*, 1976).

Spontaneous activity in the brain stem

Central projections of cardiac receptors have also been examined by searching for brain stem neurones with spontaneous activity associated with the cardiac cycle; many of the receptors in the heart (particularly Paintal-type atrial receptors) have patterns of discharge which are pulsed and related to specific phases of the cardiac cycle. A number of investigations have described such neurones (e.g. Hellner & Baumgarten, 1961; Smith & Pearce, 1961; Salmoiraghi, 1962; Humphrey, 1967; Fussey *et al.*, 1967; Koepchen, Langhorst, Seller, Polster & Wagner, 1967; Seller & Illert, 1969; Miura & Reis, 1972; Middleton, Woolsey, Burton & Rose, 1973), though many of these investigations did not differentiate between the activities of systemic baroreceptors and cardiac receptors. Most of the information about the input from particular receptors into the nucleus tractus solitarius relates to the activity in, and 'interaction' of, systemic arterial baroreceptors, and little is known of the medullary connections of myelinated fibres from atrial receptors (Kidd, 1979, 1980; Ledsome, 1979). It has been shown that vagal afferent fibres discharging with a cardiovascular rhythm enter the medulla in the more rostral rootlets of the vagal nerve (Bonvallet & Sigg, 1958) with those showing a pattern of discharge typical of atrial receptors being in the more caudal of the rostral rootlets (Baumgarten, Koepchen & Aranda, 1959). Impulse patterns from neurones suggesting that they are influenced by atrial receptors were recorded by Hellner & Baumgarten (1961) from points dorsolateral to the tractus solitarius between 1 and 3 mm rostral to the obex in the cat. Baertschi, Munzer, Ward, Johnson & Gann (1975) have investigated medullary neurones responding to small changes in blood volume or to atrial pulsation in cats and *presumed* the responses to be caused by changes in the discharge in atrial receptors (the receptors involved were not definitely identified as atrial by location in the endocardium); they found these neurones only in the nucleus of the tractus solitarius or close by in the underlying reticular formation. Since this investigation also does not provide evidence of the pattern or the profile of receptors activated by these manoeuvres it is not possible to make a useful interpretation of the specific reflex pathways to which neural changes may be related. Indeed, the possibility that some of the changes may be due to mechanical movements of the brain consequent on changes in venous pressure cannot be excluded.

Pathways from atrial receptors are said to affect the supraoptic nucleus but, as well as other criticisms, there is no evidence that there is a discrete stimulation of atrial receptors (see Chapter 10).

Pathways between the nucleus of the tractus solitarius and other 'higher centres' have also been proposed (see Chapter 9). For instance, there have been attempts (e.g. Ward, Baertschi & Gann, 1977) to define medullary areas responding to stimulation of atrial receptors and having rostral projections. Criticisms of their work in attempting to relate changes in the secretion of ACTH to stimulation of atrial receptors are presented in Chapter 9; the same criticisms (in addition to those cited above)

General background

involving possible inadequacy of the stimulus, no interruption of reflex pathways, and no evidence of discrete stimulation of atrial receptors, also apply to these experiments. It is not possible to accept this evidence as evidence that pathways from atrial receptors project to the hypothalamus.

Supramedullary influences

There is increasing evidence that neurones in supramedullary structures can affect neurones in the medulla, e.g. there is evidence that baroreceptor reflexes evoking cardiac and vasomotor activity may be modulated by suprabulbar stimulation (e.g. Uther, Hunyor, Shaw & Korner, 1970; Kent, Drane & Manning, 1971; Korner, Shaw, West & Oliver, 1972; Adair & Manning, 1975; Korner, 1979). Korner *et al.* (1972) have shown in the conscious rabbit that stimulus–response curves for pontine and thalamic animals are displaced towards a lower heart rate when compared with sham-operated animals. They suggested that anaesthesia leads to enhancement of baroreceptor-mediated sympathetic effects on the heart because these results were different from those in anaesthetised animals. Kirchheim (1976) suggests their results show that the threshold for baroreceptor activation of vagal efferent fibres to the heart is increased. As a result of these experiments it would be expected that supramedullary structures would affect reflexes from atrial receptors. In the event, Albrook *et al.* (1972) were unable to demonstrate any statistical difference between the increase in heart rate obtained by stimulating atrial receptors in the decerebrate dog and that obtained in the intact animal. These results were obtained in spite of evidence that supramedullary structures were affecting the control heart rate; the control heart rates in the decerebrate dogs were lower than those in the intact animals.

However, all this evidence is only suggestive of afferent fibres from atrial receptors terminating in the brain stem; there is no evidence that any particular nuclei were involved.

Central connections of atrial receptors

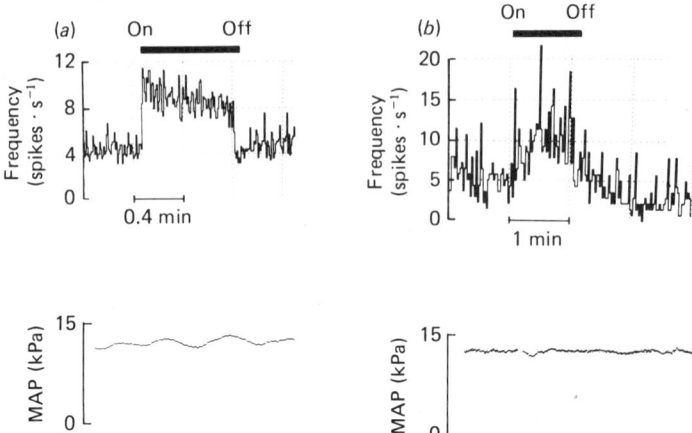

Fig. 8.1. Responses of brain stem neurones to inflation of left atrial balloons. (a) Activity of single neurone in nucleus tractus solitarius increased when the balloons are distended. (b) Activity from single neurone in the medial reticular formation increased and decreased gradually following balloon distension and removal of distension. Note the absence of any concomitant alteration in mean arterial blood pressure (MAP). (From Kidd, 1979.)

Termination of afferent fibres from atrial receptors

In this laboratory Keith et al. (1975) and Kidd (1980) have produced evidence that discrete stimulation of the left atrial receptors with small balloons in the pulmonary vein–atrial junctions leads to an increase in activity in neurones at two sites in the medulla. Neurones in the nucleus of the tractus solitarius with a cardiac rhythm increased their discharge (Fig. 8.1(a)); also another group of neurones, found in the central reticular formation near the region of the nucleus of the hypoglossal nerve, whose spontaneous activity was without a cardiac rhythm and discharging at lower frequencies, also increased their discharge (Fig. 8.1(b)). In particular, recordings were made from 40 sites at which the spontaneous activity of individual neurones or a small group of 2–3 neurones increased (Figs. 8.1 and 8.2); in no case was there evidence of inhibitory responses. The increases were abolished when the vagal nerves were cooled to 5 °C and in some instances, the spontaneous activity of neurones was reduced. Abolishing the reflex response of the increase of heart rate by blockade of sympathetic efferent nerves did not prevent the change in activity, showing that it was not secondary to such changes. The responsive sites were located between 1 mm caudal and 3 mm rostral to the obex and were distributed over superficial and deep areas (Fig. 8.2). A number of sites were in the dorso-medial area of the nucleus of the tractus solitarius while others were deeper in the medial reticular tissue adjacent to the paramedian and raphae nuclei; one neurone was located in the parahypoglossal area. The spontaneous activity of most neurones within the superficial zone had a cardiac modulation; however, this was not invariable and some had an irregular low-frequency ($1-1.5$ spikes$\cdot$s^{-1}) spontaneous discharge. The spontaneous activity of the deep neurones was invariably without an overt cardiovascular rhythm. Frequently the changes in impulse activity of the deep neurones increased and decreased more slowly than those of the superficial group following distension and release of distension of the balloons (Fig. 8.1). The observed alterations in neural activity were not the result of mechanical artefacts nor secondary to excitation of other vascular receptors. The patterns of response at both these sites were different from those characteristic of activity in systemic arterial baroreceptors. It was concluded that the neurones represent components of the neural pathways of the reflex responses evoked by stimulation of left atrial receptors (see Chapters 6 and 10). The superficial group of neurones in the nucleus of the tractus solitarius are likely to represent an 'early' synaptic linkage while the 'deep' group may represent additional interneurones cascaded in the pathway or represent cell bodies of reticulospinal connections to the sympathetic efferent motor neurones. The deep group is in the same area as those which have been implicated in the sympathetic efferent component of baroreceptor pathways (e.g. Alexander, 1946; Humphrey, 1967; Snyder & Gebber, 1973; Coote & McLeod, 1974; McCall, Gebber & Barman, 1977). However, further experiments are obviously required before the specific nature of these two groups of neurones and their interconnections can be identified.

Recently Ledsome and his group (Albrook *et al.*, 1972; Burkhart *et al.*, 1977; Ledsome, 1979) have examined the effects

Central connections of atrial receptors

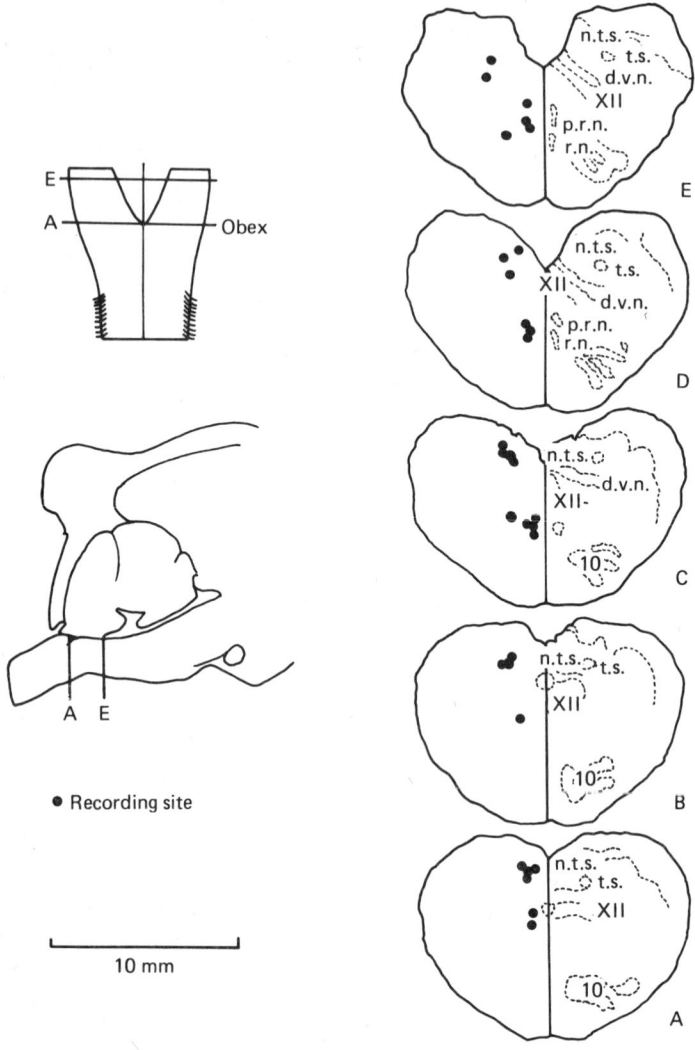

Fig. 8.2. Location of neurones in brain stem responding to stimulation of left atrial receptors. Each section is representative of a 1 mm slice of brain stem rostral to obex. Each site at which single and multi-unit activity responding to balloon inflation is shown, d.v.n., dorsal motor vagal nucleus; t.s., tractus solitarius; n.t.s., nucleus tractus solitarius; XII, hypoglossal nerve nucleus; 10, inferior olive; r.n., nucleus raphae; p.r.n., paramedian reticular nucleus. (From Kidd, 1979.)

of distending balloons in the pulmonary vein–atrial junctions on the heart rate in the anaesthetised dog decerebrated by a section of the brain stem either mid-collicular or just caudal to the inferior cerebellar peduncle. They were unable to demonstrate any statistically significant difference between the responses of the increase in heart rate in the decerebrate preparation and those in the intact animal. It was also possible by making lesions near the obex with an electro-coagulator to destroy the nucleus of the tractus and the dorsal nucleus of the vagus over a length of about 2 mm. Comparing the effects of distension of the pulmonary vein–atrial junctions and of occlusion of the carotid arteries they abolished the atrial receptor heart rate reflex but found no significant difference in the response of heart rate to carotid occlusion. It must be remembered, however, that though the extent of the lesion can be anatomically described it is probable that, acutely, the functional destruction is much greater. That care should be taken can be judged by the fact that others (e.g. Laubie & Schmitt, 1979) causing a similar lesion found that the responses to stimulation of the carotid sinus baroreceptors were also abolished. But this does not detract from the above conclusion, that the responses from the two areas, atrial and baroreceptor, were dissociated. In further experiments Burkhart et al. (1977) found that the same lesions, though having the same effects as stated above, did cause abolition of the effects of stimulating the aortic nerve, indicating that the afferent fibres from aortic arterial baroreceptors may synapse more caudally than those from the carotid sinus. Ledsome concludes that their results are consistent with a hypothesis that afferent nerve fibres from baroreceptors in the carotid sinus synapse in the intermediate nucleus of the tractus solitarius more rostral than afferent fibres from aortic baroreceptors and atrial receptors which synapse in the nucleus of the tractus solitarius closer to the obex.

Evidence which does not conflict with the hypothesis that afferent fibres from Paintal-type atrial receptors have central connections mainly in the medulla is presented fully in Chapter 10 where the reflex effects on urine flow are considered. The reflex increase in urine flow was found to be the same whether the posterior pituitary gland (and most of the hypothalamus) was destroyed or intact (Kappagoda, Linden, Snow & Whitaker, 1975).

Central connections of atrial receptors

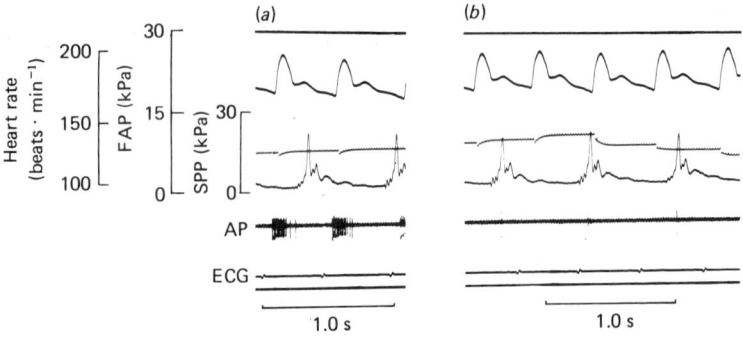

Fig. 8.3. Impulse activity of an interneurone which altered its time relationships during a period of electrical blockade of the intact ipsilateral vagal nerve. (a) Was obtained during a control period when the spontaneous activity is related to each cardiac cycle. (b) Was taken immediately after a period of high-intensity, low-frequency stimulation of the vagal nerve which produced blockade impulse transmission. The neurone now only responds to the perfused carotid sinus pressure pulse (SPP). AP, action potentials; FAP, femoral arterial pressure. (From Kidd, 1979.)

It is difficult to interpret the work of Koizumi, Nishimo & Brooks (1977) investigating centres involved in reflexes resulting from stretching the atria, in view of the nature of the stimuli used (Koizumi et al., 1975) which would have many effects other than stimulating atrial receptors (see Chapter 5).

Convergence of afferent fibres

Kidd (1979) reported that they had made repeated attempts to demonstrate convergence of afferent fibres from the carotid sinus and those in the vagal nerves. In some experiments the intact carotid sinus nerve was stimulated, in others, an isolated carotid sinus preparation was perfused with arterial blood. In each preparation, every neurone with a pulse-phased activity was tested repeatedly by brief occlusion of the common carotid artery and particular attention was placed upon transient alterations in impulse discharge immediately following occlusion and release of the carotid artery. Surprisingly, excitatory convergence was demonstrated for only three neurones. One example is shown in Fig. 8.3 where during a period of anodal blockade, which has been induced by repeated high-intensity stimulation and which had abolished the burst of action potentials associated with arterial pressure pulse, there was now a single spike in response to the oscillations in pressure within the carotid sinus. Further experiments using more subtle tests are required to define the extent of convergence effects.

In two reports of investigations where extracellular recordings of spontaneous activity in single neurones with cardiac rhythm in the medio-dorsal portion of the nucleus of the tractus solitarius (Stroh-Werz, Langhorst & Camerer, 1977a, b), it was claimed that convergence had been demonstrated between afferent fibres from various cardiovascular receptors and receptors in the lungs. The techniques for recognising the sites of origin were based on the patterns of activity of impulses, the relationship of onset to the R-wave of the ECG and the presence or absence of a relationship to the ECG. Reference to Chapter 4 will illustrate the hazards of concluding that the origin of the discharge of receptors is from the so-called 'cardiopulmonary' area or from systemic arterial sites when investigating reflex function; the same problems arise in this type of investigation and do not allow this technique to be used with certainty to differentiate between these two groups of afferent nerves. It is also not possible to recognise from the pattern of impulses and/or the relationship to the events of the cardiac cycle whether any particular activity has emanated from atrial receptors. Such possible recognition is not reliable even in the slips of nerve from the cervical vagus and even less so when considered in a second (or subsequent) order neurone in the medulla. When considering possible activity from a type B atrial receptor it does seem that the claim that the activity in one of the neurones examined 'could originate in pressoreceptors as well as atrial B receptors' was the correct conclusion (Stroh-Werz et al., 1977a). In fact there is no evidence in their report of any particular afferent fibres being responsible for any of the activity so that it is not possible to conclude whether there is convergence or not.

Thus there is no evidence from which definitely to conclude that there is or is not excitatory or inhibitory convergence between the afferent neurones from the systemic arterial baroreceptors and those from the atrial receptors at that level. However, some experiments have been completed which allow a tentative conclusion that though there is evidence of convergence somewhere in the pathways of systemic baroreceptors and atrial receptors there is no 'interaction'. The term 'interaction' is used here, not to imply specific mechanisms of action between neurones, such as occlusion and facilitation, but rather to describe changes in the effects of stimulating the two groups of receptors simultaneously, the results of which are other than the arithmetic summation of the effects of stimulating each of the systems separately. This use of the word 'interaction' is similar to that of Mancia, Shepherd & Donald (1976) who reported progressive increases in the response to vagal blockade as carotid baroreceptor inhibition was withdrawn, which became maximal at carotid sinus pressure of less than 13.3 kPa; they concluded that there was 'interaction' between baroreceptors in the carotid sinus and receptors in the chest with afferent fibres in the vagus (so-called 'cardiopulmonary receptors'). The word 'interaction' was also used in this manner by Korner (1979) who, in a review, discusses the 'resetting' of baroreceptor reflexes.

In this regard Linden, Mary & Weatherill (1979a, b, 1980a, 1981b; see also Chapter 10) examined the effects on efferent renal nerves of stimulating atrial receptors, and repeated the experiments of Karim et al. (1972) of stimulating left atrial receptors, and caused a reflex inhibition of the efferent sympathetic nerves to the kidney. By differential graded cooling of the vagi they showed that this effect was, indeed, mediated by Paintal-type atrial receptors discharging into myelinated vagal afferent fibres (see Chapter 10). In addition, a possible 'interaction' between this effect of atrial receptors and the effects of stimulating carotid sinus baroreceptors was sought (Linden et al., 1979b). In particular, anaesthetised dogs were prepared as before and small balloons were positioned in the left pulmonary vein–atrial junctions and the left atrial appendage. Both carotid sinuses were vascularly isolated and perfused with blood at constant flow. Activity in efferent renal nerves was recorded, along with the ECG and pressures in the femoral artery, carotid sinus, left atrium and trachea. The reflex increase in heart rate during balloon distension and during reduction in carotid sinus pressure was prevented by the administration of bretylium tosylate (10 mg·kg^{-1}) and atropine sulphate (0.4 mg·kg^{-1}). The reduction in activity in renal nerves caused by stimulation of atrial receptors was investigated during the steady state following stepwise changes in carotid sinus perfusion pressure.

In six dogs 10 nerve preparations were obtained; the balloons were distended 34 times at carotid sinus pressures ranging from 5.5 to 24.5 kPa. Over this pressure range the mean control frequency was 2.10 spikes·s^{-1} (range 0.45–11.20). In all 34 distensions the activity in the renal nerves was reduced. At each step the activity was expressed as a percentage of the highest frequency obtained at low carotid sinus pressure; the mean reduction was 29% (range 6–70). In the range of carotid sinus pressures of 5.5–11.9 kPa (16 balloon distensions) the response was 31% (mean; range 6–70), and in a range of 12.3–24.5 kPa (18 balloon distensions) was 27% (mean; range 6–65). There was no significant difference between the responses at low and high carotid sinus pressures ($P > 0.40$).

Since the preliminary communication this investigation has been expanded (Linden *et al.*, 1981*b*) to involve 13 single nerve fibres in eight dogs with entirely similar results; in addition similar experiments involving the stimulation of chemoreceptors and atrial receptors independently and together have been completed with similar results. From all the evidence produced it was concluded that though there was evidence of 'interaction' between different areas of baroreceptors (e.g. between right and left carotid sinus baroreceptors) as found by Gabriel & Seller (1970), and between chemoreceptors and baroreceptors (e.g. Wennergren, Little & Oberg, 1976), there was no 'interaction' between the effects of stimulating atrial receptors and baroreceptors or between atrial receptors and chemoreceptors – in spite of the fact that single efferent neurones were being examined and the activity in which was independently inhibited by each group of receptors. A simple arithmetic summation of effects explained the results; the means of assessment was checked by confirming that 'interaction' could be obtained between systemic baroreceptors from two separate areas, using the same technique. With this crude means of assessing 'interaction' it is not possible to define the mechanisms involved in either situation; but it is probable that though occlusion occurs in the pathway involved in the 'interaction' between the reflexes from different systemic baroreceptor areas, it does not when atrial receptor/baroreceptor areas are stimulated together. Explanations must await more sophisticated techniques with the examination of responses at the neuronal soma or dendritic level which could be completed when the site of the 'interaction' is found. But the possibility of two independent spike generator regions in one of the neurones of the common pathway must be considered.

This finding could explain the previous observations of Carswell et al. (1970a) who found that the reflex increase in heart rate obtained by stimulating left atrial receptors could be obtained with high and low pressures in the carotid sinus and there was little difference in the response demonstrating that there was no 'interaction' in the central nervous system between afferent nerves from these two areas or two separate pathways.

In a recent investigation yet a further difference was observed between the atrial receptor reflex pathways and the pathway of other cardiovascular reflexes; the sympathetic efferent cardiac nerve fibres which respond to stimulation of atrial receptors were shown to be separate from those responding to changes in carotid sinus pressure (Linden, Mary & Weatherill, 1980b). In six dogs, 10 single nerve preparations were studied and distension of the balloons resulted in an increase in activity in these fibres of 27% (mean; range 16–60; $n = 30$) over the activity in the control period ($P < 0.001$). But in these same single fibres there was no significant change in activity in the control periods ($P > 0.5$; paired t-test; $n = 10$) during changes in carotid sinus pressure between 9.3 kPa (mean; range 8–11) and 22.6 kPa (mean; range 19–29). The responses of the fibres to distension of the small balloon also were not different at the two carotid sinus pressures ($P > 0.5$; paired t-test; $n = 10$). Other fibres were examined which changed their activity in response to changes in carotid sinus pressure; but these fibres were unaffected by the stimulation of atrial receptors.

It seems that the atrial receptor reflex pathway has a separate efferent limb to the heart and an efferent limb to the kidney which converges with those from the baroreceptors and chemoreceptors but does not interact with them. These findings seem to emphasise the unique nature of the function of atrial receptors; possibly in the control of heart volumes (see Linden, 1975, 1976).

'Interaction' of reflex effects in man

To extend the concept of convergence of the central pathways of reflexes to investigations in man, Abboud and his colleagues (Takeshita *et al.*, 1979) have attempted to investigate what they have called the 'interaction' between systemic arterial baroreceptors and the so-called 'cardiopulmonary receptors'. 'Cardiopulmonary receptors' were supposedly stimulated by varying central venous pressure which was altered by lower body negative pressure at 3 kPa, or leg and trunk elevation. Arterial baroreceptors were stimulated by bolus intravenous injections of phenylephrine or by neck suction. None of these interventions is specific to either group of receptors. Comment has already been made in Chapter 7 on the total inadequacy of the term 'cardiopulmonary receptors'. The 'stimulus' to systemic baroreceptors will also activate other receptors and incidently will activate 'cardiopulmonary receptors'. They concluded that 'physiological variations in atrial venous pressure do not influence sinus node responses to arterial baroreceptor stimulation in man'. There are several further criticisms of this investigation. The baroreceptors were only tested over that range above a control value of stimulation – no manoeuvre involving hypotension was involved. If atrial receptors were being remotely considered by Takeshita *et al.* (1979) then an additional reason for not expecting 'interaction' in their experiments is that the effects of stimulating atrial receptors are additive at all levels of baroreceptor stimulation (Carswell *et al.*, 1970*a*; Linden *et al.*, 1979*b*; see above) and this would not be evident in their results; that the shape of their heart rate/blood pressure plot did not change is not evidence that atrial receptors were not involved.

Summary

It seems there is no evidence of 'interaction' between reflexes from Paintal-type atrial receptors and reflexes from the arterial baroreceptors. There is evidence of convergence in the central nervous pathways of the two reflexes when the reflex pathway to the kidney is involved but not the reflex pathway to the heart; the efferent sympathetic nerves to the heart activated by atrial receptors are not influenced by other afferent systems. More sophisticated investigations are required before it may be concluded that facilitation and occlusion between the two pathways to the kidney do not occur, but at the moment this would be a reasonable working hypothesis.

9 VARIOUS INTERVENTIONS AND THE KIDNEY

In attempts functionally to link together atrial receptors and the kidney various interventions have been used and various responses have been examined. Intervention has consisted of the use of techniques including negative pressure breathing, alteration of gravitational forces on the body, immersion of the body, alteration of vascular and extracellular fluid volumes, distension of the atria with large balloons and the stretching of discrete regions of the atria. The responses examined have included changes in urine flow (and sodium excretion), in blood flow to the kidney, in the renin–angiotensin system and in the concentration of steroid hormones and prostaglandins in the plasma.

In this chapter it is intended to consider these changes in response to the various interventions. With respect to the effect on the urine flow the discussion in this chapter will be confined to the response to the more generalised 'stimuli'; the effects of the more direct stimuli to atrial receptors, of distension of the atria and discrete parts of the atria on urine flow, will be discussed in the next chapter.

Changes in urine flow

Reflex effects on urine flow of stimulating receptors in the chest have been continuously proposed since 1847. Commenting on the value of hydrotherapy, Hartshorne (1847) drew attention to the increase in urine flow during immersion, hazarding that the cause of the diuresis was probably within the heart and great vessels. This interest in the intrathoracic tissues as possible sites of receptors sensing the volume of the circulating blood and causing changes in urine flow has continued through further investigations involving immersion (e.g. review by Epstein,

Various interventions and the kidney

1978), but with little success in defining precisely the receptors involved (see later). Many attempts have been made to demonstrate that stimulation of atrial receptors caused a diuresis, and thus contributed to the control of extracellular fluid volume.

A specific relationship was first proposed by Gauer, Henry, Sieker & Wendt (1954) who suggested that blood volume was regulated through the stretch of receptors in the intrathoracic circulation. Arguing from a relationship of blood volume to the control of ventricular volumes Gauer (1955) suggested the receptors most likely to be involved were atrial receptors. How such a mechanism contributes to the overall control of blood volume will be alluded to but not fully discussed; it is a large topic in its own right, at least involving the control of water and sodium intake and output. In this regard the function of the atrial receptors would have to be viewed in perspective against the possible roles of other cardiac receptors, including ventricular receptors, which discharge into non-myelinated afferent fibres in the vagi and which recently have been included in the overall 'volume-receptor' proposals (Gauer & Henry, 1976; Thorén, 1979a); presumably the function of spinal 'sympathetic' afferent fibres would also have to be considered.

However, in this section only those investigations claiming to relate the function of atrial receptors to changes in urine flow in response to the more generalised 'stimuli' will be discussed.

Negative pressure breathing

Drury, Henry & Goodman (1947) demonstrated that anaesthetised dogs subjected to positive pressure breathing showed a diminished output of urine. At that time they did not attribute the cause of the response to a diminished discharge of atrial receptors. However, later, several reports (e.g. Surtshin, Hoeltzenbein & White, 1955; Murdaugh, Sieker & Manfredi, 1959) claimed that such a response could be explained on the 'volume receptor theory', because the reduction of intrathoracic blood volume resulting from the positive pressure breathing could cause a decrease in the activity of atrial receptors (Fenn, Otis, Rahn, Chadwick & Hegnauer, 1947). However, Gauer *et al.* (1954) realising that there are many causes of a decreased flow of urine, commented that 'the evidence of any experiment

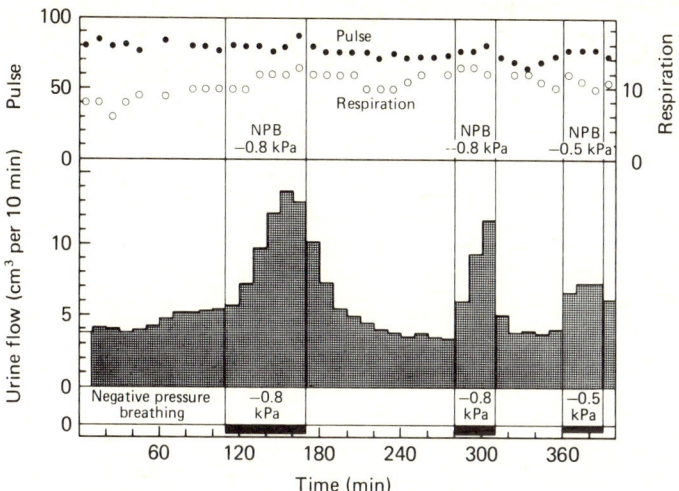

Fig. 9.1. Effect of repeated applications of negative pressure breathing (NPB) on urine flow, pulse rate and respiration. From above down, pulse rate (beats·min^{-1}), respiratory rate (breaths·min^{-1}) and urine flow (cm^3 per 10 min). Note the slow onset of diuresis and the long after-effect. In this experiment marked increases in urine flow were observed without any substantial change in pulse and respiratory rates. (From Gauer et al., 1954.)

which depends solely on reduction in urine flow was felt to be ambiguous'; a greater condemnation could have been made.

Gauer et al. (1954) therefore used negative pressure breathing in an attempt to increase the flow of urine; such a technique was used to cause an increased intrathoracic blood volume and an expected increased stimulation of atrial receptors. Gauer et al. (1954) were able to demonstrate an increase in urine flow in anaesthetised dogs (Fig. 9.1) subjected to negative pressure respiration, a finding later extended to man (Fig. 9.2) by Sieker, Gauer & Henry (1954). Although no specific mechanism was demonstrated at that time in either response, since then these workers have persistently promulgated the view that the responses were mediated by a reduction of circulating antidiuretic hormone (ADH) which resulted from the increased stimulation of atrial receptors (e.g. Chapman & Henry, 1973). This response of an increase in urine flow has also been confirmed by several other investigators (e.g. Boylan & Anthowiak, 1959; Murdaugh et al., 1959; Godley, Myers & Rosenbaum, 1967). Thus, the

Various interventions and the kidney

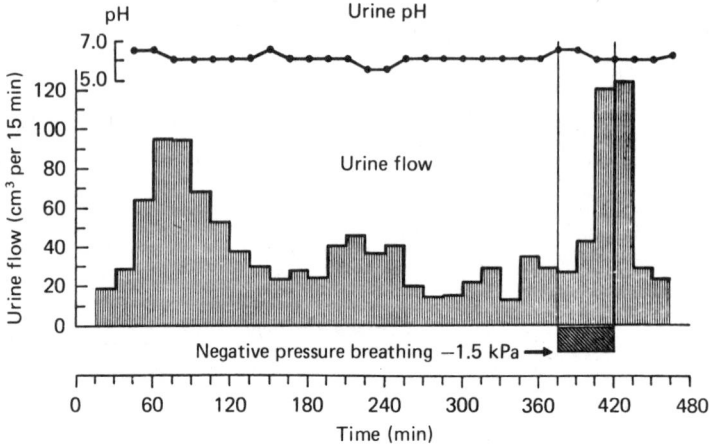

Fig. 9.2. An example of the diuresis observed with negative pressure breathing. From above down: pH in urine; urine flow (cm³ per 15 min). Note the essentially unaltered urine pH during the diuresis. (From Sieker et al., 1954.)

response of an increase in urine flow brought about by negative pressure breathing is not in dispute but the evidence in support of a reflex effect on ADH (Chapman & Henry, 1973) remains controversial.

Lenfant & Howell (1960) examined the effect of negative pressure respiration on intrathoracic pressures in anaesthetised dogs and found that intrapleural, pulmonary arterial, pulmonary venous and thoracic vena caval pressures declined during respiration at pressures down to 2.5 kPa below atmospheric. The fall in intrapleural pressure was greater than the changes in pressure in the vena cava and thus there was an increase in transmural pressure in the intra-thoracic vessels. Since Godley et al. (1967) have demonstrated a comparable fall in the right atrial pressure during negative pressure breathing, it is likely that this increase in transmural pressure would also occur in the atria. Negative pressure breathing results in an increase in venous return (e.g. Hubay et al., 1954) giving some support to explain these increases in transmural pressure and suggesting an increase in central blood volume. Accurate measurements of central blood volume are very difficult to make and such evidence as is available has failed to establish that there is a significant increase in the volume of the major vessels in the chest. But it must be borne in mind that such a failure may well reflect the inadequacies in the techniques for measuring central blood volume (e.g. Kilburn & Sieker, 1960; Paley, Leonard, Eggers, De Groot & Warren, 1960; Godley *et al.*, 1967). There is, however, circumstantial evidence indicating that the blood does pool in the pulmonary capillaries (Steiner, Frayser & Ross, 1965).

There are few measurements of cardiac output during negative pressure breathing. However, the available measurements (Gauer *et al.*, 1954; Lenfant & Howell, 1960; Godley *et al.*, 1967) indicate that the procedure is accompanied by a significant increase in cardiac output. There is also a significant increase in systemic arterial pressure (Gauer *et al.*, 1954; Godley *et al.*, 1967) and some studies have also shown an increase in glomerular filtration rate (GFR) and effective renal plasma flow (Baratz & Ingraham, 1960). The failure to demonstrate a consistent change in GFR must, however, be viewed against the background of the inaccuracies inherent in the techniques used for its measurement and the large variance of the results (see O'Connor & Summerill, 1979). However, due to the increases in cardiac output and arterial pressure consistently observed during negative pressure respiration, it must be concluded that increases in renal blood flow and GFR probably occur.

It can therefore be concluded that negative pressure breathing results in significant alterations in the circulatory system which in themselves are likely to have a direct haemodynamic effect on the function of the kidney. Thus, it is not possible to implicate exclusively any discrete reflex mechanism originating from the chest. However, it must be accepted that there is an increase in transmural pressure in the low-pressure area of the circulation. It could be argued that there is thus evidence for an increased stretch of the atrial wall and this stretch is responsible for the small increase ($+15\%$) in discharge from atrial receptors during negative pressure breathing (Henry & Pearce, 1956); but there is no evidence to suggest that these are the only receptors to be so stimulated during the procedure or to connect them with the diuresis.

Nature of the responses. The diuresis observed during negative pressure breathing has been fully described (Gauer *et al.*, 1954;

Various interventions and the kidney

Surtshin *et al.*, 1955; Boylan & Antkowiak, 1959; Murdaugh *et al.*, 1959; Baratz & Ingraham, 1960). With one exception they showed a diuresis with a consistent increase in free water clearance and a variable effect on sodium excretion. The exception was a study reported by Godley *et al.* (1967) who observed an increase in urine flow with no increase in free water clearance. This observation could have been related to the fact that they had hydrated their animals with fluids iso-osmolar compared with plasma, but the majority of other workers quoted had used hypo-osmolar fluids.

There is no evidence that this response to negative pressure breathing is reflex. No reports of the modification of the response by blocking transmission in nerves which comprise the hypothetical reflex are available.

The agent acting on the kidney, said to be responsible for this diuresis, is usually considered to be the antidiuretic hormone (ADH), a fall in the concentration of which is claimed to occur (e.g. Chapman & Henry, 1973). This aspect of the problem was investigated by Baratz and his colleagues who examined the effects of both positive and negative pressure respiration on the concentration of ADH in plasma. With positive pressure respiration the effect on the concentration of ADH appeared to depend on the precise way in which positive pressure ventilation was applied. Baratz & Ingraham (1960) studied the effect of positive pressure respiration with an end-expiratory airway pressure of 2.5 kPa and found an increase in the concentration of ADH in plasma. In a later investigation (Baratz *et al.*, 1970), used an end-expiratory pressure of zero and it was observed then that the concentration of ADH in plasma was diminished when compared with the control values. When negative pressure respiration was applied Baratz & Ingraham (1960) observed no significant changes in the concentration of ADH. Also, there is a point which may explain this variation in results; in the investigation reported by Baratz & Ingraham (1960), the blood was not examined *after* the experimental period, i.e. there was no second control value. These various results are difficult to explain as the mechanisms involved are unknown; if reflexes are involved, it is not possible, on the available evidence, to indicate which receptors are responsible.

In summary, negative pressure respiration results in a diuresis and is accompanied by increase in cardiac output and systemic blood pressure. The latter effects may well be the result of an increase in venous return for which there appear to be '*a priori*' reasons but little firm evidence. These general changes in circulatory system alone could account for the diuresis without the involvement of any discrete reflex mechanisms emanating from the low-pressure areas of the heart. There is no evidence to support the possible involvement of ADH in the diuresis.

Altered gravitational forces: centrifugation

Centrifuging the whole body has been used in several investigations to redistribute the blood volume; the precise nature of the redistribution depends solely on the position of the subject in relation to the ensuing forces and on the magnitude of the forces themselves (see Howard, 1965). These experiments have been undertaken in the expectation that when the forces are directed towards the chest there will be a redistribution of blood resulting in an increase in intrathoracic blood volume which in turn would stimulate the atrial receptors. There are however no reliable measurements of intrathoracic blood volume to support such a proposition, but it is likely that such changes in intrathoracic blood volume do occur in this circumstance. Thus it is accepted generally that when the forces act in a manner which directs blood towards the chest, there is an increase in urine flow and vice versa (Gauer, Henry & Behn, 1970).

Watson & Rapp (1962) studied the effect of forward (towards the head) acceleration on both humans and anaesthetised dogs. In man, the authors were able to demonstrate an increase in urine flow at forces of 4–5 g. They were unable to demonstrate any consistent change in the dogs at 4 and 8 g. Subsequently Rogge, Moore, Segar & Fasola (1967) studied the effect of centrifugation on the concentration of ADH in plasma of human subjects and observed an apparent diminution during acceleration. These two investigations are regarded as two important studies on this subject.

Before considering them in detail it is necessary to reflect on the changes which occur in the cardiovascular system during forward acceleration. This position is considered as being most significant in relation to the stimulation of atrial receptors (e.g.

Gauer et al., 1970). Howard (1965), quoting Wood, Sutterer & Marshall (1961), notes that at acceleration forces reaching 3.5–5.0 g there is a significant increase in cardiac output (up to 34%) accompanied by significant increments in right atrial and aortic pressures. In addition, Watson & Rapp (1962) have also shown that there are small changes in glomerular filtration rate and renal plasma flow during centrifugation. Thus it must be concluded that centrifugation results in complex changes throughout the cardiovascular system which secondarily will result in major reflex adjustments. It is not possible to determine whether specific receptors (such as atrial receptors) are, or are not, involved in the explanation of the diuresis observed during centrifugation.

The results of Rogge et al. (1967) and of Watson & Rapp (1962) are often quoted to support the volume receptor hypothesis (Gauer et al., 1970), but it must be pointed out that the position of the subjects in the two investigations differed. The differences are likely to be significant in view of the dependence of the circulatory adjustments on the position of the subject of the centrifuge (Howard, 1965).

There are two important criticisms of the methods of Rogge et al. (1967). Though it is accepted that a difference in the plasma concentration of ADH was shown between the two groups there is little information about the reproducibility of the assay in the authors' hands. However, sufficient data are supplied to suggest that there is a possibility of a large error in relation to the individual measurement; and this error is more than $1\frac{1}{2}$ times the mean value obtained in their normal subjects. The method used was attributed to Moran, Miltenberger, Shu'ayb & Zimmerman (1964) who stated that the specificity of the method in the range 0.5–2.0 $\mu U \cdot cm^{-3}$ is uncertain. The recovery rates of endogenous vasopressin quoted by Rogge et al. (1967) were $92 \pm 5\%$ from 18 trials. Such a value would provide 95% tolerance limits of approximately $\pm 56\%$ of the standard (5 $\mu U \cdot cm^{-3}$ arginine vasopressin). This information must be compared with the claim of Rogge et al. (1967) that the normal values in their subjects were 1.6 ± 0.6 (S.D.) $\mu U \cdot cm^{-3}$. Also the concentration of ADH in their experimental subjects during the initial control period was significantly greater than the concentration in normal subjects and the experimental protocol

Changes in urine flow

used was such that it did not permit the detection of a rising or falling concentration of ADH which was unrelated to the centrifugation, i.e. no samples were obtained after a lapse of an interval of time after centrifugation to constitute a final control period.

From these observations on the effects of centrifugation it must be concluded that this technique does not provide any evidence of any kind to relate the function of atrial receptors to concentrations of ADH in the plasma and the rate of urine flow. The response of an increase in urine flow observed during centrifugation could be explained solely in terms of the general changes in the circulatory system, such as the increase in cardiac output and its consequences.

Immersion

The effects of immersion of the whole body in water have been investigated extensively and have been reviewed recently (Epstein, 1978); a brief comment will be made here. Bazett, Thurlow, Crowell & Stewart (1924) showed that immersion resulted in a significant diuresis. This finding has been confirmed by several groups of investigators (e.g. Graveline & Jackson, 1962; Kaiser, Eckert, Gauer & Linkenbach, 1969; Davis & DuBois, 1977). In these experiments there is an increased free water clearance and excretion of sodium, and the extent of the increase in sodium excretion appears to depend on the degree of hydration (see Epstein, 1976, 1978 for references). It is claimed that these observations support the volume receptor thesis. The main reason for this point of view lies in the fact that immersion results in an increase in intrathoracic blood volume (e.g. Gauer & Henry, 1976; Risch, Koubenec, Beckmann, Lange & Gauer, 1978; Risch, Koubenec, Gauer & Lange, 1978) which in turn stimulates the atrial receptors. Briefly, to consider possible mechanisms involved in these responses to immersion, the effects on the cardiovascular system and the concentration of ADH in the blood will be discussed.

Changes in the cardiovascular system. Many attempts have been made to define the changes which occur in the cardiovascular system during immersion. For instance, Bazett (1924) found

Various interventions and the kidney

Table 9.1. *Circulatory changes induced by whole body immersion*

Primary effects	
Central blood volume	$+700$ cm^3
Heart volume	$+180$ cm^3
Central venous pressure	$+1.60$ to $+2.39$ kPa
Intrathoracic pressure	$+0.53$ to $+0.67$ kPa
Transmural pressure	$+1.06$ to $+1.73$ kPa
Secondary effects	
Stroke volume	$+35\%$
Cardiac output	$+32\%$
Total peripheral resistance	-30%
Peripheral venous tone	-30%
Arterial pressure	$+1.32$ kPa

From Gauer & Henry (1976).

that the changes in blood pressure encountered in subjects undergoing immersion showed a considerable individual variation. Arborelius, Balldin, Lilja & Lundgren (1972) observed that immersion of human subjects in water at 35 °C resulted in significant increase in cardiac output (mean increase 32 %) and central blood volume. These observations were compatible with the earlier findings of Kaiser *et al.* (1969) who found a significant increase in glomerular filtration rate which in turn could indicate an increase in renal blood flow.

Gauer & Henry (1976), reviewing the subject of 'plasma volume control', and commenting that immersion of the whole body 'had developed into an invaluable tool for the exploration of volume control', state that their data confirm and complement those of Arborelius *et al.* (1972). They also showed there was a considerable increase in the volume of blood in the thorax; there was an increase in central venous pressure, arterial pressure, intrathoracic pressure and 'transmural filling pressure'. The results of their work and the work of others is shown in Table 9.1 (from Gauer & Henry, 1976). That there are distensions of the heart chambers has been demonstrated by Lange, Lange, Echt & Gauer (1974) using a biplane radiographic technique (see Fig. 1, Lange *et al.*, 1974). The increase in mean heart volume on immersion, compared with the volume when standing in air, was 180.3 ± 61.8 cm^3 and this difference was statistically significant ($2P < 0.001$).

Changes in urine flow

These general and extensive changes in the cardiovascular system suggest that this technique cannot be used as an effective stimulus solely to atrial receptors; many other mechanisms capable of causing a diuresis may be involved. Such a point of view is supported by the observations of Davis & DuBois (1977) in anaesthetised dogs. They found that the response of an increase in urine flow during immersion was *not* abolished by cervical vagotomy; the response was still present. The importance of this observation was emphasised further by the demonstration that the cervical vagotomy abolished the response to distension of a balloon in the left atrium (see below).

Gilmore & Zucker (1978a) repeated these studies in anaesthetised monkeys and found that the procedure was accompanied by a significant increase in arterial pressure but no significant changes in glomerular filtration rate. In addition immersion also resulted in an increase in the urine flow and an increase in the excretion of sodium; both these responses were unaffected by cervical vagotomy. Therefore it is unlikely that the increase in urine flow which follows immersion is mediated either wholly or even in part by the stimulation of atrial receptors. The involvement of other cardiac receptors such as those discharging into sympathetic afferent fibres remains a possibility as suggested by Gilmore (1968). However, a direct effect in response to the increase in arterial pressure remains the most likely cause of the increase in urine flow observed in these studies.

Changes in the concentration of ADH. The evidence in support of a humoral agent, in particular ADH, mediating this diuresis is equally weak. There is no complete report of measurements of the concentration of ADH in plasma during immersion; a preliminary report of the concentration of ADH in the plasma of two normal subjects during immersion showed no change in concentration of ADH in spite of an increase in free-water clearance (Boasberg, Henry, Rosenbloom, Hall, Rose & Fisher, 1977).

Epstein, Pins & Miller (1975) have examined the excretion of ADH in normal subjects undergoing immersion after a period of water restriction which lasted 14 h; immersion was accompanied by a reduction in the excretion of ADH with an increase in excretion after the cessation of the immersion. In contrast

Various interventions and the kidney

Gilmore & Zucker (1978a) have shown recently that the diuresis following immersion in the monkey is unaffected by the simultaneous administration of large doses of vasopressin (50 mU·kg^{-1}·h^{-1}), and have therefore claimed that ADH is not involved in this response.

Linkenbach, Eckert & Gauer (1967) have reported that when plasma of subjects undergoing immersion was injected into water loaded rats anaesthetised with ethanol, the rats responded with diuresis. Injections of plasma from control subjects failed to produce a similar response. From these results, Linkenbach *et al.* (1967) concluded that in addition to a change of renal haemodynamics and a change in the secretion of vasopressin (in favour of which no direct evidence was presented) a humoral agent of an unknown nature was also involved in the diuresis induced by a change in the intrathoracic blood volume.

In conclusion it seems that immersion of the body in water results in a diuresis with an increase in the secretion of free water and sodium. There is no evidence to indicate that any one group of receptors, such as the atrial receptors, is involved in this response.

Alterations of vascular and extracellular fluid volume

Attempts have been made to alter the volume of the fluid compartments of the body and thus to change the stimulus to vascular receptors. Central to this concept is the idea that such changes would alter the discharge only of atrial receptors which, in turn, would lead to changes in the rate of urine flow caused by changes of ADH. Such a simple view has resulted in a large number of reports appearing in the literature purporting to provide further evidence in support of the volume receptor theory (e.g. Pearce, 1959; Sonnenberg & Pearce, 1962; Gilmore & Weisfeldt, 1965; Gilmore & Daggett, 1966; Potkay, Daggett & Gilmore, 1970); and the same idea is perpetuated in reviews. For instance, recently Gauer & Henry (1976, p. 155) particularly emphasise that they consider *all* chambers of the heart to contain receptors which participate in volume control. This opinion is sustained by Thorén (1979a) but the postulate is extended to include those receptors discharging into vagal C fibres. Both opinions ignore the evidence mustered against the theory by Goetz, Bond & Bloxham (1975).

In general the techniques used to alter the volume of the fluid compartments of the body fall into two main categories, infusion experiments and dialysis experiments.

Infusion experiments. Numerous investigations attempting to relate the effects of infusion to the rate of flow of urine have been completed, but it is not possible to review each report in detail. However, it is necessary to consider a few of them in depth to appreciate the difficulties involved in interpreting the results.

Pearce (1959) attempted to investigate the hypothesis that 'afferent vagal fibres arising in cardiac atrial stretch receptors serve as the sensory limb of a reflex mechanism sensitive to variations in blood volume and producing corresponding changes in urine flow'. The basic experimental technique consisted of infusing either Ringer–Locke solution or 6% bovine albumen in Ringer–Locke in anaesthetised dogs and determining the effects of these infusions on urine flow. Pearce (1959) observed that carotid sinus denervation and cervical vagotomy were without effect on the resultant increase in urine flow and concluded that 'receptors additional to those in the cardiac atria and the carotid sinus must contribute to the sensory component of a reflex mechanism regulating plasma volume'. In these experiments the dogs were infused with an amount approximately equal to *25% of their calculated blood volume* and such a large infusion was consistently accompanied by a significant increase in arterial pressure (see Fig. 2 of Pearce, 1959). It is obvious that such an increase in renal perfusion pressure alone could account for the changes observed in urine flow – a contention supported by the observation that cervical vagotomy and carotid sinus denervation failed to abolish the increase in blood pressure as well as the diuresis. Some support for this opinion also comes from the work of Gilmore, Peterson & Zucker (1979) who observed the same renal response to infusion in non-human primates after section of the dorsal roots, the vagi and the sino-aortic nerves. Additional effects secondary to alterations in the haemotocrit could also have caused changes in the rate of urine flow (Nashat, Scholefield, Tappin & Wilcox, 1969).

However, Sonnenberg & Pearce (1962) reported another investigation in which artificial blood was infused into anaesthetised dogs maintained at various levels of hydration. The magnitude of the response (i.e. 'diuresis and natriuresis') were related to the degree of hydration, being greatest in those dogs which were hydrated and least in dehydrated animals. In these experiments also, an amount equal to 25% of the estimated blood volume was given intravenously, and it is likely that such an infusion would have increased the blood pressure and the glomerular filtration rate. Such a suggestion is supported by the data present in Table 1 of their paper; it is not possible to arrive at any definite conclusions regarding reflex or hormonal factors mediating these responses.

Further difficulties involved in interpreting the results of infusion experiments are illustrated by the investigation reported by Johnson, Zehr & Moore (1970). In experiments conducted in conscious sheep, the authors attempted to relate concentrations of ADH in the plasma and changes in urine flow to alterations in plasma osmolarity and blood volume. Five series of experiments were performed. On the basis of their findings, the authors have suggested that 'sensitive osmo and volume receptors exist in the sheep for controlling ADH release...'. Although the conclusions appear superficially plausible, further consideration reveals several alternative explanations; each series is considered separately. In the first series the animals were infused with a solution of hypotonic saline and an unknown quantity of blood was removed at the same time to maintain a constant left atrial pressure. The volume of liquid infused was equal to approximately 12% of the estimated blood volume. This procedure resulted in an increase in urine flow (and free water clearance.). There was a significant fall in plasma osmolarity and a small fall in the plasma ADH concentration. The conclusion here is that the changes in urine flow were causally related to the changes in ADH concentration through the changes in osmolarity. Another explanation could involve changes in the haematocrit and blood flow or changes in concentration of plasma protein and glomerular filtration rate. In the second series, the authors infused isotonic liquid to cause an expansion of the blood volume, resulting in an increase in left atrial pressure, an increase in urine flow (and free water clearance) and a reduction in the concentration of ADH in the plasma. The same alternative explanations as above may be offered; in addition there was a rise in arterial blood pressure which could have contributed to an increase in glomerular filtration rate.

There is thus no obvious causal relationship between the increase in blood volume and its effect on receptors, reduction in ADH and diuresis. In the third series, the authors combined techniques of the first two series, and the same criticisms and alternative explanations apply. In the fourth series the authors bled the animals of up to 10% of an estimated blood volume, resulting in a fall in mean left atrial pressure, a reduction in urine flow and an elevation of the plasma ADH concentration. Although the blood pressure was unchanged, it would be expected, and there is evidence (e.g. Chapter 3 and Gupta *et al.*, 1966), that such haemorrhage would result in alterations in the discharge from more than one group of cardiovascular receptors. In the final series the authors combined haemorrhage with plasma hypotonicity, but the same criticisms apply.

Earlier, Zehr, Johnson & Moore (1969) had reported the results of another investigation in sheep in which they attempted to define the relationship between the concentration of ADH in the plasma, left atrial pressure and plasma osmolarity. In the two critical series of experiments (Groups C and D of Zehr *et al.*, 1969) the effect of so-called iso-osmotic infusion was studied; the relevant features in their Groups C (dehydrated) and D (normally hydrated) were that left atrial pressure rose and the concentration of ADH in the plasma fell whereas there was no change in arterial blood pressure or osmolarity of the plasma. Although at first it appears that the effect of an elevation of mean left atrial pressure is paramount in regulating the concentration of ADH in the plasma, there are certain obvious anomalies. First, the concentration of ADH in the plasma in the normally hydrated Group was considerably in excess of the control Group A (not shown above). Secondly, a so-called iso-osmotic stimulus produced a large change in plasma osmolarity. Thirdly, no attempts were made to establish whether the changes could be reversed, i.e. no final control values were established. Finally, an infusion of approximately four litres was probably in excess of the estimated blood volume and with this type of 'stimulus' it is inconceivable that only one specific type of receptor is stimulated.

In addition, it is also of interest to consider the accuracy of the assay for ADH used in both these investigations (Zehr *et al.*, 1969; Johnson *et al.*, 1970). The authors claim that the extraction procedure used by them was similar to that described by Rogge et al. (1967) the limitations of which have been discussed earlier in this chapter, where the tolerance limits were calculated as approximately $\pm 56\%$. Also the recovery rates of Rogge et al. (1967) were calculated from a concentration in the blood of $5\,\mu\text{U}\cdot\text{cm}^{-3}$ and the values obtained in the study reported (Johnson et al., 1970) were consistently lower than $5\,\mu\text{U}\cdot\text{cm}^{-3}$.

Dialysis experiments. Because of the inadequacy of infusion experiments, Share (1961) attempted to alter the volume of the extracellular fluid compartment by peritoneal dialysis. He claimed that a reduction in the volume of extracellular fluid caused an elevation of the concentration of ADH in the plasma. In two series of experiments dialysis was carried out with 100% and 0.1% glucose respectively (the electrolyte concentrations in the fluids were similar to those of extracellular fluid). A major objection to this technique is that as the stimulus is not defined no claim can be made that only the extracellular fluid volume is altered. Also the author claims that the recovery rate of the procedure was approximately 40% when 500–2000 μU of ADH was added to 10 cm³ of dog blood. In the experiments reported, the control values were of the order of 30–40 μU per 10 cm³ of blood. Clearly the recovery rates within the range 500–2000 μU per 10 cm³ of blood were not relevant when such small control values were encountered.

Therefore, *in summary*, experiments involving qualitative and quantitative changes in the fluid compartments are of no value in defining the role of atrial receptors in the regulation of urine flow. The main difficulty is that there are numerous concomitant changes which occur in these experiments which makes any reference to the interpretation of the function of atrial receptors impossible.

Injection of drugs

In an attempt to stimulate atrial receptors veratridine was used by Thomas (1967). When injected intravenously or into the left ventricle in anaesthetised dogs there was an increase in urine flow. In contrast intra-aortic injections did not increase urine flow with the vagi intact. It was concluded that atrial receptors were involved in this response. Obviously many other receptors would be stimulated and it is not valid to draw this conclusion on this evidence. However, even colder water has been poured on this investigation, which was completed in Delhi, by Paintal (1973a) who says in his review when referring specifically to the results in the paper of Thomas (1967), 'It has not been possible to confirm them (Ullman, and Paintal, unpublished observations).'

Discussion of the results of techniques involving distension of the whole atrium, or discrete regions of the atria, and their effects on urine flow and sodium excretion will be discussed fully in the next chapter (Chapter 10).

Atrial receptors and renal blood flow

Distending a large balloon (to obstruct the mitral orifice) or small balloons at the pulmonary vein–atrial junctions results, amongst other things, in an inhibition of activity in efferent nerves to the kidney as well as the diuresis (see Chapter 10). The changes in the activity in sympathetic efferent nerves to the kidney inevitably led to speculation regarding the role of these nerves in regulating the blood flow to the kidney.

Kinney & DiScala (1972) found that distending a balloon in the left atrium (i.e. partial mitral obstruction) did not affect glomerular filtration rate. Kahl, Flint & Szidon (1974) changed left atrial pressure and observed vasomotor effects in renal vessels in anaesthetised dogs. Pressure/flow curves were obtained by graded partial occlusion of the descending aorta above the renal artery and the recording of pressure and flow in the renal artery. The curves were obtained before, during and after alterations in left atrial pressure. The left atrial pressure was increased by partial mitral obstruction and decreased by snaring the venae cavae. Reduction in left atrial pressure was said to cause an increase in renal vasomotor tone but an increase in left atrial pressure was said to have little effect on renal vasomotor tone except in conditions when the tone was already high. The conclusions claiming causative relationships are not acceptable; the procedures used for altering the left atrial pressure inevitably altered the stimulus to the arterial baroreceptors (see Chapter 4) and hence the changes observed in renal vasomotor tone could not be attributed solely to the activity of atrial receptors. A similar criticism can be made of other investigations where the effects of the so-called 'cardiopulmonary receptors' have been investigated and claimed to affect renal resistance (Oberg & White, 1970a,b; Mancia, Shepherd & Donald, 1975); any reflex changes in vasomotor tone in the kidney could not arise from the pulmonary artery (Ledsome & Kan, 1977), the stimulation of receptors in which were shown to cause changes in hind-limb resistance and systemic vascular resistance but no changes in resistance in the kidney.

Examining this problem further, Mason & Ledsome (1974) investigated the effect of partial obstruction of the mitral valve and of distension of the left pulmonary vein–atrial junctions on blood flow to the kidney, perfused at constant pressure. Partial obstruction of the mitral valve so as to increase the pressure in the left atrium resulted in a small increase in blood flow to the kidney. This effect had a 'biphasic' appearance in that as the degree of mitral obstruction was increased the change in blood flow to the kidney was 'reversed' (Fig. 9.3). Repeating the experiment after cutting the vagi resulted in a response to distension of a massive reduction in renal blood flow. From these findings Mason & Ledsome (1974) concluded that the former response was dependent on the integrity of the vagi and hence on the activity of the atrial receptors. However, the renal circulation is affected by the degree of stimulation of the systemic baroreceptors (e.g. Mancia et al., 1973), and partial obstruction of the mitral orifice resulted in a fall in systemic pressure and a subsequent reduction in the stimulus to the baroreceptors. As a result there is likely to be a reduction in blood flow to the kidney. Cutting the vagi would eliminate afferent fibres from some baroreceptors, as well as atrial and other receptors (see Chapter 4) and cannot be used to eliminate only the effects of atrial receptors. However, Mason & Ledsome (1974) avoided this trap by cutting the vagi in the chest. In six dogs 'Section of the vagal nerve at the level of the upper border of the aorta on the left side and the azygos vein on the right did not cause any significant changes in the control level of heart rate or arterial blood pressure. Increases of left atrial pressure of less than (1.5 kPa) caused changes in heart rate, arterial blood pressure and hind limb pressure comparable with those observed

Renal blood flow

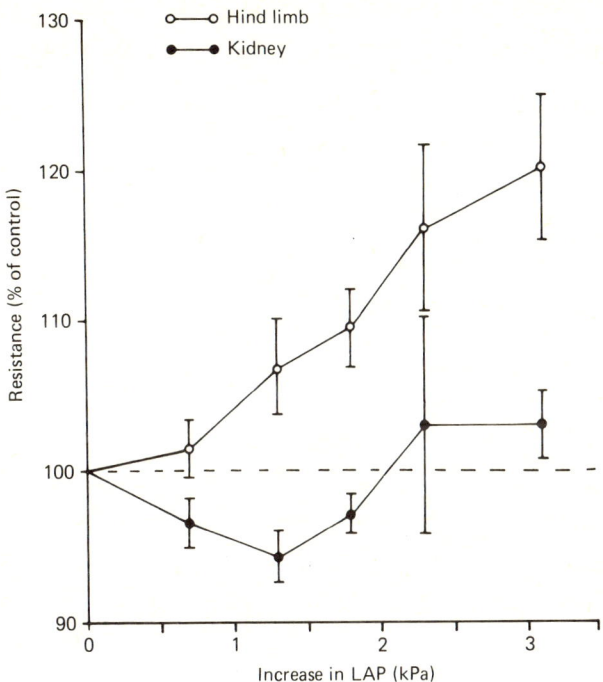

Fig. 9.3. Change in vascular resistance in the hind limb and kidney during distension of the left atrium. Abscissa shows increases in left atrial pressure (LAP). Vascular resistance is expressed as a percentage of control values (control = 100%). Averages ±S.E. from 19 dogs are given. (From Mason & Ledsome, 1974.)

before vagotomy but did not cause any increase in renal blood flow.' From the data presented (cf. top row of their Tables 1 and 2; also, 19 dogs were included in Table 1 but 6 in Table 2) it is not possible to determine whether, in these six dogs, for the same degree of atrial distension (not possible individually to determine), the changes in renal blood flow observed after thoracic vagotomy were significantly different from those observed before vagotomy; only mean and S.E.M. of data are available.

Mason & Ledsome (1974) went on to examine the changes in the renal circulation during discrete stimulation of atrial receptors by distending the pulmonary vein–atrial junctions.

Various interventions and the kidney

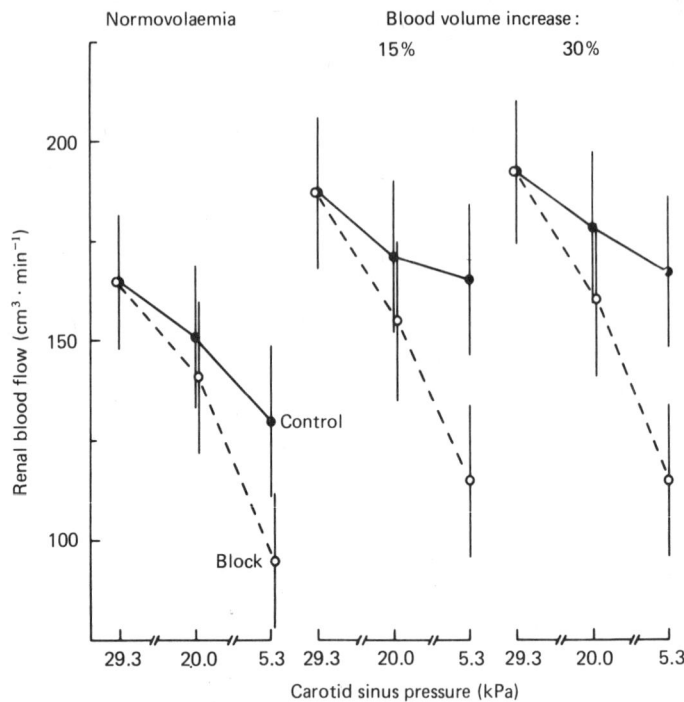

Fig. 9.4. Blood flow (mean ± s.e.) in left kidney perfused at a constant pressure of 16 kPa in 13 dogs with aortic nerves cut. Observations made in control state (●) and during vagal cold block (○) at carotid sinus pressures of 29.3 kPa (220 mmHg), 20.0 kPa (150 mmHg) and 5.3 kPa (40 mmHg) in normovolaemic state and after blood volume had been increased by 15% and 30% with dextran. (From Mancia et al., 1976.)

This procedure did not result in a significant change in systemic pressure, but did result in a small increase in renal blood flow (139 ± 7.8 cm^3 (s.e.m.) to 142 ± 7.7 cm^3 (s.e.m.)). The effect of blocking transmission in the vagi on this response was not examined. Therefore the effect of stimulating the atrial receptors on the renal circulation which is claimed to be vasodilatation, cannot be accepted with certainty on the basis of this evidence, but it is likely.

Mancia et al. (1976) studied the effect of cooling the vagi (to between −1 and 0 °C) on the renal circulation. The aortic nerves were sectioned, the carotid sinuses perfused at constant

Renal blood flow

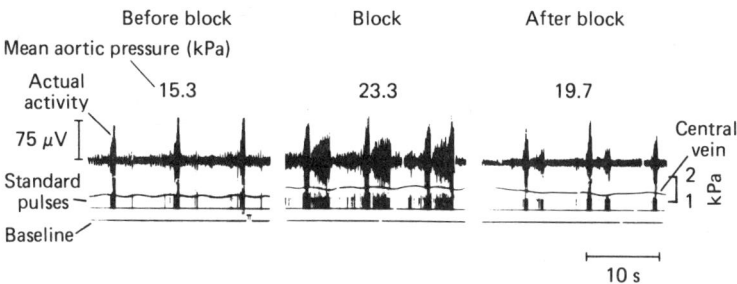

Fig. 9.5. Effect of vagal cold block on renal sympathetic activity in dog with aortic nerves cut and carotid sinus pressure at 5.3 kPa (40 mmHg). Mean renal nerve traffic was 70 spikes·s^{-1} before block, 110 spikes·s^{-1} during block, and 50 spikes·s^{-1} after block. (From Mancia et al., 1973.)

pressure and the lungs removed; they assumed that only cardiac receptors could be involved in their experiments. The techniques involved using an oxygenator and extracorporeal circulation. Cooling the cervical vagi resulted in a reduction in blood flow to the kidney perfused at constant pressure (Fig. 9.4). They also observed a rise in systemic arterial pressure and a fall in blood flow in the hind limb perfused at constant pressure. Mancia et al. (1976) showed that reduction of pressure within an isolated perfused carotid sinus also reduced the renal blood flow. Using similar techniques in an earlier investigation Mancia et al. (1973) had shown that cooling the vagi increased the discharge in sympathetic nerves to the kidney (Fig. 9.5). Thus from their investigations it was concluded that the input from receptors in the heart, conveyed in the vagi, had a tonic inhibitory effect on the renal vasomotor tone. Therefore, removal of this effect by cooling the cervical vagi resulted in a reduction in blood flow in a kidney perfused at constant pressure. In an earlier investigation, Mancia & Donald (1975) had shown that receptors in the atria, ventricles and lungs, with afferent nerves in the vagi, each have a tonic inhibitory effect on the circulation. Therefore it is reasonable to assume that afferent nerve fibres originating from the atria and traversing the cervical vagi may exert a tonic inhibitory effect on the renal circulation.

However, there is some evidence to indicate that the effects described by Mancia, Shepherd & Donald (1975) are mediated by non-myelinated fibres originating from the heart (e.g. Mancia & Donald, 1975; see Chapter 7). There is no evidence in the study by Mason & Ledsome (1974) to indicate the type of receptor they were investigating, particularly in view of the finding that both partial mitral obstruction and distension of the pulmonary vein–atrial junctions stimulates more than one type of atrial receptor (Kappagoda, Linden & Sivananthan, 1978, 1979; Chapters 3 and 6). Recently also with no evidence of the type of receptor involved in the response, Lloyd & Freidman (1977) have shown that step increases in left atrial pressure cause a decrease in vascular resistance in the kidney.

Thus, on the basis of the available evidence, it must be concluded that distension of the left atrium could exert a reflex influence on the renal circulation but the precise identification of the receptors involved must await further experiments.

Atrial receptors and the renin–angiotensin system

The factors influencing the secretion of renin by the kidney have been extensively reviewed in recent years (e.g. Zanchetti, Stella, Leonetti, Marganti & Terzoli, 1976; Ganong, 1977) and a critical examination of this evidence is beyond the scope of this book. However, there is general agreement that the secretion is affected by a variety of 'stimuli'. For instance, 'it is now well established that at least five interacting factors regulate renin secretion. Two of these factors are local: an intrarenal baroreceptor mechanism apparently operates to make renin secretion inversely proportional to the degree of stretch of the juxtaglomerular cells, and a macula densa mechanism apparently operates to make renin secretion inversely proportional to the rate of sodium or chloride transport across the cells of the macula densa. Two of the factors are humoral: renin secretion is inhibited by angiotensin II and by vasopressin. The fifth factor is sympathetic input, which is excitatory in nature and mediated by circulating catecholamines and postganglionic sympathetic nerve endings in the kidney. The sympathetic effect is mediated for the most part by way of intrarenal β-adrenergic receptors, and there is considerable evidence that these β-adrenergic receptors are located on the membranes of the juxtaglomerular cells. Thus, the juxtaglomerular cells appear to be endocrine cells that receive a direct secretomotor innervation.' (Ganong, 1977.)

In defining the role of atrial receptors experimentally any variable known to change any of the above five 'stimuli' should be controlled and a discrete stimulus applied to the atrial receptors. However, it is possible to suggest that stimulating the atrial receptors under experimental conditions could, at least concomitantly, affect the secretion of renin either through a change in the 'haemodynamic state' of the kidney or through a change in activity of renal nerves. Discretely stimulating atrial receptors (distension of the vein–atrial junctions) affects the discharge in the sympathetic nerves to the kidney (see Chapter 10). Other grosser techniques used to stimulate atrial receptors (partial obstruction of the mitral and tricuspid valves) also affect cardiac output and probably blood flow to the kidney. Some experiments involving these methods will be considered under two headings: the effect of vagal blockade and the effect of changing the volumes of liquid in various parts of the circulation.

Effect of cooling the vagi

One of the earliest attempts at linking the receptors in the low pressure areas of the circulation with the renin–angiotensin system was the investigation reported by Hodge, Low, Ng & Vane (1969). They observed that cooling the vagi to 4–6 °C in anaesthetised dogs resulted in an increase in the concentration of angiotensin in blood. Since there is a variety of afferent fibres in the vagi (see Chapter 4) these experiments yielded little information regarding the identity of the receptors involved.

Mancia, Romero & Shepherd (1975) studied the effect of cold blockade of the vagi on renal blood flow and renin production, measured by radioimmunoassay and expressed in terms of angiotensin generated in 1 cm^3 of plasma per hour. They found that cold blockade to -1 °C in an animal whose carotid and aortic sinuses were inactivated resulted in a fall in renal blood flow, an increase in systemic pressure and an increase in renin production from the 3rd–5th min. Renal denervation abolished the increase in renin production and the change in renal blood flow. The authors considered these findings as evidence for the tonic inhibition of renin release by vagally innervated receptors in the 'cardiopulmonary area'. It is important to realise that, when studying these effects, care must be taken not to allow changes in the carotid sinus reflex or renal arterial pressure, each of which affects the secretion of renin (e.g. Jarecki *et al.*, 1978).

Yun, Delea, Bartter & Kelly (1976) reported experiments in which they had studied the effect of vagotomy on systemic pressure and plasma renin activity in anaesthetised dogs subjected to sino-aortic denervation. Like Mancia, Romero & Shepherd (1975) they found that vagotomy in these animals increased the mean arterial pressure and the plasma renin activity. However, they also commented that cooling the cervical vagi to 3–4 °C had the same effect as vagotomy. No data were presented to support this proposition and the effect of rewarming the vagi was not examined in these animals. These considerations of the paper by Yun *et al.* (1976), together with the fact that the vagi were not cooled to any intermediate temperatures above 4 °C in either investigation, makes it impossible to ascribe this effect on renin secretion to either myelinated or non-myelinated afferent nerve fibres. Also no evidence of which receptors were involved was offered by Brosnihan & Bravo (1978) when they concluded that release of renin following graded reductions in atrial pressure was of neural origin.

Regarding the efferent component of this response, it could be concluded from other studies of the Mayo Clinic Group (e.g. Mancia *et al.*, 1973; Mancia, Shepherd & Donald, 1975) that cooling the vagi to -1 °C increases the sympathetic discharge to the kidney and that it is likely to decrease overall blood flow to the kidney and even (by implication) alter the distribution of the blood flow within the kidney. The renal denervation *per se* does not help to delineate the precise efferent mechanism for the renin release.

In summary, even though the conclusion that receptors in the 'cardiopulmonary area' could exert a tonic inhibitory effect on the release of renin from the kidney is probably valid, there is no evidence from these cooling experiments to link the complex unencapsulated nerve endings in the atria or any other specific group of receptors with renin release.

Effect of changing volumes of various parts of the circulation

Brennan, Malvin, Jochim & Roberts (1971) investigated the effects of distending balloons in the left and right atria on the secretion of renin. They found that distension of a balloon in the left atrium had little effect while distension of a balloon in the right atrium decreased the secretion of renin. These experimental techniques would cause changes in the systemic circulation which in turn would indirectly influence the release of renin.

Zehr, Hasbargen & Kurz (1976) in anaesthetised dogs, stimulated receptors within the atria by distending a balloon in the left atrium so as to increase the mean left atrial pressure by approximately 0.6 kPa. Distension of the left atrium was accompanied by a decrease in the secretion of renin but there were no significant changes in mean arterial pressure or renal blood flow. This response was abolished by cervical vagotomy and by renal denervation. In these experiments the rate of renin secretion was measured before and during stimulation of atrial receptors but not after cessation of the stimulus. Even though the authors point out that multiple tests were done on individual animals, it is not possible to judge from the experiment whether: (a) a reduction in renin secretion occurred in each test, and (b) the reduction in the secretion of renin was reversed by the release of the balloon distension. With these restrictions, it may be concluded that there is some evidence to suggest that renin secretion may be influenced by the stimulation of receptors in the left atrium; but which of the three groups of receptors are involved cannot be judged from this type of experiment. However, no change in plasma renin activity was observed in normal dogs or dogs with heart failure by Zucker, Share & Gilmore (1979) when they distended a balloon in the left atrium with 10–20 cm^3 saline; changes in the urine flow and the concentration of ADH in the plasma were observed.

Fisher & Malvin (1980) claimed that their experiments do not support the hypothesis that the renin–angiotensin system is an efferent limb of 'a cardiopulmonary reflex'. Volume expansion with isotonic iso-oncotic solution containing 3% dextran in dogs anaesthetised with chloralose resulted in a 50% decrease in renin secretion. However, the same volume expansion performed after bilateral cervical vagotomy also suppressed renin release – and again, even with a single denervated kidney. They conclude that a combination of intrarenal factors may have been responsible for the suppression of renin secretion. Such experiments do not exclude an effect of atrial receptors on renin secretion; the experiment could not disprove such an hypothesis because an animal after vagotomy does not necessarily provide an adequate base line to compare with one before vagotomy – but the results do suggest it is not necessary to erect the hypothesis.

Another attempt to investigate this problem was made by Thames, Zubbair-Ul-Hassan, Brachett, Lowe & Kontos (1971). They studied the effect of haemorrhage upon the concentration of renin in peripheral plasma. In a group of anaesthetised normal dogs haemorrhage resulted in an increase in the concentration of renin in the plasma. In a second group of dogs, subjected to previous cardiac autotransplantation, a response which was qualitatively similar to the above, although attenuated, was observed. In both groups the control concentration of renin and the changes in blood pressure following the haemorrhage were not significantly different. The authors claimed that the cardiac transplantation was carried out in such a manner that the posterior wall of the atrium (i.e. the region containing the complex unencapsulated nerve endings) was left intact. Thus they attributed the above effects on renin concentration to the activation of receptor endings in the heart other than the complex unencapsulated nerve endings. In fact, they could just as easily be attributed to extracardiac receptors. Again, though changes in the concentration of aldosterone and in plasma renin activity accompanied hypovolaemia in rats induced by the extravascular administration of polyethylene glycol (Stricker, Vagnucci, McDonald & Leenen, 1979), no attempts were made to elucidate the mechanisms; no conclusions as to which receptors were involved, if indeed any at all were involved, can be drawn.

Finally, the effects of positive and negative pressure on the lower body, on the concentration of renin in plasma were studied by Bevegard, Castenfors & Lindblad (1977). They found that negative pressure to the lower body resulted in a fall in cardiac output, pulse pressure and central venous pressure. These changes were accompanied by an increase in plasma renin activity. Lower body positive pressure resulted in a significant increase in mean arterial pressure; the other changes in haemodynamic variables were not significant. The accompanying changes in plasma renin were not significant. Even though the authors claim that these results corroborate the findings published previously by Mancia, Romero & Shepherd (1975), relating to 'cardiopulmonary receptors', there is little or no justification for so doing.

In summary, these investigations regarding the release of renin present a confusing picture which in itself is not surprising when one considers the various factors which potentially could effect a secretion of renin (Ganong, 1977). It is not possible to conclude that stimulation of any particular cardiac receptors affects the release of renin.

Atrial receptors and steroid hormones

Anderson, McCally & Farrell (1959) studied the effect of stretching both atria (by external ligatures) on rates of secretion of aldosterone and hydrocortisone. The experimental protocol was such that comparisons were only made between groups; they observed that the test group had a lower secretion rate of hydrocortisone (when stretching both left and right atria) than control animals. Stretch of the left atrium was observed to be without effect on the secretion of aldosterone but stretch of the right diminished the rate of secretion. No evidence regarding the involvement of a reflex mechanism was presented and there was also no evidence to indicate that this method of stimulation did provide an adequate stimulus to receptors in the atrial wall. However, there was evidence of a lower mean arterial pressure in the animals subjected to the crude atrial stretch than in the control animals. It is just not possible to interpret these results in terms of any receptors or reflex responses.

Baisset, Douste-Blazy & Montastruc (1959) reported the effect of distending a balloon in each atrium on the secretion of aldosterone. Once again, distension of the left atrium was without effect whilst distension of the right atrium was said to diminish the secretion of aldosterone. This response was abolished by vagotomy and by placing lesions in the posterior hypothalamus. Lesions of the anterior hypothalamus and hypophysectomy were said to be without effect. A final control sample was not obtained in each experiment. Yet again it has to be commented that distending the atria in this way constituted a complex stimulus to the circulatory system because changes in cardiac output, and consequently systemic baroreceptor activity as well as activity of other cardiovascular receptors, are inevitable.

Little support for the atrial receptors being involved in the secretion of aldosterone was provided by the study of Cox, Davies-Jones, Leonard & Singer (1963), who showed that positive pressure breathing was accompanied by an increase in aldosterone secretion. Assuming a diminished central blood volume, and hence the degree of stretch of intrathoracic baroreceptors, it could be argued that it is opposite to the response described by Baisset et al. (1959). However, again many other receptors, e.g. baroreceptors, would have changed their discharge and no one group of receptors could be implicated by the intervention.

Producing hypovolaemia in rats in a study contributing to sodium and water balance (Stricker et al., 1979) showed that there was a rise in the concentration of aldosterone and corticosterone in the plasma. No attempt was made to elucidate mechanisms so that no claims were made that any cardiac receptors were involved; indeed with the technique of injecting polyethylene glycol extravascularly to produce the hypovolaemia, many other receptors would also have to be eliminated from the argument.

The investigations of Gann and his colleagues have yielded a large number of publications claimed to involve atrial receptors in the regulation of the secretion of adrenocortical steroids (e.g. Cryer & Gann, 1973, 1974; Cryer, Grayson & Gann, 1974). To investigate the function of right atrial receptors Cryer & Gann, (1974) first demonstrated an increase in the rate of secretion of cortisol in response to a haemorrhage of $5 \text{ cm}^3 \cdot \text{kg}^{-1}$ body weight. This response was considerably diminished when the haemorrhage was repeated with the simultaneous distension of a balloon in the right atrium. It was implied that distension of the balloon prevented the reduction in receptor activity which in turn prevented a large increase in the secretion of the hormone. A response qualitatively similar to the above was obtained in a second group of experiments where a balloon was distended in the left atrium (Cryer *et al.*, 1974) but this stimulus seems unlikely to influence the discharge from receptors in the right atrium. In neither of these investigations was any evidence presented to indicate the nature of the effect of this stimulus on the discharge from atrial receptors: changes in atrial pressure were not given. In addition there was also no information regarding any other concomitant effects, e.g. systemic arterial pressure, in the circulation. This information is of importance for the interpretation of the results, because Gann (1966) has shown that receptors in the carotid artery exert an influence on the secretion of ACTH.

Baertschi, Ward & Gann (1976) have made a further study of this problem by attempting to define the receptor endings involved in these responses. They inserted small balloons into the cavities of the atria and injected them with a volume of ± 1 cm^3 in a sinusoidal fashion at a frequency of 1 Hz. This volume constituted approximately $\pm 35\%$ of the atrial volume. Measurements were then made of the concentration of ACTH and cortisol during these procedures. In addition they also attempted to define the nature of the receptor endings activated by this procedure by recording action potentials in vagal afferent fibres.

They found that this stimulus activated not only Paintal-type atrial receptors but also some baroreceptor fibres as well. Indeed there is evidence in their report to indicate that the stimulus caused an obstruction at the atrio-ventricular valves in such a manner as to cause changes in mean arterial pressure, particularly when the stimulus was applied to the left atrium. It is also surprising that the authors encountered no evidence of non-myelinated vagal afferent fibres activated by this stimulus.

To link the right atrial receptors (type B receptors) with the secretion of ACTH and cortisol, as the authors intended, it is necessary to measure the concentrations of these hormones in blood during control periods before and after the application of the stimulus as well as during the period of stimulation. As the authors described, their stimulus is 'pseudo random' and it is not possible to obtain the above information. However, considering their Fig. 3, it appears that the right atrium was distended twice for approximately 10 min; the concentration of the hormone showed a peak approximately 5 min after the onset but returned virtually to control levels well before the cessation of the stimulus. In two other distensions of the atrium which lasted 3 min an entirely different time course was evident. It is possible that these changes in concentration were random, but it is not possible definitely to draw this conclusion because of the way the data are presented.

Distending the left atrium produced a substantial fall in blood pressure (Fig. 3, Baertschi et al., 1976), unlike the effect on the right atrium. It is therefore not possible to attribute any response solely to changes in activity of left atrial receptors. Also a criticism of this work is that no potential nervous pathways were investigated, therefore no discrete reflexes could be implicated; the 'statistical' evidence of correlation may be only concomitant variation.

Grizzle, Johnson, Schramm & Gann (1975) attempted to examine the central nervous connections of atrial receptors (see also Chapter 8). In a previous investigation Grizzle, Dallman, Schramm & Gann (1974) had demonstrated that stimulating areas of the medial dorsal hypothalamus resulted in changes in ACTH. Subsequently the authors were able to demonstrate a group of neurones in this region (Grizzle et al., 1975) which responded to distension of a small balloon located on the external surface of the superior vena caval–right atrial junction. The responses in the cells were classified as an increase, a decrease or complete cessation of activity. The authors implied that these cells mediated the corticosteroid response to balloon distension described previously (Cryer & Gann, 1974). However, the volume of saline injected in the balloon was only 0.5 cm^3 and such a volume was unlikely to distort the superior vena caval–right atrial junction in a fashion likely to stimulate receptors attached either to the myelinated or non-myelinated afferent fibres from the atria (cf. Kappagoda, Linden & Snow (1973) for the stimulus to receptors attached to the myelinated afferent fibres). The authors provided no evidence to show that atrial receptors could be stimulated by this manoeuvre. Once again they did not make use of vagal blockade to establish whether the responses in these cells were caused by receptors discharging into the vagi. Similar criticisms can be made of the more recent publications from this group (Baertschi et al., 1975;

Conclusion

Ward *et al.*, 1977) in which they describe attempts to define medullary areas responding to inputs from the atria and having rostral projections.

Thus *in summary*, it is concluded that the link between the atrial receptors and either ACTH or the steroid hormones is at best tenuous and the existence of such a link must await the results of more detailed carefully controlled experiments.

Atrial receptors and prostaglandins

It was inevitable that, with such an intervention as distending a balloon in the left atrium being available, its effects on prostaglandins would be examined. Recently, Wiberg, Vaage & Scott (1979) have distended a balloon in the left atrium of anaesthetised cats and shown an increase in prostaglandin-like activity in arterial blood and the response was blocked by a prior dose of indomethacin. As hydrostatic pressure was raised throughout the lungs and systemic arterial blood pressure fell it is not possible to implicate any particular receptors or even establish a reflex. Other relevant evidence relating 'cardiopulmonary' vagal afferent fibres to renal prostaglandins arises from the work of Mancia, Romero & Strong (1974), who showed that cold blockade of the vagi resulted in a two-fold increase in the concentration of renin and prostaglandin E2. However, the secretion of renin and prostaglandins may be closely linked; Romero, Dunlop & Strong (1976) provided some evidence for this concept by showing that blockade of prostaglandin synthesis inhibits the secretion of renin. Although renal prostaglandins may play an important role in intrarenal mechanisms, the evidence to incriminate them as systemic humoral agents is not available.

There is thus no evidence that stimulation of atrial receptors causes the release of prostaglandins.

Conclusion

Throughout this chapter it has repeatedly been pointed out that the attempts to 'stimulate' various receptors with several blunderbuss techniques have not provided results from which it could be concluded that atrial receptors were responsible for

Various interventions and the kidney

any of the responses described. Though again, the proposed link has not been disproved; the definitive experiments have just not been completed.

The effect of discretely stimulating the atrial receptors will be considered in the next chapter.

10 ATRIAL RECEPTORS AND URINE FLOW

In discussing the effects on the kidney of various interventions, the techniques of applying a stimulus to the receptors in the atria by distending balloons, both large and small, were mentioned but the responses to these distensions were not fully discussed. This chapter will be concerned closely to examine the evidence from investigations using these methods. Briefly, two approaches to stimulation of atrial receptors are made. One consists of distending a large balloon in the atrium to obstruct the mitral orifice, which raises the left atrial pressure but causes a fall in cardiac output with various consequences (e.g. Henry, Gauer & Reeves, 1956; Ledsome, Linden & O'Connor, 1961). The other method involves distending small balloons at the vein–atrial orifices (e.g. left atrium, Ledsome & Linden, 1968; right atrium, Kappagoda *et al.*, 1973; see Chapter 4), with the veins tied off in such a manner that distension of the balloons distends the junctions without causing an obstruction to blood flow through the atrium and therefore there are no changes in atrial pressure, cardiac output or systemic arterial pressure.

Distension of the left atrium: obstruction of mitral orifice

The investigations examined in Chapter 9 have, at best, only provided indirect evidence to link receptors in the low-pressure areas of the circulation with a response of an increase in urine flow. Attempting to identify the receptor areas involved in this response, Henry *et al.* (1956) distended various regions of the central circulation in anaesthetised dogs (these techniques were described earlier by Reeves, Henry & Gauer, 1956). The pulmonary arterial pressure was raised by the injection of plastic beads into the jugular vein; an increase in mean pulmonary arterial pressure from 1.5 to 3.0 kPa was obtained but no significant changes in urine flow were observed. Snaring the pulmonary veins to increase the pressure in the pulmonary veins and arteries also did not cause changes in urine flow. However, distending a balloon in the lumen of the left atrium resulted in an increase in left atrial pressure, a small decrease in systemic arterial pressure and a significant increase in urine flow. Henry & Pearce (1956) later also obtained similar responses.

Over the next 20 years, experiments essentially the same as those described above have been performed in anaesthetised dogs during the course of other investigations and the main aspects of the response of the diuresis have been established (e.g. Ledsome et al., 1961; Arndt et al., 1963; Lydtin & Hamilton, 1964; Ledsome & Linden, 1968; Kinney & DiScala, 1972; Ledsome & Mason, 1972; Gillespie et al., 1973; Lawrence et al., 1973; Kappagoda, Linden, Snow & Whitaker, 1974). However, Gilmore & Zucker (1978b) were unable to obtain a response which was statistically significant in monkeys: there was an increase in urine flow in only five of the ten experiments. In Leeds in the course of investigating the mechanisms of this response in anaesthetised dogs since 1961, several investigations have been completed. Distending the large balloon to obstruct the mitral orifice in intact anaesthetised dogs resulted in an average increase in urine flow of 131.4% (84 distensions in 69 dogs; Table 10.1); distension of similar balloons in dogs in which there was also extra surgical intervention averaged 98.2% (36 distensions in 27 dogs; Table 10.2).

In the majority of the investigations listed above the urine was collected and measured at 10 min intervals. The protocol consisted of an initial control period of 30–40 min, a period of 30 min during which the balloon was distended, followed by release of the distension and a further collection of urine for 40–50 min. The initial 30–40 min formed the first of the two control periods; the test period was taken to be the final 20 min of the period of distension and the first 10 min following the release of the distension; the second, post stimulus, control was taken as the final 30–40 min of collection. These criteria were initially adopted by Henry et al. (1956) and the same format will be followed in this review unless stated otherwise.

Evidence allowing a description of the diuretic response to the

Table 10.1. *Increase in urine flow in response to distension of balloons*

Site of distension	No. of dogs	No. of distensions	Percentage response of increase in urine flow mean (range)	References
I. Left atrium				
Large balloon	16	16	105 (9–236)	Kappagoda, Knapp, Linden, Pearson & Whitaker (1979)
	16	19	100.6 (9–390)	Kappagoda, Linden & Sreeharan (1979)
	6	6	113 (4–283)	Kappagoda, Linden, Snow & Whitaker (1974)
	8	10	130 (64–480)	Ledsome & Linden (1968)
	5	9	170 (10–500)	
	18	24	170 (0–850)	Ledsome et al. (1961)
II. Pulmonary vein–atrial junctions	8	12	63.3 (8–142)	Kappagoda, Linden & Sreeharan (1979)
	5	6	69 (25–128)	Kappagoda, Linden, Snow & Whitaker (1974)
Small balloons	10	14	20 (0–128)	
	5	9	50 (0–130)	Ledsome & Linden (1968)

Table 10.2. *Increase in urine flow in response to distension of balloons (with extra surgical or pharmacological intervention)*

Site of distension	No. of dogs	No. of distensions	Percentage response of increase in urine flow mean (range)	References
I. Left atrium Large balloon				
(a) pituitary ablation + bretylium tosylate	4	10	74.7 (19–148)	Kappagoda, Linden, Snow & Whitaker (1975)
(b) ansae cut	3	3	141 (105–210)	Ledsome & Linden (1968)
(c) denervated kidney	4	4	90 (5–200)	Ledsome et al. (1961)
denervated kidney	16	19	87.2 (5–314)	Kappagoda, Linden & Sreeharan (1979)
II. Pulmonary vein– atrial junctions Small balloons				
(a) denervated kidney	8	12	52.9 (5–75)	Kappagoda, Linden & Sreeharan (1979)
(b) pharmacological denervation	8	11	33 (5–110)	Linden & Sreeharan (1979)

Distension of the left atrium

stimulation of atrial receptors will be presented first before describing the reflex mechanisms; mostly experiments on anaesthetised dogs will be discussed without describing the anaesthesia, but special emphasis will be made of experiments in unanaesthetised animals where that is relevant.

Time course of the response

Distension of a balloon in the lumen of the left atrium, in the manner of the investigations referred to above, so as to elevate the mean left atrial pressure by 1.5–2.0 kPa causes an increase in the volume of urine within 5–10 min after completion of the distension. A small increase in urine flow is usually evident in the first of the three 10 min collections made during distension. Thereafter the urine volume increases over the next 20 min. After release of the distension, the urine flow begins to wane only after 5–10 min. Thus the urine flow during the 10 min immediately following the release may be less than, equal to or even greater than that immediately before (some of the increase may be the result of the 'rise' in arterial pressure, see later). Over the next 30–40 min the urine flow gradually returns to the control values. Thus there is clearly a delay in the onset and decay of the response in relation to the distension of the balloon (Fig. 10.1).

Distension of the balloon for a period longer than 30 min results in the urine flow decreasing from the peak flow attained towards its control value after about 30 min. This observation was initially recorded by Henry *et al.* (1956) and was subsequently confirmed by Ledsome *et al.* (1961). The data presented by Lydtin & Hamilton (1964) also appear to support such a finding. This particular aspect of the problem was investigated more recently by Lawrence *et al.* (1973) who studied the effect of distending a balloon in the left atrium for 90 min. They also observed that the magnitude of the response diminished after 30 min but it did not return to the control level until the distension was released. However, when the urine flow, solute excretion, urinary osmolarity and free water clearance were considered separately, it was found that the solute excretion returned to control values after 40 min and was independent of any concurrent changes in the dilution of urine. When the free

Atrial receptors and urine flow

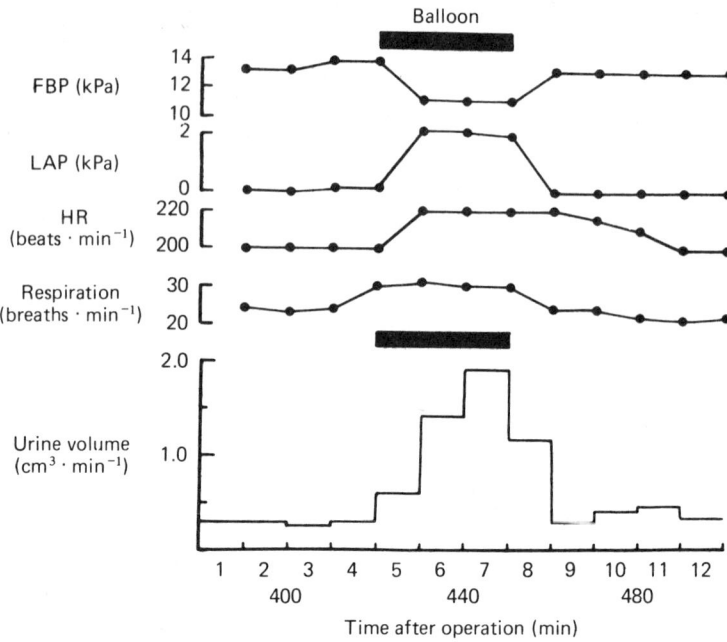

Fig. 10.1. Effect of inflating a balloon in the left atrium, for the 30 min indicated by the solid bar. From above downwards, femoral arterial pressure (FBP), left atrial pressure (LAP), heart rate (HR), respiratory rate and urine volume. Numbers 1–12 indicate 10 min periods of urine collection. (From Ledsome et al., 1961.)

water clearances were examined it was found that the increase in free water clearance reached its peak approximately 40 min after the distension and was still present after a period of 90 min, i.e. the apparent diminution in the response as indicated by the overall urine flow tended to obscure the effect on free water clearance which continued at an increased rate. Nevertheless, even free water clearance decreased towards, but did not attain, control values before the distension was released. From these results Lawrence et al. (1973) concluded that the response had two components – a transient one responsible for the increase in solute excretion and a more prolonged one responsible for the increase in free water clearance (see later for evidence of three efferent limbs to this reflex response).

Nature of the response

The concentration of solutes in the urine produced during distension of a balloon in the left atrium is more dilute than that in urine produced during the control periods; there is an increase in free water clearance but a small increase in the excretion of solutes. Ledsome et al. (1961) found an increase of approximately 20% in the solutes excreted – which presumably consisted of urea, sodium and potassium salts – whilst the urine volume increased by 350%; an analysis of sodium and potassium excretion in some experiments showed 'small changes in the excretion of these ions even when the diuresis was 2 to 6 times the control flow'. The data obtained from several laboratories on sodium excretion show consistent results if the comparisons are made between experiments when the protocols are approximately the same. For example, Arndt et al. (1963) obtained overall small and inconsistent changes in sodium excretion; however, in some of their experiments they found a considerable increase in the excretion of sodium and postulated the possibility of a haemodynamic mechanism as a causative factor (see later). Ledsome & Linden (1968) did not express the increase in sodium excretion numerically, but calculation from their figures suggests an increase in sodium excretion of up to 10% during distension with small balloons and up to 20% using mitral obstruction; however, they commented that some of the large changes in urine flow were associated with significant increases in sodium excretion. Ledsome & Mason (1972) found small but significant increases in osmolar clearance, unaffected by exogenous infusions of vasopressin; but this was not accompanied by consistent and significant increases in sodium and potassium excretion. Gillespie et al. (1973), however, observed significant increases in osmolar clearance as well as sodium and potassium excretion during distension of the left atrium in dogs with and without exogenous vasopressin. Lawrence et al. (1973), during a longer period of distension of the left atrium, demonstrated significant increases in osmolar clearances in 11 of 18 tests. These increases in the 11 experiments were associated with a mean increase in sodium excretion of approximately 8%. Kappagoda, Linden, Snow & Whitaker (1974) reported that in five experiments there was a mean increase of 8% in sodium excretion. Carswell et al. (1970b), in studying the effect of distension of the left atrium on urine flow from an isolated perfused kidney, noticed an increase in sodium excretion in 12 out of 18 tests with a mean increase of 38%; the mean increase in urine flow being 57%. However, a closer analysis of the results show that because of the variation in sodium excretion during the control periods, a firm conclusion cannot be made as to the existence of a natriuretic response in the perfused kidney. On the other hand, Kinney & DiScala (1972) and de Torrente, Robertson, McDonald & Schrier (1975) during similar experiments involving distension of a balloon in the left atrium, did not observe any change in sodium excretion during distension of a balloon in the left atrium.

Thus, distension of a balloon in the left atrium, partially obstructing the mitral orifice and raising left atrial pressure, results in inconsistent changes in solute excretion. This variability in response probably reflects the variable and non-specific nature of the stimulus and the secondary effect of the accompanying haemodynamic changes in solute excretion.

However, it is pertinent to comment here that experiments involving the distension of small balloons, at the pulmonary vein–atrial junctions and in the appendages which discretely stimulate atrial receptors, shows a more consistent effect on solute excretion. Distension of atrial appendages (Kappagoda, Linden & Snow, 1972c) resulted in a mean increase in sodium excretion of 11% during an increase in urine flow of 23%; both increases were statistically significant. Significant increases in mean urine flow (26%) and sodium excretion (16%), similar to the above, were observed when the right atrial receptors were stimulated (Kappagoda et al., 1973). Distension of the pulmonary vein–atrial junctions (Kappagoda, Linden, Snow & Whitaker, 1974) caused a mean increase in urine flow of 70% and sodium excretion of 19% (Whitaker, 1977).

Therefore, unlike the atrial distension experiments involving distension of a large balloon to block the mitral orifice, discrete stimulation of atrial receptors results in a small but significant increase in the excretion of sodium. Although Ledsome & Linden (1968) did not quantitate the changes in sodium excretion, it is of interest that distension of the pulmonary vein–atrial junctions with the ansae subclaviae cut (preventing

Distension of the left atrium

any increase in heart rate) resulted in an increase in urine flow but the sodium excretion remained 'relatively constant'.

The experiments on conscious dogs present an entirely different picture as regards solute excretion. Lydtin & Hamilton (1964) were the first to study the effect of distension of the left atrium in conscious animals. They observed a mean increase of 217% (S.E. 86.5%; $n = 29$) in sodium excretion, with an increase in urine flow (mean of 64%). To quote from their paper, 'This value represents the mean difference between the average of three subsequent 10 min samples of the control period and the average of all the 10 min samples of the period of increase LAP (left atrial pressure). The increase in total sodium excretion occurred with or without anaesthesia and with or without prehydration. There was no significant difference between the increases in prehydrated and nonprehydrated animals.' The increase in sodium excretion is substantially greater than the values observed in anaesthetised animals. It is not possible fully to explain this result; there may be many contributory factors. Comment must be made on the method of calculation of the response: control values before and after distension were not used for the calculation; again, the very large range of 'sodium responses' (S.E.M. $\pm 86.5\%$, $n = 29$) must indicate that sodium excretion did decrease on occasion. The experimental protocol used was also different from the acute experiments in anaesthetised animals. In addition, distension of the left atrium was associated with an increase in mean arterial pressure of 2 kPa, which could well have contributed to the enhanced natriuresis (e.g. Selkurt, Womak & Dailey, 1965).

The workers from the Freie Universität Berlin (1975–8) also found enhanced natriuretic responses in conscious dogs on high as well as low salt intake (Reinhardt, Kaczmarczyk, Eisele, Reidel, Kuhl & Gatzka, 1975; Kaczmarczyk, Eigenheer, Gatzka, Kuhl & Reinhardt, 1978) and in dogs on low salt diet undergoing highly stimulated tubular reabsorption of sodium by the administration of deoxycortisone acetate (Reinhardt, Kaczmarczyk, Eisele, Arnold, Eigenheer & Kuhl, 1977). Again, the mean arterial pressure was found to be increased by 2 kPa during distension of the atrium (Reinhardt et al., 1977) and 2.5 kPa (Kaczmarczyk et al., 1978); the arterial pressure was not measured by Reinhardt et al. (1975). Since renal blood flow, as measured using an electromagnetic flow meter, did not change during distension of the atrium (Kaczmarczyk et al., 1978), it was argued that the natriuretic response seen in conscious dogs occurred independently of renal blood flow. The contribution of the increase in renal perfusion pressure to this natriuresis still remains a possibility; though it is likely to play a smaller part than hitherto suspected because Reinhardt, Kaczmarczyk, Mohnhaupt & Simgen (1980a) have obtained the natriuresis with a constant mean renal perfusion pressure, though there may be changes in pulse pressure (see later in this chapter). They have also concluded that their post-prandial water and sodium diuresis is not related to the concentration of ADH in the blood (Kaczmarczyk, Kuhl, Riedel, Arnold, Gatzka, Eigenheer & Reinhardt, 1976; Kaczmarczyk, Reinhardt, Riedel, Eisele, Gatzka & Kuhl, 1977).

The atrial tamponade experiments of Goetz, Hermreck, Slick & Starke (1970) offer indirect evidence to incriminate the atrial receptors in the enhanced natriuresis seen in conscious dogs. It was observed that reduction in the atrial transmural pressure by atrial tamponade results in a decrease in urine flow and sodium excretion both of which return towards normal values on release of the tamponade. This effect is seen in the absence of any change in cardiac output or arterial pressure. However, as discussed previously (see Chapter 9), the stimulus applied cannot be ascribed solely to the atrial receptors.

In conclusion, distension of the left atrium in anaesthetised dogs causes a variable increase in solute excretion; but it must be clearly appreciated that the sodium excretions quoted above have been derived from experiments in which a balloon has been distended in the lumen of the left atrium so as to cause mitral obstruction and thereby increase the atrial pressure; but as cardiac output and blood pressure fall (see below), there may be secondary effects on sodium excretion. Application of a discrete stimulus to atrial receptors results in a small but significant increase in sodium excretion. The high natriuretic response seen in conscious dogs cannot be directly attributed to atrial receptors; there is usually an associated increase in arterial pressure. Experiments in which additional surgical procedures were performed for other reasons (e.g. renal denervation, hypo-

Distension of the left atrium

physectomy, etc.) will be discussed in subsequent sections, and the effects on sodium excretion fully discussed.

Effect on the cardiovascular system

Distension of a balloon in the left atrium so as to cause partial obstruction of the mitral valve results in large changes in the cardiovascular system. There is an increase in heart rate and a fall in blood pressure – an observation which has been consistently observed during all such investigations. Such measurements of cardiac output as have been made (e.g. Henry et al., 1956) indicate that distension of the balloon was accompanied by a reduction in cardiac output – which is not wholly unexpected. The truly remarkable feature is that the above procedure results in a diuresis in spite of a fall in cardiac output and systemic arterial pressure. However, some of the increase in urine flow observed in the final 10 min period after removal of the distension (the last 10 min of the test period) may be attributable to the increase in systemic arterial pressure following removal of the mitral obstruction.

Evidence of the reflex nature of the diuresis

Henry & Pearce (1956) observed that this diuresis was abolished by cooling the cervical vagi. These findings were confirmed subsequently by Ledsome et al. (1961). Ledsome & Linden (1968) also established that section of the ansae subclaviae was without effect on this response; an important conclusion, remembering that the efferent limb to the atrial receptor reflex from Paintal-type atrial receptors causing an increase in heart rate, was only in the sympathetic nerves to the heart (see Chapter 6). A detailed discussion of the afferent and efferent limbs of this reflex is presented later in this chapter.

Conclusion

The evidence discussed so far has indicated that distension of a large balloon in the left atrium of anaesthetised dogs results in an increase in urine flow. This response is dependent on the

Atrial receptors and urine flow

integrity of the vagi. It is also evident that this partial obstruction of the mitral orifice results in haemodynamic change which is accompanied by several other reflex adjustments in the dog so that it is not possible to attribute this reponse to any one particular reflex mechanism – though Henry & Pearce (1956) did suggest that the atrial receptors may play a major role in it.

Distension of the right atrium: obstruction to flow

Atrial receptors have been described in the right atrium (see Chapters 2, 3, 6) and several attempts have been made to stimulate these receptors in order to ascertain whether such a procedure would affect urine flow. Mills & Osbaldiston (1968) reported that stretching the right atrium in anaesthetised dogs resulted in no significant changes in urine flow, rates of sodium and potassium excretion and the clearance of inulin and para aminohippuric acid. However, it is difficult to take such an investigation seriously; the experiment involved pulling on strings attached to the right atrial wall and the sole evidence of the involvement of receptors and reflexes was section of the vagi. Subsequently Brennan *et al.* (1971) attempted to stimulate right and left atrial receptors by distending balloons in the lumina of the two atria. Distension of a balloon in the right atrium resulted in a reduction in the concentration of ADH in the plasma. Subsequently in a similar experiment (with a distension sufficient to increase mean right atrial pressure by approximately (0.5–0.7 kPa) Stitzer & Malvin (1975) examined the effect on urine flow, sodium excretion, renal plasma flow and glomerular filtration rate. Distension of a balloon in the right atrium resulted in a small fall in mean arterial pressure, reduction in urine flow, sodium excretion, renal plasma flow and glomerular filtration rate – all findings which are entirely consistent with a reduction in renal blood flow brought about by a fall in cardiac output in an areflexic animal. Though the authors speculate on the possible reflex mechanisms involved in this response, there is no evidence in their report to indicate that the authors were dealing with a reflex.

From this sort of experiment, where it is suspected that flow through the atrium has been impeded, and there is no evidence to the contrary, it is not possible to eliminate other causes completely; it is not possible confidently to implicate atrial receptors.

Distension of localised regions of the atria: no obstruction to flow

Stimulation of left atrial receptors using small balloons

Since partial occlusion of the mitral orifice results in the primary and secondary activation of several cardiovascular reflexes, it was necessary to use a discrete stimulus applied only to the vein–atrial junctions to examine the role of atrial receptors in this reflex increase in urine flow; Ledsome & Linden (1964b) had already observed a reflex increase in heart rate using this technique (see Chapter 6); Ledsome & Linden (1968) found that such a procedure, as well as increasing the heart rate also increased urine flow in anaesthetised dogs. In addition, it was found that when mitral occlusion and distension of the pulmonary vein–atrial junctions were applied alternately in the same animal, the responses (i.e. increases in urine flow) were qualitatively the same (Figs. 10.2, 10.3). The response to distension of the pulmonary vein–atrial junctions was, however, smaller than that evoked by partial occlusion of the mitral valve. More recently Kappagoda, Linden, Snow & Whitaker (1974), Kappagoda, Linden & Sreeharan (1979), Linden & Sreeharan (1979) have confirmed these observations that distension of the vein–atrial junctions alone results in an increase in urine flow (see Table 10.1). In all the investigations using the small balloons but without extra surgical intervention there was an increase in urine flow averaging 50.6% (41 distensions in 28 dogs; Table 10.1) and in investigations with extra intervention, of 43.0% (23 distensions in 16 dogs; Table 10.2).

In the experiments reported by Ledsome & Linden (1968) distension of the pulmonary vein–atrial junctions did not result in any changes in left atrial pressure. In addition, the response of an increase in urine flow was abolished by cooling the cervical vagi. These findings taken in conjunction with the observations that distension of the pulmonary vein–atrial junctions results in stimulation of atrial receptors (Kidd *et al.*, 1966, 1978; Kappagoda, Linden & Sivananthan, 1977, 1979) suggests that

Atrial receptors and urine flow

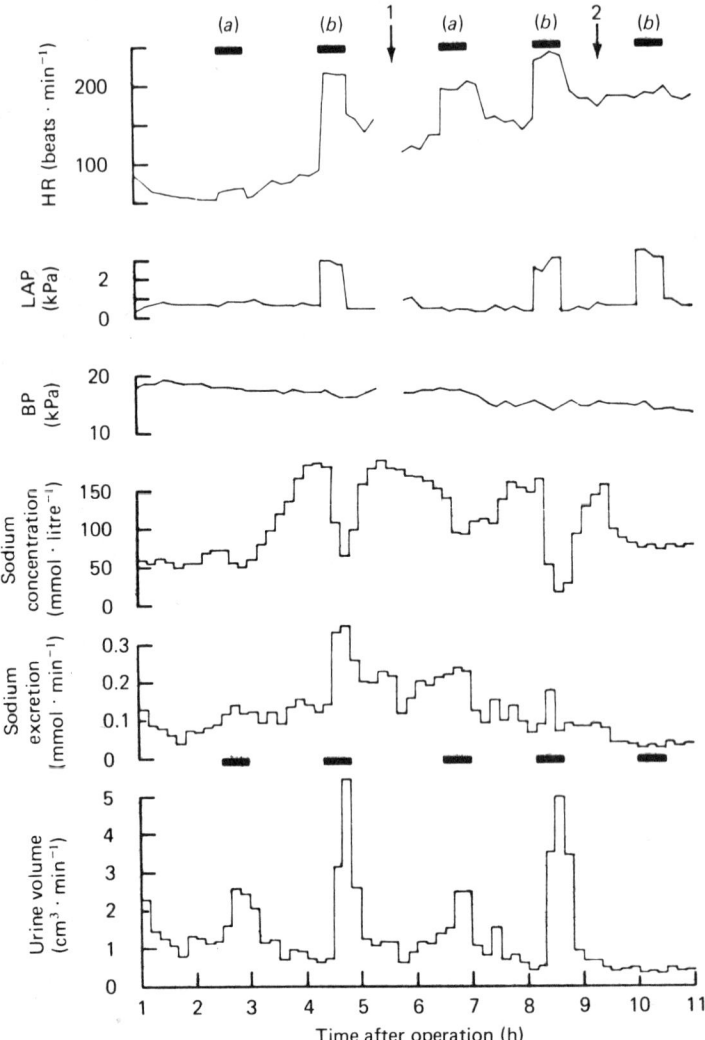

Fig. 10.2. Changes occurring in measured variables during one experiment. During (a) small balloons were distended in the pulmonary vein–atrial junctions. During (b) a balloon was distended in the left atrium to cause mitral obstruction. There is a break in the record at '1', when the atrial balloon was replaced because it leaked. At '2' the right vagus nerve was cut in the neck and the left vagus nerve was cut at the level of the upper border of the aorta. HR, heart rate; LAP, left atrial pressure. (From Ledsome & Linden, 1968.)

Distension of localised regions of the atria

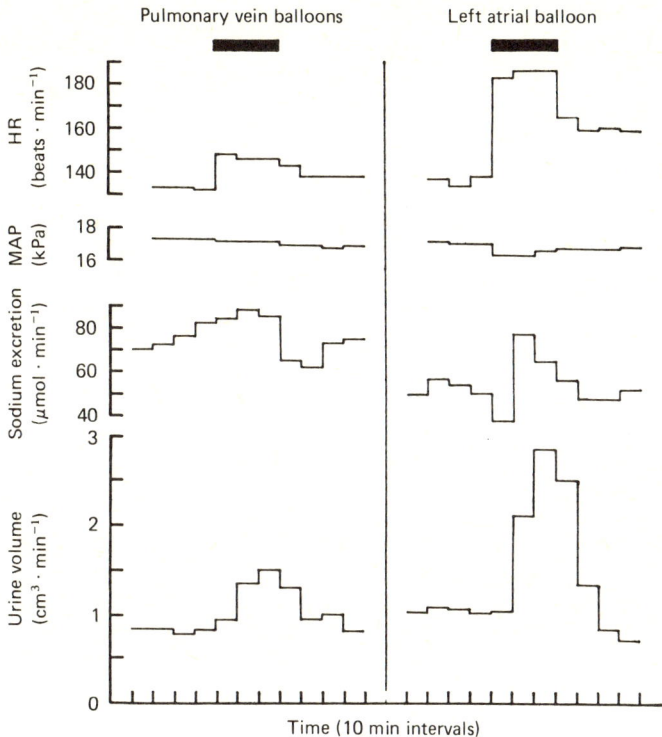

Fig. 10.3. Changes in heart rate (HR), mean arterial pressure (MAP), sodium excretion and urine volume produced by distension of the pulmonary vein–atrial junctions and by mitral obstruction caused by inflating a balloon in the left atrium. Each horizontal line is the average of nine individual values from five dogs. (From Ledsome & Linden, 1968.)

the increase in urine flow is mediated by the atrial receptors. Although the diuretic response to stimulation of atrial receptors by distension of small balloons was small compared with the responses obtained by occluding the mitral orifice with a large balloon, it was nevertheless concluded that a reasonable hypothesis would be that only atrial receptors were involved and responsible for the response (Ledsome & Linden, 1968); the small balloons were stimulating only *some* of the receptors on the left side of the left atrium (see Fig. 10.4 & Table 10.1).

Subsequently, Kappagoda, Linden & Saunders (1972b) found that distension of the atrial appendages alone resulted in

Atrial receptors and urine flow

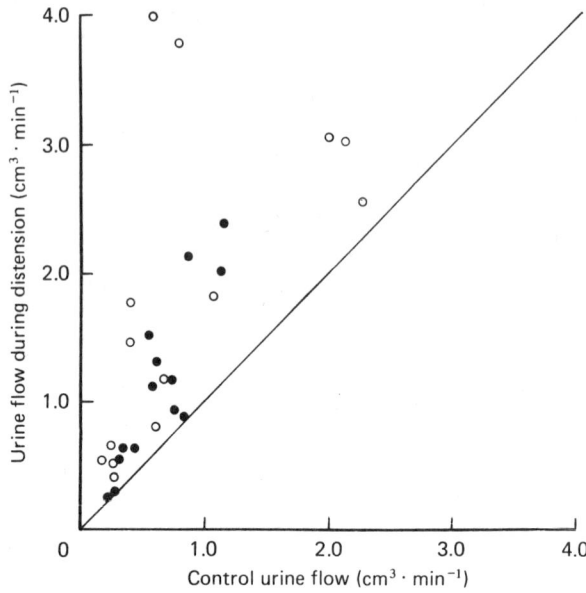

Fig. 10.4. Plot of urine flow during stimulation of left atrial receptors (●, small balloons) and occlusion of mitral orifice (○, large balloon), against control values of urine flow. (From Linden, 1976.)

a reflex increase in heart rate which was qualitatively similar to the response elicited by distension of the pulmonary vein–atrial junctions (Chapter 6). Later, Floyd, Linden & Saunders (1974) observed that the endocardium of the appendages also contained atrial receptors (i.e. complex unencapsulated nerve endings). More recently Kappagoda, Linden & Sivananthan (1979) have established from an electrophysiological study that distension of the left atrial appendages does stimulate atrial receptors. Thus it appears that distension of the atrial appendages alone (without causing obstruction to the atrioventricular valves) constitutes a qualitatively similar stimulus to that of distension of the pulmonary vein–atrial junctions. Therefore we can consider the investigations of Kappagoda, Linden & Snow (1972c) who studied the effect on urine flow of distending the atrial appendages alone in anaesthetised dogs; there was an increase in urine flow which was again abolished by cooling the vagi and by crushing the base of the atrial appendages. These results therefore further

Distension of localised regions of the atria

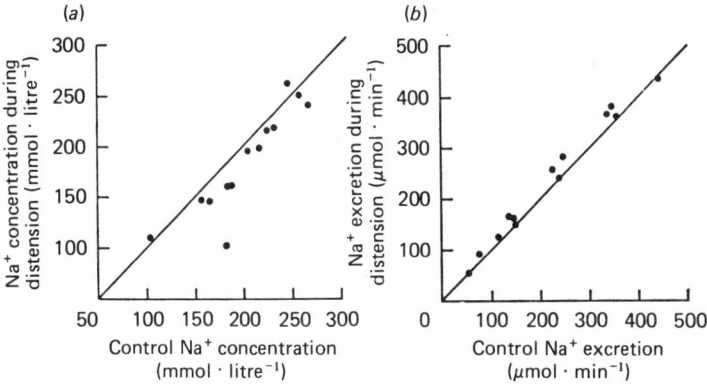

Fig. 10.5. (a) The effect of distension of atrial appendages on urinary sodium concentration. The urinary sodium concentration (mmol·litre^{-1}) during the period of distension is plotted against the urinary sodium concentration (mmol·litre^{-1}) during the control periods. (b) The effect of distension of the atrial appendages on the urinary excretion rate of sodium. The urinary sodium excretion (μmol·min^{-1}) during distension is plotted against the urinary sodium excretion (μmol·min^{-1}) during the control periods. Each point represents a single test and the continuous line is the line of no change. (From Kappagoda, Linden & Snow, 1972c.)

support the claim that stimulation of atrial receptors results in a reflex increase in urine flow and indeed it is not necessary, on quantitative grounds, to involve any other receptors.

Features of the increase in urine flow. In general, the increase in urine flow observed in response to distension of small balloons is evident 5–10 min after application of the stimulus. It begins to wane 5–10 min after removal of the stimulus (see Fig. 10.3), features which are similar to the response seen after partial occlusion of the mitral valve (see earlier in this chapter).

During the period of stimulation the concentration of sodium in the urine is less but there is, however, a small inconsistent increase in sodium excretion as shown, for example, in Fig. 10.5 where the increase in sodium excretion was 11 % and statistically significant (e.g. Kappagoda, Linden & Snow, 1972c). This response of an increase in sodium excretion to discrete stimulation with small balloons is similar to that where distension of a large balloon was used to obstruct the mitral orifice (e.g.

Atrial receptors and urine flow

Kappagoda, Linden, Snow & Whitaker, 1974) (see earlier in this chapter).

Though in both investigations statistical significance (5 % level) was attained, the biological significance of this finding remains a matter for conjecture. The efferent mechanism causing this response is discussed at length later in this chapter.

Stimulation of right atrial receptors using small balloons

Kappagoda *et al.* (1973) stimulated the right atrial receptors in one of two ways without obstructing flow into or out of the right atrium and without raising right atrial pressure. The first method was to stretch the superior vena cava–right atrial junction and the second to distend a small balloon in the lumen of the right atrial appendage; both procedures did not alter either the right atrial pressure or the mean arterial pressure. In these experiments it was found that distension of the balloon in each system resulted in an increase in urine flow. The characteristics of the response were qualitatively similar to those observed from stimulation of the left atrial receptors. Kappagoda *et al.* (1973) also found that cooling the right vagus resulted in a consistent reduction in the response to distension of a balloon in the right atrial appendage. From these results it was concluded that stimulation of right atrial receptors also results in a reflex increase in urine flow in the same manner as the atrial receptors in the left atrium.

Reflex nature of the responses

The afferent path

As described in Chapter 3 there are three types of receptor in the atrial wall and, though only one has been described histologically (see Chapter 2), three types of receptor can be recognised by the fact that two receptors discharge into the vagal nerves and one into the sympathetic rami. Of the two vagal pathways one is in myelinated fibres and one in non-myelinated (Chapter 3). In Chapter 6, when considering the heart rate reflex obtained by stimulating atrial receptors a technique was described which allowed the function of Paintal-type atrial receptors discharging into myelinated fibres to be distinguished from the function of receptors discharging into the other two pathways. The same technique has been used to examine the urine response to stimulation of atrial receptors and this will be described here.

The evidence presented so far has shown that the response to partial obstruction of the mitral valve by distending a balloon in the lumen of the left atrium produces a response which is qualitatively similar to that of stretching the pulmonary vein–atrial junctions. Stretching the pulmonary vein–atrial junctions by distending small balloons was shown to stimulate receptors discharging into myelinated and non-myelinated fibres in the vagi and into 'sympathetic' afferents (see Kappagoda, Linden & Sivananthan, 1979, and Chapter 6 for references), and the increased activity in these fibres could be differentiated by graded cooling of the vagi between temperatures of 20 and 8 °C (Kappagoda, Linden & Sivananthan, 1979; Chapter 6).

Using the same technique the effect of distending a large balloon to evoke the diuresis and then cooling the vagi was examined (Kappagoda, Linden & Sivananthan, 1978; Sivananthan, Kappagoda & Linden, 1981).

Three groups of experiments were completed: the effects of cooling the vagi on, first, the urine response, second, the response in myelinated fibres and third, the response in non-myelinated fibres were examined.

The urine response was obtained and calculated as described earlier. The response at any cooled temperature of the vagi was then expressed as a percentage of the average of the responses at 37 °C obtained before and after the cooled response. The responses of the activity in the two groups of nerve fibres to cooling the vagi were calculated in the same way (cf. the calculation in Chapter 6 and Kappagoda, Linden & Sivananthan, 1979).

In the event, the investigations confirmed that the increase in urine flow produced in response to the distension of a large balloon in the left atrium is reduced by cooling the vagi but in addition there was a graded response. Cooling the vagi to 18 °C resulted in a reduction in the response to 65% of that obtained at 37 °C; the response at 12 °C was reduced to 35% (Fig. 10.6). Cooling the vagi between 8 and 12 °C also abolished the diuretic

Atrial receptors and urine flow

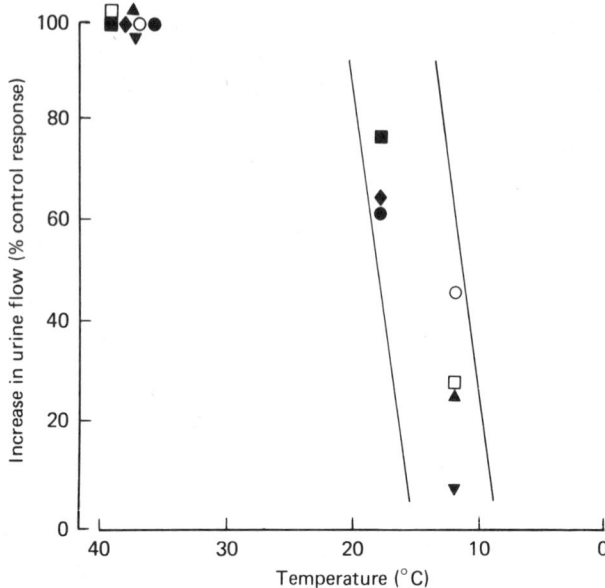

Fig. 10.6. Response of the increase in urine flow resulting from distension of a balloon in the lumen of the atrium, to cooling the vagi to 18 and 12 °C. Each point represents the reponse of the increase in urine flow at each temperature expressed as a percentage of the control responses obtained with the temperature at 36–37 °C; the control responses were obtained before and after the cooled responses. Each symbol represents the results from one dog. The responses at 36–37 °C were rated 100 % response. The continuous lines are the same as in Figs. 10.8 and 10.9 and were drawn by eye to aid comparison. (From Sivananthan et al., 1981.)

response in six experiments of Henry & Pearce (1956); an example from their work is shown in Fig. 10.7 where it is seen that the urine response was abolished during cooling at 9 °C. Also shown in Fig. 10.7 is the effect of cooling on conduction in two left atrial fibres; conduction during the resting state was reduced at 12 °C and blocked at 6 °C. No evidence was provided of the effect on the conduction of cooling the vagus during distension of the balloon. Because at that time (1956) there was no evidence that activity in non-myelinated fibres also increased during distension of a balloon in the left atrium, no attempt was made to distinguish between the two groups of fibres. In fact Henry & Pearce (1956) pointed out that 'Conclusions from this

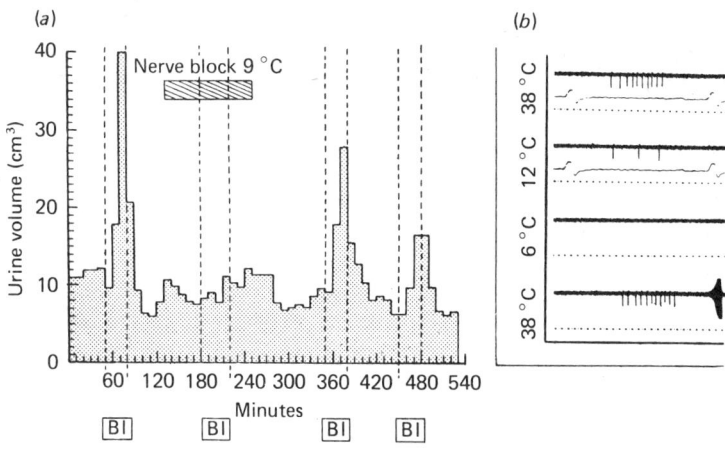

Fig. 10.7. (a) The increase in urine flow (ordinate, cm^3 per 10 min) in response to distension of a left atrial balloon (BI) is abolished by cooling the vagi to 9 °C. (b) Conduction in two left atrial stretch fibres is blocked at about 12 and 6 °C. The spikes have been retouched. The blocking temperature range is approximately the same as that which prevents the diuretic response to distension of the atrial balloon. (From Henry & Pearce, 1956.)

finding must be drawn with caution, however, in the light of Paintal's demonstration (1953c) of the wide range of conduction rates of fibres of a given origin, and evidence of the wide range of blocking temperatures of fibres of a given function (Widdicombe, 1954).' But the investigation reported here (Kappagoda, Linden & Sivananthan, 1978; Sivananthan, Kappagoda & Linden, 1981) completely differentiated between the effects in myelinated and non-myelinated fibres.

The response in myelinated fibres was similar to that reported by Kappagoda, Linden & Sivananthan (1979) when distending the small balloons. Both Paintal type A and type B receptors were stimulated by distension of the large balloon and the discharge resembled the responses to large intravenous infusions (Kappagoda, Linden & Mary, 1977b). The response in the myelinated fibres to distension was also attenuated in a graded manner: at 18 °C the response to distension was reduced to 65%, and at 12 °C to 30% of the value attained at 37 °C (Fig. 10.8). This result is similar to that of the urine response.

Atrial receptors and urine flow

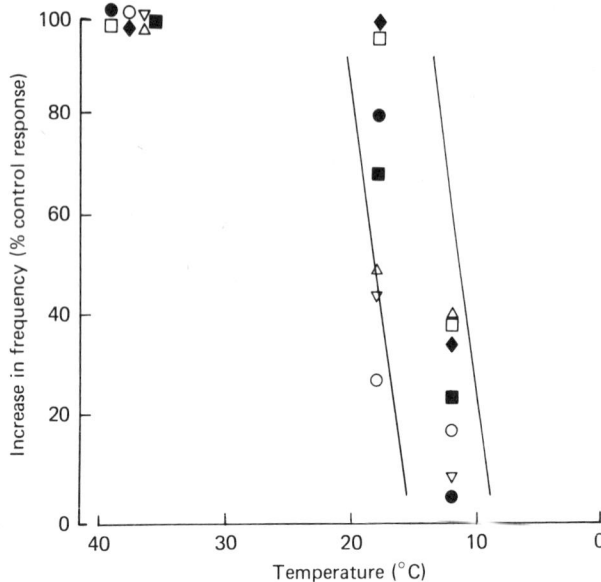

Fig. 10.8. Response of the increase in action potentials in myelinated fibres resulting from distension of balloons in the lumen of the left atrium, to cooling of the vagus at 18 and 12 °C. Each point represents the response of the increase in action potentials (mean frequency) expressed as a percentage of the response with the vagus at 36–37 °C. Each symbol represents the response in one nerve fibre. Seven fibres with conduction velocities of 6.0–27.1 m·s^{-1} were examined in four dogs. The two continuous lines were drawn by eye and are the same as in Figs. 10.6 and 10.9. (From Sivananthan et al., 1981.)

With the non-myelinated fibres cooling the cervical vagus resulted in a reduction in the response to distension, but the temperature at which this reduction occurred was different from that observed with the myelinated fibres; the increased discharge in four receptors was not at all affected by cooling the vagi to 12 °C, one was slightly less at 12 °C, whereas in the sixth receptor the increased discharge was abolished by cooling to 17 °C (Fig. 10.9). These results are entirely similar to those obtained during examination of the heart-rate reflex (Kappagoda, Linden & Sivananthan, 1979; Chapter 6); compare Figs. 10.6, 10.8 and 10.9 with Figs. 6.8, 6.6 and 6.11 respectively.

Since as well as the similarity of the urine response and the

Reflex nature of the responses

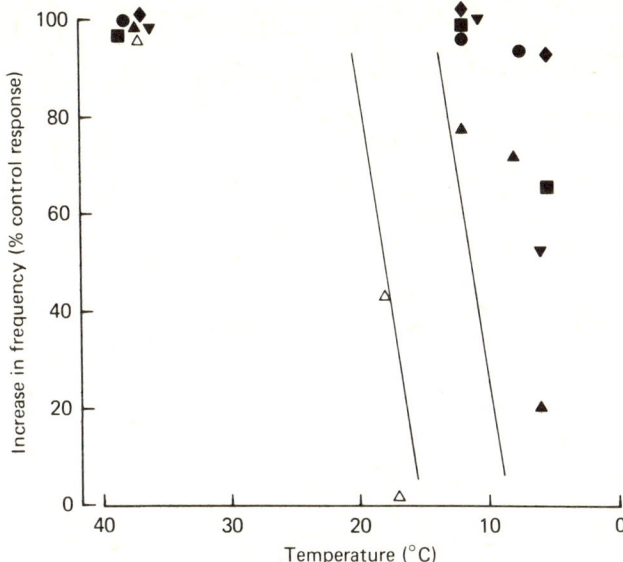

Fig. 10.9. Response of the increase in action potentials in non-myelinated fibres resulting from distension of balloons in the lumen of the left atrium, to cooling of the vagus at 18 and 12 °C. Each point represents the response of the increase in action potentials (mean frequency) expressed as a percentage of the response with the vagus at 36–37 °C. Each symbol represents the response in one nerve fibre. Six fibres with conduction velocities of 0.9–1.8 m·s^{-1} were examined in four dogs. The two continuous lines were drawn by eye and are the same as in Figs. 10.6 and 10.8. (From Sivananthan, et al., 1981.)

response in the myelinated fibres to vagal cooling, it is known that the urine response is abolished by vagal section (e.g. Ledsome et al., 1961) it is possible to conclude that receptors attached to the sympathetic afferent fibres are unlikely to be involved.

Thus Paintal-type unencapsulated atrial receptors discharging into myelinated fibres in the vagi are solely responsible for urine response as well as the response of increase in heart rate.

The efferent path

The efferent pathway of the response of an increase in urine flow obtained during stimulation of atrial receptors is still controversial and the problems involved will be discussed below. With evidence based mostly on investigations completed in Leeds it is proposed that there are two efferent limbs to the reflex, a humoral agent and a nervous pathway; in addition there is a secondary haemodynamic effect. Certainly there is a humoral component which is not ADH, and is possibly a diuretic substance. The question of whether, in addition, ADH is released still awaits firm evidence. The evidence on which these opinions are based is discussed below.

The blood-borne agent: is it ADH? There is a considerable body of evidence which supports the proposition that surgical denervation of the kidney does not abolish the response of an increase in urine flow (e.g. Ledsome *et al.*, 1961; Kappagoda, Linden, Snow & Whitaker, 1975; Kappagoda, Linden & Sreeharan, 1979). The diuresis was also obtained with the animal and its kidney 'pharmacologically denervated' (Linden & Sreeharan, 1979). This proposition is supported further by observations of Carswell *et al.* (1968, 1970b) that the response also occurred in an isolated kidney, perfused with blood obtained from a dog whose atrial receptors were stimulated. These findings indicate that the renal nerves are not necessary in eliciting this response (see later).

The identity of this humoral agent has remained controversial but the current opinion is that the response is mediated by a reduction in the concentration of circulating antidiuretic hormone (see Gauer & Henry, 1963; Gauer *et al.*, 1970; Goetz *et al.*, 1975; Gauer & Henry, 1976; Donald & Shepherd, 1978; Epstein, 1978; Schrier, Berl & Anderson, 1979; Zucker, Share & Gilmore, 1979). It is not possible fully to discuss all the evidence presented for and against this view but some important aspects will be described and the results of some pertinent investigations critically discussed, so that adequate judgements on the conclusions can be made.

The earliest evidence thought to support the belief that ADH was involved in this reflex was provided by the observation of Henry *et al.* (1956) and Henry & Pearce (1956) that the urine passed during the period of stimulation was considerably more dilute than that passed during the control periods. These early findings have been elegantly confirmed by the observations of

Lawrence et al. (1973). But such evidence does not demonstrate a link between atrial receptors, ADH and urine flow.

Two major conditions have to be met: (1) stimulation of atrial receptors has to be consistently associated with an increase in urine flow and a fall in the concentration of ADH; (2) it must be shown that the changes observed in the concentration of circulating ADH are capable of eliciting those changes in urine flow.

The evidence does not fully support the contention (see Kappagoda, Linden, Snow & Whitaker, 1974, for review). Measurement of the concentration of ADH in the plasma during distension of the left atrium has been used in a number of investigations to evaluate the role of the hormone in the urine response. Baisset & Montastruc (1957) observed a 50% reduction in the concentration of the hormone during distension of a balloon in the lumen of the left atrium. However, no measurements of the hormone were made after the release of distension and since individual experimental results were not presented, it was not possible to conclude whether the observed reduction in ADH was the cause of the diuresis during atrial distension. Share (1965) distended the left atrium against a background of carotid occlusion. Although a reduction in the concentration of ADH was observed in six out of the eight experiments, no statistical analysis was carried out and it could also be argued with some justification that the results refer solely to the particular situation prevailing during carotid occlusion. Shu'ayb, Moran & Zimmerman (1965) showed a mean reduction in ADH concentration during atrial distension. However, such a decrease was not obtained during every distension nor was a diuresis consistently obtained. Johnson, Moore & Segar (1969) observed a small but significant decrease in plasma ADH concentration and an increase in urine flow during small changes in transmural left atrial pressure brought about by distending a balloon in the left atrial appendage. However, the individual results were not given so that it is not possible to determine whether the changes noted occurred in all the experiments. In addition, the mean difference in ADH concentration between the test and control periods was $1.9\ \mu U \cdot cm^{-3}$ and since the random error of the assay technique was not given, the biological significance of this small change in ADH concentration cannot be determined. The decrease in ADH concentration reported by Brennan et al. (1971) during distension of balloons in the left and right atria was neither statistically significant nor related to changes in urine flow. All the evidence mentioned above has only shown inconsistent and small reductions in concentration of ADH during atrial distension without any correlation with the changes in urine flow. These particular aspects of the problem were investigated by Kappagoda, Linden, Snow & Whitaker (1974, 1975). In the first of these investigations it was found that stimulation of atrial receptors consistently produced an increase in urine flow but failed to produce a consistent reduction in the antidiuretic activity of plasma as detected by water-loaded ethanol-anaesthetised rats. In the same investigation it was also shown that anaesthetised dogs were far less sensitive to ADH than conscious dogs, thus supporting the proposition that changes in urine flow mediated by ADH should be accompanied by large changes in the concentration of the hormone. Such changes were large enough to be detected by rats anaesthetised with ethanol and yet were *not* observed during stimulation of atrial receptors. Although this is the only evidence against the ADH hypothesis where the atrial receptors have been stimulated discretely and no secondary effects were likely, Goetz, Bond, Hermreck & Trank (1970) arrived at a similar conclusion after showing that the antidiuresis occurring during reductions in atrial transmural pressure by atrial tamponade was not accompanied by any increase in the concentration of ADH as assessed by a bioassay technique. Later, Kappagoda, Linden, Snow & Whitaker (1975) demonstrated an increase in urine flow following stimulation of atrial receptors in dogs subjected to hypophysectomy (Table 10.2); this response was also unaffected by surgical denervation of the kidney (Figs. 10.10 and 10.11). Thus it was concluded that ADH was unlikely to be involved in the response observed in this preparation.

The claim that the antidiuretic hormone is involved in this reflex diuresis was reviewed by de Torrente et al. (1975) who reported that distension of a balloon in the lumen of the left atrium resulted in an increase in urine flow which was accompanied by a consistent reduction in the concentration of antidiuretic hormone as measured by radioimmunoassay. Also the diuresis in hypophysectomised dogs was prevented by an

Reflex nature of the responses

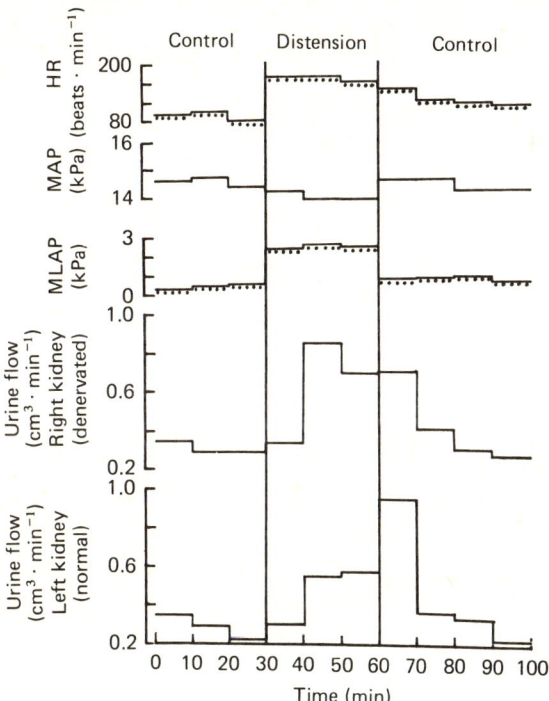

Fig. 10.10. The effect of distension of a balloon in the lumen of the left atrium after destruction of the pituitary gland. The right kidney alone was denervated and bretylium tosylate was administered in a dose of 10 mg·kg^{-1}. From above down: heart (HR); mean arterial pressure (MAP); mean left atrial pressure (MLAP); urine flow (cm^3·min^{-1}) in the denervated right kidney; urine flow (cm^3·min^{-1}) in the intact left kidney. The urine was collected over 10 min periods and the values for heart rate, mean arterial pressure and mean left atrial pressure refer to the average values during the corresponding collection periods. Dots under lines are for ease of identification. (From Kappagoda, Linden, Snow & Whitaker, 1975.)

infusion of vasopressin. In view of the difference between these results and those described above their experiments will be considered in detail, and an argument, modified from Whitaker (1977), presented to suggest that their claim is not supported by their observations. Their experimental protocol was different. In the majority of investigations described in this chapter the

Atrial receptors and urine flow

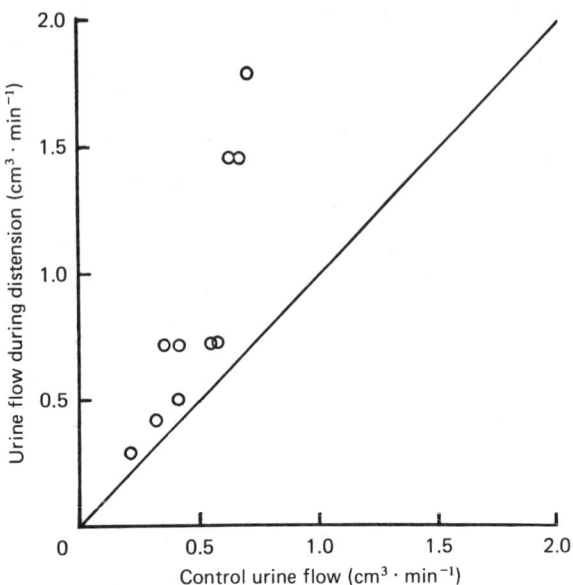

Fig. 10.11. The effect of distension of a balloon in the lumen of the left atrium on urine flow, after destruction of the pituitary gland. The urine flow ($cm^3 \cdot min^{-1}$) during the period of distension is plotted against the urine flow ($cm^3 \cdot min^{-1}$) during the control period. Each point represents a single test and the continuous line is the line of no change. (From Kappagoda, Linden, Snow & Whitaker, 1975.)

experimental protocol included an initial control period of 30 min, a test period of 30 min and a final control period of 30 min. In the investigation reported by de Torrente et al. (1975) a different protocol was adopted. The initial control period varied between 15 and 30 min, followed by an equilibrium period of 20–30 min, which in turn was followed by a test period varying from 15 to 50 min; distension of the balloon was then ended and the preparation was left for 15–30 min for 'equilibration', followed by a final control period of 15–30 min. The first criticism of this protocol is its variability. The second is that the length of control period, 15 min, is too short to allow the variability of urine flow and concentration of ADH to be estimated. The third is that the blood samples were collected during alternate collection periods with no reference to the state of the urine response. With such variability in protocol it is clearly impossible to define an association between stimulation of atrial receptors, the urine response and the concentration of the antidiuretic hormone. It is not possible even to comment on trends observed in individual experiments because the results were presented as single mean values for the control and test periods. The presentation of individual data is essential, particularly where there are significant variations in experimental protocol.

Even when it is hypothetically assumed that the changes in plasma concentration of the antidiuretic hormone could be associated with distensions of the balloon, it is still not possible from the data of de Torrente *et al.* (1975) to attribute the diuresis solely to the changes in concentration of the antidiuretic hormone. The relationship between the changes in concentration of ADH in the plasma and the changes in urine flow in anaesthetised dogs should be considered; one way is to take the argument from published results, as follows. Orloff, Wagner & Davidson (1958) have shown in conscious dogs that a water diuresis was suppressed by the infusion of vasopressin at a rate of $1.5 \text{ mU} \cdot \text{kg}^{-1} \cdot \text{h}^{-1}$. This suppression was achieved in dogs which showed an osmolar clearance of approximately $2.5 \text{ cm}^3 \cdot \text{min}^{-1}$, i.e. a state similar to that of the anaesthetised dogs described by de Torrente *et al.* (1975). Subsequently, Perlmutt (1961; Fig. 1, Table 1; $50 \text{ mU} \cdot \text{h}^{-1}$ in four dogs) showed that in dogs anaesthetised with Nembutal (as were those of de Torrente *et al.*, 1975), the suppression of a water diuresis was achieved by an infusion of approximately $3.8 \text{ mU} \cdot \text{kg}^{-1} \cdot \text{h}^{-1}$. This suppression was also achieved in dogs having an osmolar clearance of 2–$2.5 \text{ cm}^3 \cdot \text{min}^{-1}$. It must be emphasised that in both groups of experiments, the suppression of the diuresis (i.e. the positive water clearance) was achieved with no change in the osmolar clearance. Lauson & Bocanegra (1961) have shown that when a steady state is achieved during an infusion of antidiuretic hormone the concentration in plasma can be obtained by dividing the rate of infusion by the plasma clearance of the hormone. The value of the plasma clearance has been calculated by Lauson & Bočanegra (1961) to be approximately 16% of plasma volume. If these values are accepted, and the plasma volume of dogs calculated on the basis of a blood volume of 80 cm^3 of blood per kg body weight, the concentration of ADH in the plasma in the experiments on conscious dogs quoted above (Orloff et al., 1958) would be 3.5 μU·cm^{-3} of plasma. Using the same assumption a comparable value for the dogs anaesthetised with Nembutal (Perlmutt, 1961) would be 8.9 μU·cm^{-3} of plasma. On this basis, it would be reasonable to expect dogs anaesthetised with Nembutal to be sensitive to antidiuretic hormone in a manner which yields a dose response curve over a range of concentration from zero to 9 μU ADH·cm^{-3} of plasma. It is equally reasonable to expect such dogs to have a positive free water clearance when their kidneys are operating within this range.

When the experiments of de Torrente et al. (1975) are considered with these calculations in mind, it becomes apparent that the diuresis could not have been solely caused by changes in plasma concentration of ADH. For instance, in the control state these dogs, which were anaesthetised with Nembutal, were clearly hydrated, but nevertheless had a 'negative' free water clearance and an osmolar clearance of 2.5 cm^3·min^{-1}. Such a position can only be consistent with a nearly complete suppression of water diuresis by antidiuretic hormone, if indeed this hormone was responsible for that state of affairs. The concentration of ADH in plasma of approximately 10.5 μU·cm^{-3} during control periods as reported by de Torrente et al. (1975) appears to support this proposition. However, during distension of a large balloon in the left atrium, the concentration of the hormone in plasma fell to 5 μU·cm^{-3}, a value which should result in incomplete suppression of a water diuresis in a hydrated dog anaesthetised with Nembutal as the relationship will now be operating about the middle of the dose–response curve. Thus one would expect to observe a positive free water clearance. However, the data of de Torrente et al. (1975) indicate that the urine volume was increased but the free water clearance remained 'negative'. On this basis it appears doubtful whether the concentration of antidiuretic hormone was the only determinant of the increases in urine flow in these dogs. Similarly, Yaron & Bennett (1978) are also critical of this work of de Torrente et al. (1975) complaining that, 'at all times the urine remained hypertonic to plasma and the levels of ADH found so high (10 times higher than the present study), even after the rise in left atrial pressure, that the study is difficult to interpret'.

An added criticism of the work of de Torrente et al. (1975) is that no control sham operation, with which to compare a negative response obtained in the hypophysectioned animals, was completed. It may be significant that their Fig. 2 shows a small, but not significant, increase in mean urine flow, and a small difference in urine osmolality, in the animals subjected to hypophysectomy.

De Torrente et al. (1975) also suggested that in the experiments quoted in this chapter (Kappagoda, Linden, Snow & Whitaker, 1975) the hypophysectomy was inadequate because the animals did not show any evidence of diabetes insipidus following the procedure. On the other hand, in their animals subjected to hypophysectomy it was claimed that diabetes insipidus was observed. However, after the hypophysectomy the animals were given an infusion of vasopressin. During this infusion the left atrium was stimulated in precisely the same manner above. At the conclusion of the distension experiment the infusion of vasopressin was stopped and the urine was collected and examined for a further 1–2 h at the end of which period the dogs were said to produce urine of an osmolality less than 100 mosm·kg^{-1} H$_2$O. The authors put this information forward as evidence of diabetes insipidus and therefore adequate hypophysectomy in their experiments. However, it is significant that in each experiment, which covered a period of nearly 6 h, the dogs had a 'positive balance' of approximately 1350 cm^3 of fluids (infusions minus urine volume) composed mainly of 0.6% saline. It is a matter of common laboratory experience that an infusion of this magnitude would produce a urine having an osmolality of less than 100 mosm·kg^{-1} H$_2$O, a finding wholly unconnected with the adequacy of the hypophysectomy. The important question as to the reason why classical diabetes insipidus is not seen in these acute experiments is also highlighted by this argument. It is suggested that this finding is related in part to the effect of the anaesthetic (Warren & Ledingham, 1975, 1978); for instance, there is evidence of increased sympathetic activity to the kidney during anaesthesia (see Chapter 9).

This work cannot be accepted as evidence, at least in support of a predominant role of the antidiuretic hormone in the mediation of the diuretic response.

In another similar investigation reported recently, Zucker,

Share & Gilmore (1979) also have suggested that distension of a balloon in the lumen of the left atrium of dogs anaesthetised with pentobarbitone resulted in a reduction of plasma concentration of ADH, measured by radioimmunoassay. However, again this report can be criticised. First, yet another different protocol was used in obtaining blood samples. For instance, a single sample was obtained during each of the three periods, initial control, test and final control periods. In the final control period a blood sample was taken 25 min after recovery from distension (an unknown period of time following removal of distension) and the test sample was taken at varying periods between 20 and 25 min from distension, with the period of distension itself varying between 30 and 50 min. Secondly, whilst the known effect of vagotomy on the urine response was studied, the effect of such a procedure on the response of ADH was not supplied. Finally, individual data on the urine response and the ADH response were not given. In fact from their Table 1 (Zucker, Share & Gilmore, 1979) it is obvious that only a selected number of data during the final control period were used for analysis.

It may also be argued that assessment of plasma ADH by radioimmunoassay alone in the manner of de Torrente *et al.* (1975) and Zucker, Share & Gilmore (1979) provides a more sensitive method than a bioassay. However, whilst few antisera have sufficient sensitivity to detect immunological activity in plasma (e.g. Forsling, 1974), the results of radioimmunoassay do not necessarily reflect biological activity of ADH. Therefore the reports of de Torrente *et al.* (1975) and Zucker, Share & Gilmore (1979) cannot be used as unequivocal evidence that stimulation of atrial receptors affects the release of ADH.

The evidence given above by Kappagoda, Linden, Snow & Whitaker (1974, 1975) and the arguments presented in these two publications suggest that the dog, anaesthetised in this way, has a high concentration of ADH in the plasma and, in addition, the kidney responds only to large changes in the concentration of ADH. In this regard it is interesting that Zucker, Share & Gilmore (1979) use this sort of evidence to explain why, although the dog with heart failure shows a decrease in ADH concentration in the plasma in response to distension of the balloon in the left atrium, there is no change in urine flow; but an alternative explanation could be that ADH is not responsible for the decrease in their comparable normal dogs – another substance could have been responsible. This explanation would save them the embarassment of having also to explain away why their dogs with heart failure showed a decrease in ADH concentration *at all*. They suggest that in dogs with heart failure, not only is there electrophysiological evidence of decreased sensitivity of atrial receptors (Greenberg, Richmond, Stocking, Gupta, Meehan & Henry, 1973; Zucker, Earle & Gilmore, 1977), but also evidence from post mortem histology of thickening and calcification of the atrial wall. If this evidence is correct then the atrial receptors in dogs with heart failure should have responded less, or not at all, to the same stretch as used in normal dogs, and thus some other explanation of the decrease in ADH concentration in the dogs with heart failure must be sought. One could conclude from these experiments that a substance other than ADH is responsible for the diuresis resulting from stimulation of atrial receptors (see below).

Thus there is little evidence to support the hypothesis that the response itself is mediated by ADH. However, it is conceivable that stimulation of atrial receptors under certain circumstances is accompanied by a reduction in the concentration of circulating ADH although such an effect does not confirm a causative role for the hormone. For instance, it is possible that there was a small change in the concentration of ADH in the plasma during stimulation of atrial receptors in the investigation of Kappagoda, Linden, Snow & Whitaker (1974). Though there was no statistical difference between the concentration during the distension period and that during the control periods, the variance was large; all that can be concluded is that no statistical difference could be demonstrated. Again even if an effect were to be shown, it would still be necessary to show which receptors were involved; such receptors would be unlikely to be the Paintal-type atrial receptors, mainly stimulated by the small balloons. A possible role for non-myelinated receptors and ADH release has been postulated recently (Thorén *et al.*, 1976; Thorén, 1979a) and could explain the findings of Thames & Schmid (1979) who searched for a cause and effect relationship between the ubiquitous 'cardiopulmonary' receptors and the concentration of ADH in the plasma of various groups of dogs;

in one group with sino-aortic denervation vagotomy resulted in a rise in the concentration of ADH, but no particular receptors were implicated.

Recently groups of experiments have been reported in which the activity in hypothalamic neurones has been examined (e.g. Koizumi & Yamashita, 1977, 1978; Menninger, 1979; Menninger & Frazer, 1972). The basis of the argument is that changes in the electrical activity of 'identified' neurosecretory cells in the supraoptic nuclei of the hypothalamus reflect an increase or a decrease in neurophypophyseal hormone release (Brooks & Koizumi, 1974; Hayward, 1977). This in itself must be in doubt unless discerned on every occasion; the sample of cells is too small. However, it is difficult to take the work of Koizumi & Yamashita (1977, 1978) seriously as their stimulus involves tying threads directly to the right or left atrium and then attaching weight to the threads. Criticism of this technique has been made in Chapter 5 but it must be even more relevant here where no attempts were made to make sure secondary haemodynamic changes did not occur; changes which are well known to affect the supraoptic nucleus. Similar techniques were used by Menninger (1979) who sutured silk threads to the atrial wall and attached the threads to a micromanipulator; changes in blood volume used as a stimulus by Menninger & Frazer (1972) are far removed from a discrete stimulus to atrial receptors. These sorts of experiments contribute nothing to the very important question as to whether atrial receptors affect the secretion of ADH.

It is easy to agree with Donald & Shepherd (1978) when they conclude, 'It would appear that resolution of the problem would demand a model in which the stimulus was confined to the left atrium and did not cause circulatory changes which could be held responsible for an alteration in ADH secretion. Also blood levels of ADH should not be markedly different in control and recovery periods and each should be significantly different from the value obtained during the test period (Kappagoda et al., 1974). The matter of circulatory changes acquires importance in view of the observations that reduction in atrial transmural pressure by distension of a previously prepared pericardial pouch still caused decreases in renal sodium excretion and urine flow in dogs with acute cardiac denervation (Goetz et al., 1976).'

This latter point is emphasised by study of Linden & Sreeharan (1979, 1981; also see end of this chapter).

Thus, in conclusion, there could be a small change in ADH as a result of stimulating atrial receptors but its possible demonstration awaits carefully controlled investigation.

An alternative hypothesis. It is possible that the response is mediated by a blood-borne agent of unknown nature – and this hypothetical agent may be a naturally occurring diuretic substance.

The Leeds group drew this conclusion because they first decided that the blood-borne agent which they were observing in response to either distension of a large balloon or small balloon, in the left atrium, was not ADH in their preparation. Destruction of the post-pituitary gland and most of the hypothalamus did not abolish the response (Kappagoda, Linden, Snow & Whitaker, 1975), whether the response was observed in innervated kidneys or denervated. The small balloons at the pulmonary vein–atrial junctions were shown to be a discrete stimulus to atrial receptors (Chapters 3 and 6); whether the small balloons were distended or the large balloons, they could not detect a change in the concentration of ADH in the plasma (Kappagoda, Linden, Snow & Whitaker, 1974). They also demonstrated that a concentration of ADH higher than in the unanaesthetised dog would be required to cause antidiuresis and that both these amounts could easily be assayed by their assay preparation. This assay preparation has recently been improved by a factor of 5–10 times (Kappagoda, Linden & Pashley, 1979). The fact that the plasma obtained during a diuretic response does not inhibit the urine flow of the water-loaded ethanol-anaesthetised rat (the ADH assay preparation) suggested the agent may be diuretic (Kappagoda, Linden, Snow & Whitaker, 1974).

In seeking the identity of such an agent, Kappagoda, Knapp, Linden & Whitaker (1976) and Kappagoda, Knapp, Linden, Pearson & Whitaker (1979) reported the use of Malpighian tubules of *Rhodnius prolixus* as a means of detecting differences in the plasma of anaesthetised dogs, obtained during control periods and during periods of stimulation of atrial receptors. It was shown that Malpighian tubules suspended in 'control

Atrial receptors and urine flow

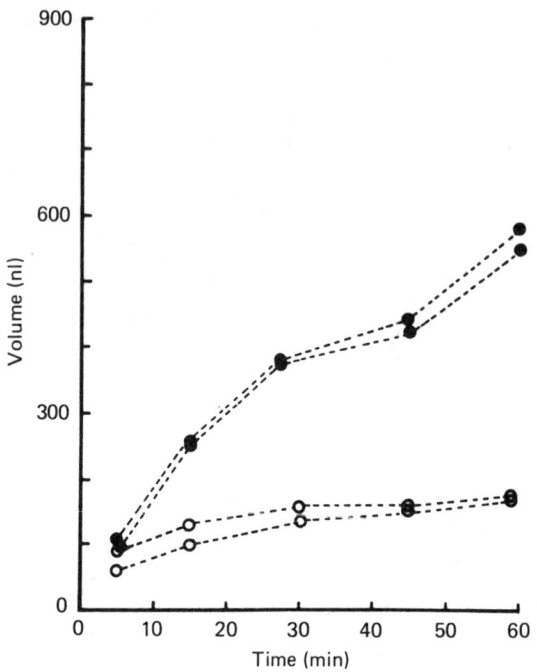

Fig. 10.12. Secretions of four Malpighian tubules from one Rhodnius, suspended in n-butanol extracts of plasma. Ordinate: cumulative volume of fluid secreted (nl). Abscissa: time (min); ●, secretion of tubules suspended in test extract; ○, secretion of tubules suspended in control extract. (From Kappagoda, Knapp, Linden, Pearson & Whitaker, 1979.)

plasma' secreted at a considerably faster rate than those suspended in test plasma. These differences in plasma and the increases in urine flow were abolished by cooling or cutting the cervical vagi. In addition it was found that the differences in plasma were preserved by extracting the plasma in butanol (Fig. 10.12) and these differences were also abolished by cooling or cutting the cervical vagi. The only claim made is that these differences in the plasma as detected by the behaviour of the Malpighian tubules may reflect the presence of the hypothetical diuretic agent.

The blood-borne agent 'recognised' by the tubules may be a concomitant variable; but it is not ADH. First, this preparation does not respond to ADH. Secondly, incubation of an extract

Reflex nature of the responses

of plasma, obtained during the diuresis, with sodium thioglycollate does not affect the blood-borne agent which still has an effect on the tubules; and such treatment would destroy ADH (Linden, 1979b; Knapp, Linden & Pearson, 1981).

All this evidence suggests the blood-borne agent with which we are dealing is not ADH, but some other substance, possibly diuretic.

Efferent renal nerves: background. The effect of stimulating atrial receptors on the activity in renal nerves has been investigated by several groups of workers. The earliest and perhaps the most conclusive investigation was that reported in Leeds by Karim et al. (1972), who found a reduction in the activity in efferent renal nerves in response to discrete distension of the pulmonary vein–atrial junctions, using the technique shown in Fig. 10.13. Before discussing these results further it is important to realise that there is a vast literature about the effects of efferent nerves on the kidney. It is not possible fully to discuss all reports but a brief survey will help the discussion on the function of atrial receptors better to be understood.

The kidney is a richly innervated organ, nerves emanating from a renal plexus on and around the surface of the extra-renal portion of the renal artery (e.g. Mitchell, 1950; Christensen, Lewis & Kuntz, 1951). The innervation of the renal blood vessels is derived mainly from the plexus and is said to be solely sympathetic (Christensen et al., 1951). Aström & Crafoord (1968) recorded action potentials in renal efferent nerves and demonstrated rhythmic inhibition during systole identical to that in splanchnic nerves. They also showed that the rhythmic discharge could be affected by the carotid sinus.

Many studies have shown that the renal efferent nerves have an effect on the functions of the kidney. Only examples of reports of investigation in this field can be given. Denervation diuresis has been recognised since 1859 (Bernard, 1859). It was left to Berne (1952), using anaesthetised and unanaesthetised dogs, to conclude that the higher urinary volume and sodium excretion observed in the denervated kidney in the anaesthetised animal was due to a prior vasoconstriction resulting from the anaesthetic. In the unanaesthetised dog the glomerular filtration rate and urinary sodium excretion were the same in innervated and denervated kidneys. There has been dispute concerning the statement that the increase in sodium excretion resulting from the stimulation of renal nerves in anaesthetised animals is mediated by an increase in glomerular filtration rate alone; some evidence is reviewed in an excellent article on the control of sodium excretion by de Wardener (1973). It is now apparent that the renal nerves can affect other kidney functions as well as glomerular filtration rate (e.g. Bonjour, Churchill & Malven, 1969). Pomeranz, Birtch & Barger (1968) have produced reflex responses (from carotid sinuses) or direct responses (stimulating splanchnic nerves) and were able to obtain a reduction in blood flow in the outer cortex, an increase in blood flow in the medulla with no alteration in total renal blood flow. Thus there was a redistribution of blood flow; but de Wardener (1973) thinks it possible that this does not represent changes in true blood flow. More recently DiBona (1977) has reviewed the evidence showing, and he accepts, that there is nervous control of renal tubular sodium reabsorption.

Renin can be released on stimulation; by using an intensity of stimulation of renal nerves which did not reduce total renal blood flow or glomerular filtration rate, there was a response of a release of renin and a reduction in sodium excretion (LaGrange, Sloop & Schmid, 1973); stimulation in a non-filtering kidney releases renin (Johnson, Davis & Witty, 1971), the release of renin in response to stimulation of the renal plexus can be inhibited by propranolol (Johns, Lewis & Singer, 1976), and the renin response to slow haemorrhage was altered by renal denervation (Tanigawa, Dua & Assaykeen, 1974); all these effects were found in anaesthetised animals.

As well as the example by Kidd and his group above (Karim et al., 1972) others have shown that renal efferent nerves can be involved in reflexes originating in the cardiovascular system. Occlusion of the carotid arteries in anaesthetised animals so as to lower the pressure in the carotid sinuses and lessen the stimulus to baroreceptors resulted in vasoconstriction in the kidney (Oberg & White, 1970a, b; Mancia, Shepherd & Donald, 1975; Chapter 7), and an increase in carotid sinus pressure decreased renal resistance (Little, Wennergren & Oberg, 1975; Chapter 7). These same authors (Oberg & White, 1970a, b; Little et al., 1975; Mancia, Shepherd & Donald, 1975) have shown that an increase in activity in afferent nerve fibres from the 'cardiopulmonary area' also affects the efferent renal nerves to decrease renal resistance. It is also pointed out that these two sets of afferent nerves interact, with the nerves from the 'cardiopulmonary area' having a larger effect on renal nerves, and preferentially over their effects in other parts of the body. Both sets of afferent nerves also affect renin release (Little *et al.*, 1975; Chapter 7). Stimulation of receptors in the ventricles depresses renin release (Thames, 1977). A fuller discussion of the interaction of these groups of receptors may be found in recent reviews (Donald & Shepherd, 1978; Thorén, 1979*a*).

Earlier in this chapter during discussion of the nature of the response to stimulation of atrial receptors it was noted that there was a small increase in sodium excretion. All the evidence suggests that efferent nerves to the kidney can cause changes in sodium excretion, though some of the mechanisms are in dispute. Nashat (1974) has enumerated the mechanisms in the kidney known to affect sodium excretion and which could be affected by renal nerves as follows:

1. glomerular filtration and hence the filtered load;
2. the intrarenal distribution of blood flow between groups of nephrons that retain or lose sodium;
3. the reabsorption capacity of the tubular cells brought about by:
    (a) neural mechanisms,
    (b) the presence of specific or non-specific hormones capable of altering tubular function, and
    (c) the physical environment of the tubular cells.

However, there is dispute about the significance of renal nerves in the excretion of sodium, as most experiments have been completed in anaesthetised dogs. But the prevailing opinion is that given by de Wardener (1973) when he concludes, 'it appears that renal function in a denervated kidney in a conscious animal is not distinguishable from that in a normal kidney'. Many reports hold the view that in the conscious animal and man the renal nerves have no function. An argument in favour of this view is that anaesthesia causes an increase in sympathetic 'tone' to the kidney and this allows reductions of this tone to have an effect. For example the most recent investigation with this viewpoint examines renal responses in conscious dogs under stresses of volume expansion and volume depletion (haemorrhage) and concludes that 'renal nerves do not have a significant role in the regulation of sodium excretion in conscious animals' (Lifschitz, 1978).

However, searching in conscious animals which possess many and various mechanisms for the control of sodium excretion by removing one, the renal nerves, appears to be fruitless. Who would remove one of five thermostats from a waterbath and expect the temperature not still to be controlled? Instead it is better to look for examples of evidence which suggest the nerves do have an effect.

There is evidence in conscious animals that psychologically stressful situations lead to profound renal vasoconstriction, which is often abolished or reduced during habituation but may persist in spite of repetition (e.g. Gross & Kirchheim, 1978; Seal & Zbrozyna, 1978) and the effect of carotid occlusion depends on the resting activity in renal nerves (Gross & Kirchheim, 1978). A series of investigations into patients with autonomic failure by Wilcox (Wilcox, Aminoff & Slater, 1977) suggests that their inadequate sodium homeostasis may in part be a result of the diminution of renal nerve activity. An augmented sympathetic tone to the kidneys is said to be a major determinant of salt retention in dogs with congestive heart failure (e.g. Barger, Muldowney & Liebowitz, 1959), with vena caval constriction (e.g. Gill, Carr, Fleischmann, Casper & Bartter, 1967; Azer, Gannon & Kaloyanides, 1972; Slick, DiBona & Kaloyanides, 1974) and in patients with heart failure (e.g. Brod, 1972). These examples are adequate to sustain an argument that renal nerves may have some function in normal sodium homeostasis. Certainly two reviewers (Nashat, 1974; DiBona, 1977) believe that the finding of nerves supplying the proximal and distal tubules and the demonstration, using fluorescence histochemical and electron-microscope techniques, of adrenergic nerve terminals in direct contact with tubule basement membranes, furnishes anatomical evidence to support a neural control of tubular reabsorption.

Thus there is a dispute about the effects of the efferent nerves to the kidney and suggestions that there are no effects which are relevant. But in anaesthetised dogs it appears that efferent renal nerves affect both urine flow and sodium excretion. The reflex effects on these two parameters during the stimulation of atrial receptors will be considered in the next section.

Atrial receptors and efferent renal nerves. With this background it is now possible to consider the effects of atrial receptors on efferent renal nerves. All the investigations to be described have been completed in anaesthetised animals as techniques of stimulating atrial receptors in the conscious animal or man are not yet available.

General experiments, with no specific stimulus to any particular receptors, have been completed by various workers in a similar manner to those experiments in which a heart-rate reflex was sought (see Chapter 5) with similar inconclusive results. For example, Clement, Pelletier & Shepherd (1972) investigated the role of vagal afferent fibres on the regulation of renal nerve activity in anaesthetised rabbits. Both the carotid and aortic sinuses were denervated and action potentials were recorded from the multifibre preparations of efferent sympathetic renal nerves. The blood volume was then altered either by bleeding or infusing dextran – in each instance up to 10% of an estimated blood volume. An increase in blood volume was accompanied by a reduction in renal nerve activity and a decrease in volume, an enhancement of nerve activity. Sectioning the vagi below the diaphragm left the response unaffected but cooling the cervical vagi to 2–5 °C or cutting the cervical vagi abolished the response. The authors concluded that the changes in blood volume affected receptors in the 'cardiopulmonary region' which reflexly altered the sympathetic outflow to the kidney; the afferent path of the reflex(es) lay in the vagi. Though the techniques adopted by Clement *et al.* (1972) did not permit a more definite location of the receptor endings, it was possible that they were investigating in the rabbit a mechanism similar to that described previously by Karim *et al.* (1972) in the dog; however, the limitations of investigation into so-called 'cardiopulmonary receptors', rendering the results of such experiments valueless (except as pilot experiments for laboratory notebooks) have been pointed out in Chapter 3. Claims that the decrease in renal nerve activity resulting from atrial distension causes changes in tubular sodium reabsorption (Prosnitz & DiBona, 1978) should be viewed with caution considering the

Atrial receptors and urine flow

difficulty in completely eliminating secondary haemodynamic changes (see end of this chapter).

Using a discrete stimulus to left atrial receptors, as pointed out above, Karim et al. (1972) recorded action potentials in slips of efferent cardiac nerves, renal nerves, splenic nerves and nerves in the lumbar region as shown in Fig. 10.13. They found that distension of the pulmonary vein–atrial junctions in anaesthetised dogs resulted in a reduction in activity in efferent sympathetic nerves to the kidney, and this response was abolished by cooling the cervical vagal nerve to 5 °C. The activity in the same multifibre preparation was increased by carotid occlusion. A further significant finding was that distension of the vein–atrial junctions resulted in an increase in activity in cardiac sympathetic nerves but no change in activity in sympathetic nerves to the spleen and lumbar region (Fig. 10.14). Since the observations on the renal sympathetic nerves were made in multifibre preparations, the investigation was repeated on single fibre preparations of nerves to the kidney by Scott (1975); the results of Karim et al. (1972) were confirmed. In addition Scott (1975) concluded that the same sympathetic efferent fibre was capable of decreasing its activity in response to stimulation of atrial receptors or systemic arterial baroreceptors. This effect has been confirmed by Linden, Mary & Weatherill (1979b); but an important finding, when the receptors in the two areas were stimulated simultaneously, was that the responses in the renal nerves caused by stimulating atrial receptors were not influenced by changes in carotid sinus pressure (see also Chapter 8).

Recently, Ricksten, Noresson & Thorén (1979) observed a difference in the inhibition of activity in efferent renal nerves in response to volume loading in spontaneously hypertensive rats as compared with normal rats; and claimed that this was a result of resetting of the atrial receptor reflex. This conclusion was not valid. There were no attempts made by location to determine which receptors were involved; the techniques used were occluding the aorta or the pulmonary artery and section of the vagi. At best it may be suggested that cardiac receptors on the left side of the heart *may* be involved.

Before concluding that stimulation of atrial receptors is responsible for the changes observed in the discharge in the renal nerves, it is necessary to consider the nature of the

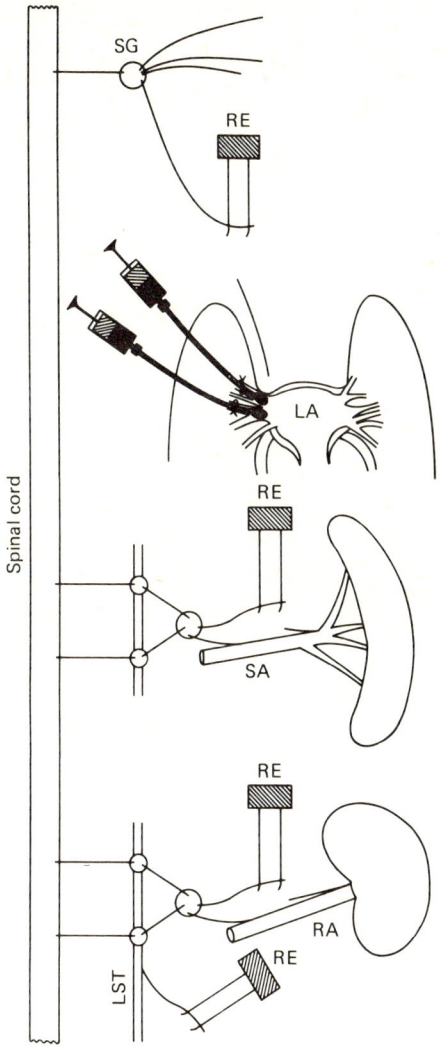

Fig. 10.13. Schematic diagram of the preparation showing position of the balloons and the different sympathetic efferent nerves used for recording. Recording electrodes (RE); stellate ganglion (SG); left atrium (LA); splenic artery (SA); renal artery (RA); lumbar sympathetic trunk (LST). (From Karim et al., 1972.)

Atrial receptors and urine flow

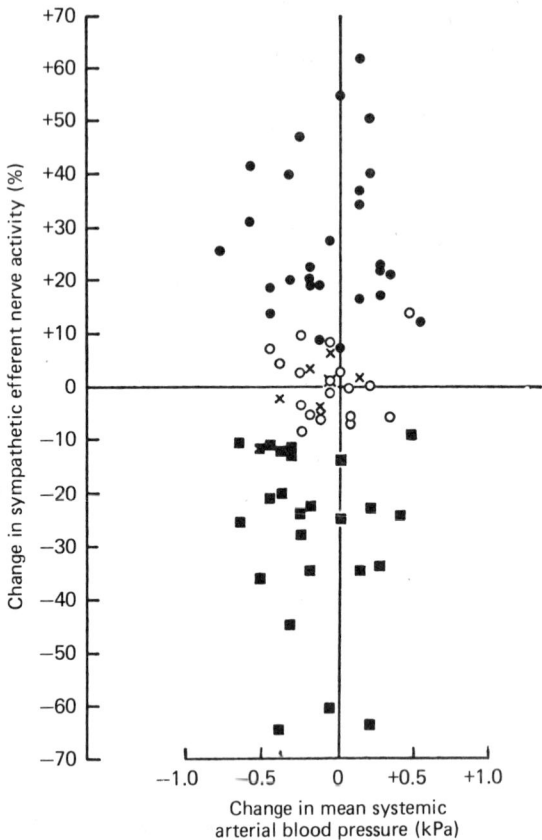

Fig. 10.14. Relationship between sympathetic efferent impulse activity and mean systemic arterial blood pressure during distension of the pulmonary vein–left atrial junctions. Each symbol indicates responses of a group of sympathetic strands; ● cardiac, ○ lumbar, × splenic and ■ renal. (From Karim et al., 1972.)

stimulus in some detail (cf. Chapter 6 when considering the heart-rate reflex). Distension of pulmonary vein–atrial junctions in the manner of Ledsome & Linden (1964b) clearly stimulates the complex unencapsulated nerve endings, i.e. the atrial receptors which discharge into myelinated nerves in the vagi (Kidd et al., 1978). Recent evidence shows that this stimulus also activates nerve endings which discharge into the non-myelinated nerves in the vagi (Kappagoda, Linden & Siva-

Reflex nature of the responses

nanthan, 1977, 1979) and nerve endings which discharge into fibres conveyed in the afferent sympathetic nerves (see Chapter 3 and 6; Holton, 1977). Since cutting the cervical vagi abolished the response in renal nerves to distension of the balloons (Karim *et al.*, 1972) and to changes in blood volume (Clement *et al.*, 1972) it is possible to conclude that in their experiments the sympathetic afferent fibres were not involved in the response elicited in the renal nerves (see below). The only means available at present for separating the effects of distending the pulmonary vein–atrial junctions on myelinated and non-myelinated vagal afferent fibres is graded cold block of the cervical vagi (Kappagoda, Linden & Sivananthan, 1977, 1979; see Chapter 6); earlier in this chapter the technique was referred to, and comments were made on investigations in which it was used to show that Paintal-type atrial receptors discharging into myelinated fibres were the only receptors involved in the reflex diuresis. This technique was not used by either Karim *et al.* (1972) or Clement *et al.* (1972). Both groups of workers cooled the cervical vagi to 5 °C or below and observed that the response was abolished. This temperature would not only block the myelinated fibres but would also block a proportion of the increase in activity in the non-myelinated fibres (Kappagoda, Linden & Sivananthan, 1977, 1979).

The response in renal nerves elicited by Karim *et al.* (1972) was re-investigated using the cold block technique (Kappagoda, Linden, Mary & Weatherill, 1978; Linden *et al.*, 1980*a*). The atrial receptors were stimulated by distending small balloons positioned at the pulmonary vein–atrial junctions. The application of this stimulus was found to reduce the activity in the renal sympathetic nerves as before (Karim *et al.*, 1972). On setting up, the response of an increase in heart rate was first obtained to demonstrate the viability of the preparation and then abolished by the injection of bretylium tosylate (Chapter 6). Linden *et al.* (1979*a*, 1980*a*) examined a total of 111 preparations of renal nerves in 17 dogs. First they demonstrated that the response of an inhibition of activity in renal nerves brought about by stimulating atrial receptors could be maintained for 30 min; thus such a finding showed that this effect could be causally related to the increase in sodium excretion and urine flow (see earlier in the chapter).

Atrial receptors and urine flow

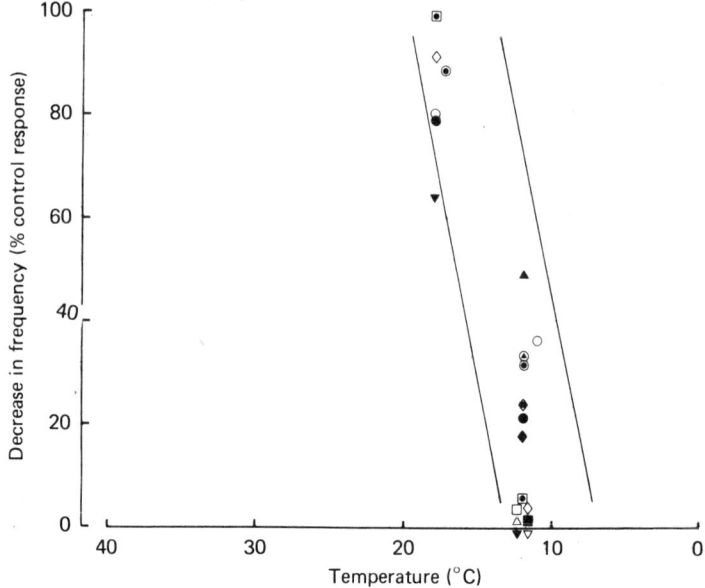

Fig. 10.15. The effect of cooling the vagi on the response in renal nerves during stimulation of atrial receptors. The ordinate shows the magnitude of the response expressed as a percentage of the mean control response with the vagi warm; the abscissa shows temperature of the vagi. The oblique lines are the same as those in Fig. 5 in Kappagoda, Linden & Sivananthan (1979), enclosing most responses in afferent myelinated vagal fibres. Each symbol represents results from one preparation of renal nerve. The response was slightly reduced by cooling the vagi to 18 °C; on cooling to 12 °C the response was markedly reduced or abolished. (From Linden *et al.*, 1980*a*.)

Using the same means of calculation of the effect of graded cooling on the response as that used by Kappagoda, Linden & Sivananthan (1979) (also described earlier in this chapter in relation to the response of the diuresis and in Chapter 6 in relation to the heart-rate reflex), it was shown that the reflex response in the renal nerves at 18 °C was 82 % and at 12 °C was 14 % of the average of the responses with the vagi warm (37 °C) as shown in Fig. 10.15. These effects of cooling were the same as those found in myelinated fibres by Kappagoda, Linden & Sivananthan (1979) (Chapter 6) when examining the heart-rate reflex and when examining the urine response (see earlier in this chapter), but totally unlike the responses of non-myelinated fibres. Thus it was concluded that, as with the heart-rate response and the urine response, the reflex inhibition of renal efferent nerves was caused solely by Paintal-type atrial receptors discharging into vagal myelinated fibres.

To confirm this conclusion Linden et al. (1979a, 1980a) completed a further series of experiments. In six dogs a total of 54 preparations of renal nerve were examined with the vagi at 9 °C – no responses to stimulation of atrial receptors were observed. It is known that at 9 °C the increase in activity in non-myelinated fibres resulting from distension of the small balloons is not affected – these experiments confirmed the above conclusion. The role of these fibres in the response elicited by Clement et al. (1972) remains to be resolved. However, it must be emphasised that neither response appeared to be mediated by afferent fibres conveyed in nerves other than the cervical vagus.

'*Sympathetic*' *afferent fibres and renal nerves.* In anaesthetised dogs, Purtock et al. (1977) studied the effect on renal nerve activity of stimulating electrically the sympathetic chain below the stellate ganglion and above the level of T5 ramus communicans. The vagi were first sectioned and the arterial pressure was maintained at 6.7 kPa to enhance sympathetic activity. The strength of the stimulus was such (6–8 V, 3 ms duration) that it was likely to have activated both myelinated and non-myelinated fibres (see Chapter 7; Peterson & Brown, 1971). When this stimulus was applied at 3 Hz the renal activity in the nerves was diminished and the renal vascular resistance was also reduced. However, when the stimulus was applied at 30 Hz the activity in the renal nerve was diminished transiently and then increased. There were also corresponding changes in renal vascular resistance. In cats, Weaver (1977) also studied the effect of electrical stimulation of sympathetic afferent fibres on the activity in sympathetic nerves to the kidney. The strength of the stimulus applied was 4.0–15.0 V and the duration 0.5 ms. When this stimulus was applied at low frequencies (1–2 Hz) the predominant effect was a reduction in activity in the sympathetic nerves. When the frequency was increased to 10–20 Hz the effect was one of enhanced sympathetic activity. These findings therefore corroborated the findings of Purtock et al. (1977)

above. Weaver *et al.* (1979) in cats with vagal and glossopharyngeal nerves sectioned, and using crude stimuli such as tying sutures to the atria and ventricles, stimulation of nerves, infusion and perfusion, stretching the aorta, have again examined the changes in activity in efferent renal nerves. The biphasic response of excitation followed by inhibition was previously thought to be caused by a single afferent input into long latency supraspinal reflexes (Weaver, 1977); Weaver *et al.* (1979) now accept the more likely explanation that the response may be caused by inputs from the different receptors in the chest having opposite effects. Such findings again emphasise the folly of using the word 'cardiopulmonary' – even with reference to sympathetic afferents (see Chapter 7). Equally difficult to interpret in terms of specific reflex responses and their interaction is the investigation of Reimann & Weaver (1980) where the administration of bradykinin or potassium chloride to the epicardium or within the coronary arteries provoked changes in activity in efferent renal nerves. Using different groups of animals with and without section of vagal and sympathetic afferent nerves it was concluded that 'cardiac sympathetic afferent neurones could have significant excitatory influences on the cardiovascular system' even in the presence of 'inhibitory afferent groups'. The stimuli to receptors would obviously be so diffuse, and at various sites, not demonstrably the same under the various conditions, that it could be argued that possible interaction between reflexes had not occurred; it is not possible to conclude that interaction has taken place from observation of multifibre preparations (see Chapter 8). There were no criteria on which to accept even that reflex pathways were involved. The observations, under these conditions, seem particularly valueless.

Weaver (1977) also examined the effect of increasing the blood volume on the activity in renal nerves in these animals. It should be appreciated that these animals had denervated baroreceptors and hence were comparable to rabbits investigated by Clement *et al.* (1972). Weaver (1977) found that increasing the plasma volume by 20–25% resulted in an increase in central venous pressure (approximately 0.4 kPa) and a reduction in renal nerve activity by 20–30%. This response was not correlated with the concurrent increments in systemic pressure. Sectioning the 'cardiopulmonary' sympathetic afferent nerves (T1–T6) abolished this effect. There is a contradiction between these findings in the cat and those described by Clement et al. (1972) who observed no response in renal nerves to infusion following cervical vagal cooling or section in the rabbit with sino-aortic denervation even though there has been a decrease in activity in efferent renal nerves before section of 41 %. Weaver (1977) has suggested that this apparent discrepancy was probably not attributable to a species difference but could have arisen as a result of the experimental protocol adopted, claiming that insufficient time had elapsed after vagotomy in the experiments of other workers for the reflexes mediated by sympathetic afferents to become operational. One other explanation could be that the stimulus applied by Clement et al. (1972) (i.e. infusion of $5.4 \text{ cm}^3 \cdot \text{kg}^{-1}$ in a rabbit) was inadequate though such an explanation seems unlikely because the blood pressure increased by approximately 4 kPa in these experiments. Thus there is no explanation readily available at the moment to account for this discrepancy. Recently Echtenkamp & Gilmore (1980) have stated in the cat that 'No evidence was found for a significant contribution from sympathetic afferent nerves.' Unfortunately this investigation does not seem to carry the subject much further. They studied anaesthetised cats and investigated the effects of noradrenaline, blood volume expansion and of veratrine on the activity in the renal nerves before and after vagotomy and sino-aortic denervation. They concluded that there is no evidence for a significant contribution from sympathetic afferent nerves to changes in renal nerve activity caused by the three interventions used. However, these conclusions are not justified by the results presented. First, efferent activity of the whole left renal nerves was recorded and zero level of activity in the renal nerves was determined at the end of the experiment by crushing the central end of the nerve. The sensitivity of this technique in detecting small changes in renal nerve activity is unknown; a small change relative to the activity of the whole nerve is not easy to measure. Furthermore, no evidence was presented that the 'noise' level of activity in the nerve will remain constant throughout the experiments. Therefore small changes, though undetected, can still occur in preparations with an intact afferent sympathetic nerve. Secondly, the distinction drawn by the report between stimulation of 'high-pressure receptors' and 'low-pressure receptors' is less than meaningful. During the different stimuli applied, the pressures in the chambers of the heart were not measured. In fact a multitude of different receptors could be involved as a result of the stimuli used and the interaction or summation of the effects of many of these receptors is unknown.

However, whether or not the sympathetic afferent fibres activated by Purtock et al. (1977) and by Weaver (1977) originated in the atria cannot be determined from their experiments using electrical stimulation. That it is unlikely that atrial receptors could be involved is indicated by some experiments of Holton (1977). Distension of balloons located at the pulmonary vein–atrial junctions was shown to activate fibres traversing the rami communicantes in T1–T4; also these fibres increased their activity during intravenous infusions of fluid. The changes in atrial pressure required to cause this increased activity were greater than those noted by Weaver (1977) – a finding which was supported by investigations described by Kostreva et al. (1975). Therefore it is unlikely that the afferent fibres involved in the response evoked by infusions (Weaver, 1977) were the same as those examined by Holton (1977). This proposition is also consistent with the inability of Karim et al. (1972), Kappagoda, Linden, Mary & Weatherill (1978) and Linden et al. (1980a) to demonstrate a reduction in the activity in sympathetic nerves to the kidney after blocking transmission in the cervical vagi. Further evidence against the proposition of Purtock et al. (1977) and Weaver (1977) was obtained from Linden et al. (1980a) who studied a fourth group of dogs. These anaesthetised dogs were prepared as the others but were given atropine. Following the demonstration of a reduction in activity in renal nerves in response to stimulation of atrial receptors, the vagi were sectioned in the neck and the effect of distension of the balloons on activity in renal nerves was studied. In the 24 preparations of renal nerves the inhibition was not present after vagal section; this observation eliminates the 'sympathetic' afferent pathway as a potential part of this reflex. In addition in 21 of the preparations the abolition of the response was tested again at various times up to 6 h after vagotomy and no response was ever observed. This result refutes the suggestion of Weaver

(1977) that changes in activity in 'sympathetic' afferents from the 'cardiopulmonary region' may have been masked by the immediate effects of these techniques; in this study no influence of the activation of sympathetic afferent nerves was observed any time up to 6 h after vagotomy.

These results also refute the conclusion of Thorén (1979a) that, 'Activation of the atrial C-fibres is likely to contribute to the renal sympathetic nerve withdrawal because of the pronounced inhibitory effect the latter receptors have on the sympathetic nerve traffic to the kidney even at the very low level of activation (Little et al., 1975).'

Conclusion. From the investigations discussed above, it is possible to draw the following conclusions in relation to the atrial receptors and the renal nerves:
  1. Stimulation of the complex unencapsulated nerve endings (Paintal-type) which discharge into the myelinated vagal fibres results in a reflex inhibition of the activity in the sympathetic nerves to the kidney.
  2. There is, as yet, no direct evidence to indicate that stimulation of receptors which discharge into non-myelinated vagal afferents exerts a similar influence on the sympathetic nerves to the kidney – though such a role could be expected as a part of the generalised vasomotor inhibition attributed to these nerves (cf. Thorén, 1979a, b).
  3. A relationship between the 'sympathetic' afferent fibres originating in the atria and the renal sympathetic nerves has not been demonstrated.

Atrial receptors, renal nerves and the urine response

Recent evidence obtained by Kappagoda, Linden & Sreeharan (1979) shows that the renal nerves could yet play a role in modifying the response by altering the excretion of sodium when atrial receptors are stimulated. In this preliminary report Kappagoda, Linden & Sreeharan (1979) used large balloons to block the mitral orifice and small balloons to stimulate only the atrial receptors and the urine responses were evoked; again in chloralose-anaesthetised dogs. The dogs were prepared with one kidney denervated and one remained innervated (Kappagoda,

Linden & Sreeharan, 1979). The urine was collected every 10 min from a cannula in each ureter.

Interim results suggest that with the large balloon (19 experiments) there was an increase in urine flow in the innervated kidney of $100\% \pm 19.4$ (S.E.M.) and in the denervated of $87\% \pm 18.8$ (S.E.M.); and the difference was statistically significant ($P < 0.01$). Sodium excretion increased by 74% (± 22.5) in the innervated and 43.8% (± 21.4) in the denervated kidney. Though the change in the denervated kidney was not in itself significant, the difference between the two responses of the two kidneys was significantly different ($P < 0.01$). Thus the innervated kidney excreted more water and more sodium than the denervated kidney.

With the small balloons (12 experiments) and thus less stimulus, the responses were smaller but similar. There were significant ($P < 0.001$) increases in urine flow of $63\% \pm 11.1$ (S.E.M.) and $53\% \pm 8.5$ (S.E.M.) in the innervated and denervated kidneys respectively. The respective increases in sodium excretion of $30\% \pm 8.2$ (S.E.M.) and $14\% \pm 6.4$ (S.E.M.) were also statistically significant ($P < 0.05$). The differences in the diuretic and natriuretic responses between the two kidneys were statistically significant ($P < 0.05$). However, though the changes in sodium excretion in the innervated kidney were always in a positive direction those in the denervated kidney varied about the line of no change. We concluded that the renal nerves contribute significantly to the increase in urine flow and sodium excretion that result from stimulation of left atrial receptors; but nevertheless the main efferent pathway is humoral.

In a series of experiments in conscious animals Reinhardt and his group (Reinhardt, Kaczmarcyzk, Eisele, Arnold, Eigenheer & Kuhl, 1977; Kaczmarczyk et al., 1978) have increased the left atrial pressure by tightening a purse string around the mitral orifice. Having fed groups of dogs on high and low sodium diets they claimed that their results allowed the conclusion that stimulation of intrathoracic receptors augments renal sodium excretion even in a state of high tubular reabsorption, that intrathoracic receptors are involved in regulation of body fluids and these mechanisms operate independently of renal blood flow. It was not possible to control relevant variables in these experiments. For example, the mean arterial blood pressure rose during atrial distension by 2.0 kPa (Reinhardt et al., 1977) and 2.5 kPa (Kaczmarczyk et al., 1978); since renal blood flow did not change (Kaczmarczyk et al., 1978) it was argued that the natriuretic response seen in conscious dogs occurred independently of renal blood flow. However, changes in renal perfusion pressure or differential changes in flow in renal medulla and cortex are possible explanations. Recently Reinhardt, Kaczmarczyk, Mohnhaupt & Simgen (1980a, b) have claimed that distending the left atrium whilst maintaining renal perfusion pressure constant still results in a natriuresis. They investigated four unanaesthetised dogs kept on high sodium intake and measured the natriuresis associated with distension of the left atrium by narrowing the mitral annulus, first when the renal perfusion pressure was allowed to increase with the arterial blood pressure as a result of left atrial distension and secondly after preventing changes in renal perfusion pressure. Reinhardt et al. (1980a) concluded that the response of natriuresis 'is not mediated by an augmentation of renal perfusion pressure'. However, first, it is not yet known whether this urine response to the intervention of Reinhardt et al. (1980a), involves atrial receptors at all and particularly those attached to myelinated vagal fibres, as described by Sivananthan et al. (1981). Secondly, there were significant differences in the baseline values of urine flow (which were used in the calculation of sodium excretion) and in heart rate (i.e. during the control period before distension) between the two experiments with and without constant renal perfusion pressure; also, the values of arterial blood pressure are not fully given. Therefore it is not possible to exclude an effect of changing baseline values on the responses studied. Thirdly, in their Table 1 Reinhardt et al. (1980a) state that in the dogs with mean body weight of 10.9 kg, the mean value of sodium excretion during elevation in renal perfusion pressure (112.27 μmol·min^{-1}) was greater by 10.9 μmol·min^{-1} than that when the renal perfusion pressure was constant (101.37 μmol·min^{-1}). In fact if the period after release of distension of the left atrium was included in the analysis, to constitute an average control period (before and after), then the response of an increase in sodium excretion with constant perfusion pressure would be further reduced relative to that when renal perfusion pressure was allowed to increase. Fourthly, in keeping the renal perfusion pressure constant, pulsatile pressure was markedly reduced, a state incomparable with that involving pulsatile renal perfusion pressure.

Finally, it is not surprising that any contribution to the natriuretic response attributable to renal perfusion pressure *per se* would be small in the experimental setting of Reinhardt *et al.* (1980*a*); many other variables are involved in changes in sodium excretion e.g. the neuro-humoral mechanisms associated with increase in heart rate and blood pressure. In a recent review article the Reinhardt group suggest that humoral mechanisms involving the renin–angiotensin system are involved in natriuretic responses observed in their experiment (Reinhardt *et al.*, 1980*b*). Therefore, the report of Reinhardt *et al.* (1980*a*) first, does not provide evidence that the atrial receptors are involved in the natriuresis in response to distension of the left atrium; this response is likely to involve various mechanisms other than atrial receptors. Secondly, although the mechanism attributable to the increases in renal perfusion pressure would be a minor one, the report of Reinhardt *et al.* (1980*a*) does not unequivocally exclude this factor.

These experiments provide little evidence for or against the mechanisms involved in reflexes from atrial receptors. As it is not possible to control all the necessary variables in conscious animals it is difficult to provide evidence adequate to demonstrate mechanisms. But it is probable that all the mechanisms involved following stimulation of atrial receptors, blood-borne agent, renal nerves and haemodynamic factor, were operative in these animals – plus the stimulation of many other receptors.

However, in Leeds, we were not sure that the variable but statistically significant increase in sodium excretion we had observed in the denervated kidney was biologically significant or whether it could be caused by the preparation not being fully 'controlled'. Having the distinct impression that small variations in blood pressure and heart rate caused large changes in sodium excretion we (Linden & Sreeharan) formed a hypothesis that only water was excreted as a result of stimulating atrial receptors. The hypothesis was tested in a series of experiments (Linden & Sreeharan, 1979, 1981). The investigation was made solely to examine the humoral nature of the diuretic and natriuretic responses to stimulation of atrial receptors; the heart and kidney were 'pharmacologically denervated' and the blood pressure and heart rate remained constant throughout each experiment.

Dogs were anaesthetised with chloralose and the chest opened on the left side. The following drugs were administered intravenously, bretylium tosylate 10 mg·kg^{-1}, atropine 0.5 mg·kg^{-1} and atenolol 2 mg·kg^{-1}. The left atrial receptors were stimulated by distending small balloons located in the pulmonary vein–atrial junctions and the left atrial appendage. The urine was collected through ureteric cannulae over 10 min periods and the concentration of sodium in the urine was analysed using an Atomic Absorption Spectrophotometer (Perkin & Elmer, Model 103).

The balloons were distended eleven times in eight dogs. The left atrial pressure, femoral arterial pressure and heart rate during the test period were 0.8 ± 0.20 kPa, 15.8 ± 1.91 kPa and 110 ± 22.1 beats·min^{-1} respectively (mean$\pm$S.D.); in each animal they did not change significantly ($P > 0.1$; t-test for paired data) from the respective control values of 0.8 ± 0.19 kPa, 15.9 ± 1.86 kPa and 110 ± 21.5 beats·min^{-1} (mean$\pm$S.D.).

The urine flow increased significantly ($P < 0.001$, t-test for paired data) from 0.5 ± 0.24 cm^3·min^{-1} (mean$\pm$S.D.) during the control periods to 0.7 ± 0.26 cm^3·min^{-1} (mean$\pm$S.D.) during the test period (Fig. 10.16); the urinary sodium concentration decreased significantly ($P < 0.005$, t-test for paired data) from 133.4 ± 85.55 mmol·litre^{-1} to 106.9 ± 83.66 mmol·litre^{-1} (mean $\pm$S.D.) (Fig. 10.17) while the sodium excretion did not change significantly ($P > 0.7$; t-test for paired data) during the control (72.2 ± 65.09 μmol·min^{-1}) and test periods (72.9 ± 70.65 μmol·min^{-1}) (mean$\pm$S.D.) (Fig. 10.18).

Thus when changes in the haemodynamic state of the animal were prevented, as evidenced by the constancy of heart rate, arterial pressure and atrial pressure, stimulation of atrial receptors resulted only in an increase in excretion of water – there was no increase in sodium excretion. Looking back through our records from previous experiments it is now possible to recognise a positive correlation between concomitant changes in heart rate and sodium excretion, adding a point in favour of the above conclusion. A conclusion from the above evidence is that a change in the haemodynamic state causes a change in sodium excretion and probably in urine flow; such a haemodynamic factor has been suggested before (Arndt et al., 1963).

Atrial receptors and urine flow

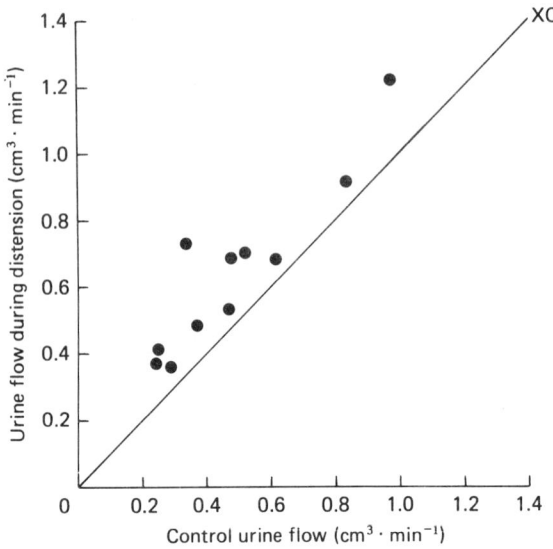

Fig. 10.16. Effect of distending small balloons on urine flow. Ordinate: urine flow during distension, $cm^3 \cdot min^{-1}$. Abscissa: urine flow during control periods, $cm^3 \cdot min^{-1}$. (From Linden & Sreeharan, 1981.)

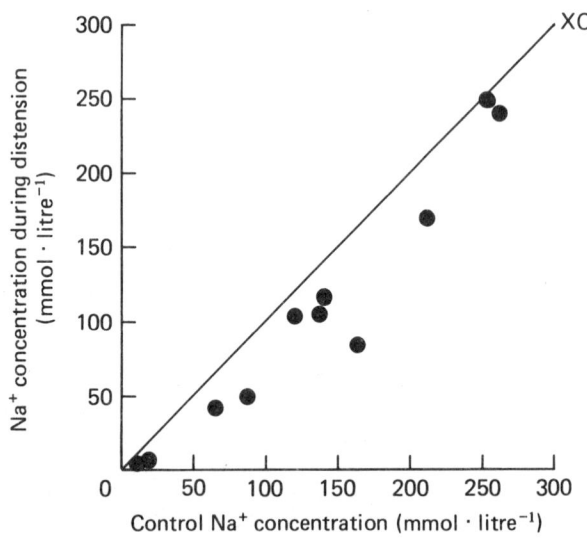

Fig. 10.17. Effect of distension of small balloons on sodium concentration in urine of dogs with results shown in Fig. 10.16. Ordinate, sodium concentration during diuresis, $mmol \cdot litre^{-1}$. Abscissa, sodium concentration during control periods, $mmol \cdot litre^{-1}$. (From Linden & Sreeharan, 1981.)

Note on 'volume receptors'

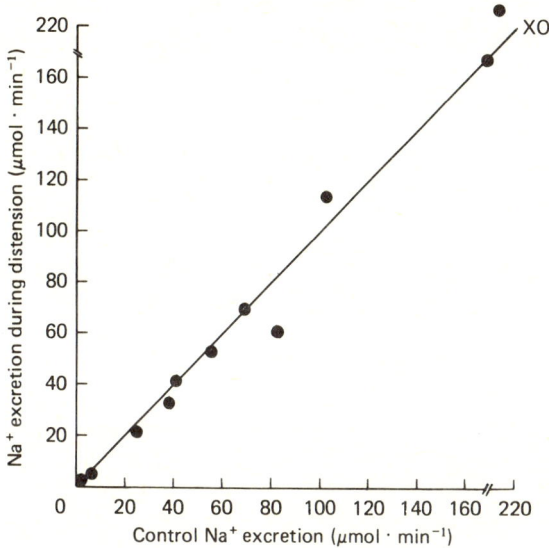

Fig. 10.18. Effect of distension of small balloons on sodium excretion in urine of dogs with results shown in Fig. 10.16. Ordinate: sodium excretion during diuresis, μmol·min^{-1}. Abscissa: sodium excretion during control periods, μmol·min^{-1}. (From Linden & Sreeharan, 1981.)

Conclusions

Thus in summary of evidence presented in this chapter, we conclude that stimulation of Paintal-type atrial receptors results in an increase in urine flow and sodium excretion with the afferent nerves solely myelinated nerves in the vagi; the efferent limb of the reflex consists of a humoral agent, possibly diuretic, affecting only water excretion and efferent sympathetic nerves to the kidney affecting both water and sodium excretion. There is a haemodynamic contribution to water and sodium excretion secondary to the change in heart rate (which is itself brought about by activity solely in efferent cardiac sympathetic nerves; see Chapter 6).

Note on 'volume receptors'

As pointed out in Chapter 9 'volume receptors', as part of a mechanism for the control of blood volume, have been postulated (e.g. Gauer & Henry, 1963, 1976). Consideration of the control of blood volume is too large a topic to discuss here but must at least involve consideration of the intake and output of salt and water. So far we have considered the role of atrial receptors as they affect salt and water excretion, but this does not necessarily demonstrate a control mechanism; some negative feedback on blood volume must eventually be demonstrated. The evidence from the examination of the receptors themselves is inadequate. For instance there is no basis for the oft repeated claim that the frequency of discharge of atrial receptors signals blood volume (e.g. Gauer & Henry, 1956; Henry & Pearce, 1956). In investigating this problem, little is to be gained by a comparison of discharges of atrial and systemic baroreceptors during infusion and bleeding (Gupta et al., 1966; Knutsson & Sjöstrand, 1974) because there is no information as to the quantitative effects at second-order neurones; it is almost incidental that, in addition, there was no certainty that either group was examining atrial receptors; they did not locate the endings.

However, this complex reflex response *could* be included in theories involving control of the functions of the heart and kidney. For instance, and first, to repeat, stimulation of atrial receptors involves two responses: an increase in heart rate resulting from the changes only in efferent sympathetic nerves (and no positive inotropic response) and an increase in urine flow, but no sodium excretion, caused by a blood-borne diuretic substance and involving changes in activity in efferent sympathetic nerves to the kidney possibly involving renal blood flow, but affecting both water and sodium excretion. The functional significance of this reflex has been postulated (Linden, 1973, 1975) as possibly being involved in the control of heart volumes in that an increase in atrial receptor discharge increases heart rate and this in turn decreases heart volumes; the increase in receptor discharge also causes an increase in urine flow which would cause a decrease in extracellular liquid, blood volume, and thus heart volume. Such a hypothesis would envisage the atrial receptors as being the first link in the negative feedback on heart volumes.

This hypothesis does not completely deny the working hypothesis of Gauer & Henry (1963) in which they insist that the atrial receptors are involved in the control of blood volume, but it must be remembered that there are no cause and effect relationships existing which would provide the evidence that blood volume is regulated by atrial receptors. It is difficult not to hold the view that extracellular fluid is not regulated by a single mechanism but by many mechanisms; the atrial reflex may be only one part of a complex group of mechanisms and its importance is certainly not known. However, the fact that atrial receptors may not influence the concentration of antidiuretic hormone in the blood as claimed by Gauer & Henry (1963) and others, but possibly cause an increase in a 'diuretic substance' (see above) does not alter the argument for or against the atrial receptors being a possible control mechanism related to blood volume.

As opposed to the control of the output of salt and water the intake of water has received little attention in investigations of the function of atrial receptors. Fitzsimons (e.g. 1972, 1979) has often stated that atrial receptors affect thirst, an increase in discharge causing inhibition of drinking; there is no evidence definitely to support such a statement. The literature relating to the mechanisms of thirst, whether thirst is important to the intake of water and the psychology of thirst, have led to an enormous amount of literature too vast to review here, but reference to Epstein, Kissileff & Stellar (1973) and Fitzsimons (1979) would illustrate the magnitude of the concept which has arisen out of a paucity of evidence. However, recently Fitzsimons & Moore-Gillon (1980) have produced preliminary evidence that the left atrial receptors may be involved in the thirst mechanism by distending balloons in the pulmonary vein–atrial junctions of conscious dogs and inhibited drinking. They have not fully excluded the participation of other receptors in this response, e.g. systemic baroreceptors could be involved. Indeed Fitzsimons (1979, pp. 525–6) suggests stretch receptors in the walls of the 'low pressure thoracic circulation', 'stretch receptors elsewhere in the body and arterial baroreceptors' and 'chemoreceptors in various parts of the body' may be involved in the thirst mechanism; there is little evidence in support of any of these suggestions. A marvellous thought is that, if the suggestion that atrial receptors affect thirst could be confirmed, the evidence would be beginning to suggest that atrial receptors *could* provide a major component in the control of water balance and therefore in the control of extracellular liquid and blood volume.

11 ATRIAL RECEPTORS IN DISEASE

Of necessity, because there are no adequate models of diseases of the heart and circulation, all the discussion in this chapter will be speculative – there is little or no evidence. Most of the experiments and comment rightly concern receptors from the ventricle, and again mostly concern receptors discharging into non-myelinated fibres. For more extensive reviews and further comments on the difficulties of extrapolation, see Goetz et al. (1975), Donald & Shepherd (1978) and Thorén (1979a). It is difficult not to agree with Donald & Shepherd (1978) who conclude, 'From the foregoing analysis, it is evident that the present knowledge of cardiovascular perturbations caused by cardiopulmonary receptors in human disease is rudimentary.'

There is a temptation to extrapolate too extensively from the findings in experimental animals in order to explain the clinical manifestations of heart disease. But an attempt will be made here to explore the possible links between disturbances in the function of the complex unencapsulated nerve endings in the atria and certain pathological changes in the circulation which involve changes in heart volumes.

For reasons discussed fully in Chapter 3, changes in the volume of the atria will influence the number and frequency of the action potentials generated by the receptor endings in the atrial wall. There is some evidence in the 'normal' dog that changes in the size of the chamber affect the discharge from these receptors and some extrapolation from this data may be allowed. As already indicated in Chapter 3, the natural stimulus to the complex unencapsulated nerve endings (Paintal-type atrial receptors) is a function of the tension generated in the tissues underlying the receptors. For instance, Kidd et al. (1978) examined the electrophysiological behaviour of receptor endings in the atrial wall when this part of the wall was in the whole

Atrial receptors in disease

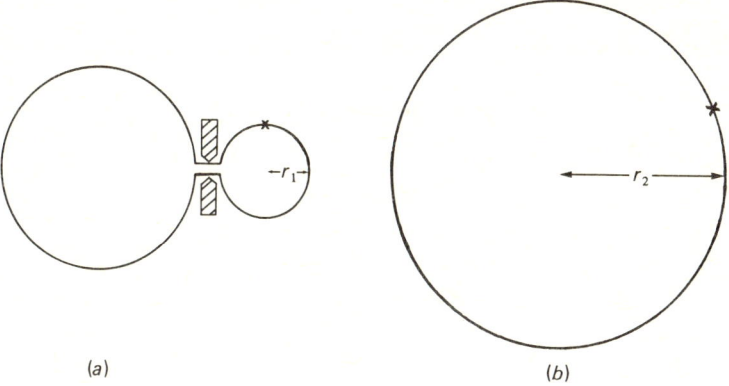

Fig. 11.1. Diagram representing the left atrium as a cylinder cut transversely. (a) with a clamp isolating a pouch of the left atrium; (b) with clamp removed. The ratio $r_1:r_2$ is 0.4:1.5. The tension in the atrial wall at the point × in each figure is proportional, at equivalent pressure, to the radius. (From Ledsome & Linden, 1967.)

atrium and when it was incorporated into a smaller atrial pouch; the same receptor being examined in both chambers. It was shown that receptors examined under the latter condition generated action potentials at a considerably greater threshold. These findings are in accordance with the Law of Laplace (see Chapter 3). The atrial wall when forming part of the pouch requires a greater internal pressure in the chamber to attain a given tension than it does when forming a part of the intact atrium; the diameter of the pouch being smaller than that of the whole atrium (Fig. 11.1).

Apart from generalised changes in the tension of the atrial wall, it is possible also for the tension to alter in a localised manner in the immediate environment of the receptor ending – either due to a change in the shape and size of the atrium or due to the influence of inotropic agents (see Chapter 3).

Therefore extrapolating from the evidence obtained in the heart of the normal animal it is expected that there will be an increase in discharge from atrial receptors with increasing dilatation of the heart, unless the atrial receptors are defective as a result of the disease process.

Atrial receptors in heart failure

Left ventricular failure usually results in an increase in pressure in and size of the left atrium. As pointed out above if such a change were to occur acutely it is likely that the discharge from the complex unencapsulated nerve endings would increase. On the other hand in congestive heart failure, a more insidious change may not necessarily produce similar increments in the activity in these nerves. The conditions immediately around the receptor are not necessarily the same as in the normal endocardium, e.g. when staining for atrial receptors in the human appendage, removed at operation for mitral stenosis, it was evident that the penetration of the stains was much more difficult to obtain, due to thickened endocardium; and the tissues were disordered (Saunders, 1979). Thickening of the endocardium with age has also been reported by MacMillan & Lev (1959) and by Zehr, Hawe, Tsakiris, Rastelli, McGoon & Seger (1971) who showed fibrosis and calcification of the atrial wall in chronic mitral stenosis in dogs. Such thickening might damage atrial receptors and lead to a different pressure/stretch relationship of these receptors.

Also, Greenberg et al. (1973) and Zucker, Earle & Gilmore (1977) have shown that in dogs in a chronic state of congestive cardiac failure there is a reduction in the discharge from the complex unencapsulated nerve endings in response to increments in left atrial pressure (Fig. 11.2) at higher atrial pressures than in the normal dog. Thus there has been a change in the 'transducer properties' of the atrium as a result of damage to the receptor itself or an alteration in the compliance of the atrium. Zucker, Earle & Gilmore (1977) have claimed that some changes in compliance and destruction of atrial receptors do occur. The changes in atrial compliance were based on observations in four dogs (two normal and two in heart failure) and were limited to the atrial appendage alone. From compliance curves published in Fig. 3 of their paper it appears that in the control animals the appendage had a diameter of less than 2 mm whilst in the animals in heart failure, the appendage had a diameter of 18 mm – the diameters being measured by microsonometry. If the atrial receptors were functioning normally, the discharge from them should have been greater in the

Atrial receptors in heart failure

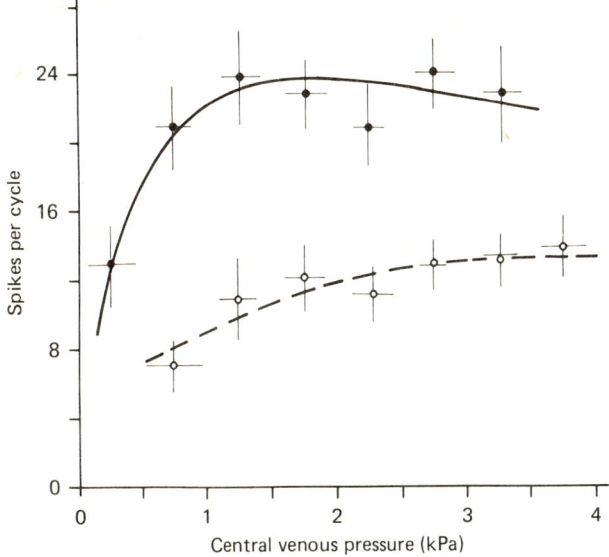

Fig. 11.2. Frequency of atrial receptor discharge in spikes per cardiac cycle plotted against mean central venous pressure; observations grouped in increments of 0.5 kPa. Broken line, experimental group; solid line, controls. Vertical and horizontal bars indicate ±s.e. (From Greenberg et al., 1973.)

diseased dogs. However, Zucker, Earle & Gilmore (1979) claimed that there was some destruction of atrial receptors. Because of difficulties in obtaining comparable areas of atrial tissue for histology and of the capricious nature of the methylene blue staining technique, it is doubtful whether this claim can be sustained. But in spite of this criticism it is likely that the compliance of the atrial wall was less in the diseased animals and the discharge was less at higher atrial pressures (see above). Therefore the basic proposition that chronic heart failure is accompanied by changes in the transducer properties of the atrial receptors appears to be a likely mechanism to explain the impairment of their function.

It is a matter of speculation to suggest that these changes in transducer properties of atrial receptors can relate to the retention of liquid in patients with chronic heart failure. It has been suggested that the above observations are compatible with such claims and it is an even greater speculation to link atrial receptors further with the failure in the regulation of the secretion of ADH in patients with chronic mitral stenosis (see Zucker, Earle & Gilmore, 1977 for discussion). As indicated in Chapter 10, the link between the atrial receptors and the secretion of ADH remains to be established. Pursuing this topic further Zucker, Share & Gilmore (1979) have examined the renal effects of distending a balloon in the left atrium in normal dogs and dogs with chronic congestive heart failure, measuring the concentration of ADH in the plasma by a radioimmunoassay. This investigation has been criticised in Chapter 10, and though the data are suggestive, there is certainly doubt that this cause and effect relationship has been established. It is sufficient to add here that though in the heart failure dogs they were unable to demonstrate a diuresis in response to distension of the balloons (they were successful in the normal dogs), they did obtain a fall in the concentration of ADH. It is interesting to note these responses in view of the fact that this group claimed malfunction of atrial receptors with histological evidence of deformity, and yet continue to claim a relationship between stimulation of atrial receptors and the release of ADH. As pointed out in Chapter 10, at least one other explanation of that finding is that a substance other than ADH is responsible for the diuresis in their normal dogs and is not released during distension of the balloon in the dogs with heart failure.

Yaron & Bennett (1978) re-investigated the mechanism of impaired water excretion in acute right ventricular failure in conscious dogs. They obstructed the flow of blood through the pulmonary artery by distension of a chronically implanted balloon and observed an increase in end-diastolic pressure in the right ventricle, a fall in left atrial pressure, and an increase in mean arterial pressure. These haemodynamic changes were accompanied by a reduction in both the flow of urine and the free water clearance, with an increase in the concentration of ADH. The authors concluded that the fall in the pressure in the left atrium was causally related to the changes in urine flow and ADH concentration.

However, many reflexes from the 'cardiopulmonary area' could have been involved other than in atrial receptors in the left atrium (see Chapter 7). As one example, receptors which could have been stimulated directly by the balloon, regardless of secondary effects, have been described in the pulmonary artery (Bianconi & Green, 1959; Coleridge & Kidd, 1960) and these receptors when stimulated have been shown to cause changes in vascular resistance in the limb (Ledsome & Kan, 1977). The entire experiment was performed against a background of an infusion of Ringer lactate at a rate of approximately 16 cm$^3 \cdot$min^{-1} during the initial control period and 12 cm$^3 \cdot$min^{-1} during the test period. The obstruction to the flow of blood through the pulmonary artery was accompanied by an increase in systemic pressure indicating a massive increase in sympathetic activity. It is not possible from this evidence to link the activity of receptors in the chest with the regulation of ADH in chronic heart failure.

The question of the relationship of atrial receptors, ADH and disease is taken up in anecdotal reports which claim to demonstrate the effect of destruction of reflex pathways involving atrial receptors and ADH. For instance, Boasberg et al. (1977) correlated concentration of vasopressin in the plasma with renal water handling during immersion in two normal subjects and in two patients with advanced intrathoracic carcinoma and evidence of disordered autonomic function including orthostatic hypotension. The normal subjects showed an increase in free water clearance during immersion in spite of no change in the concentration of vasopressin assayed by radioimmunoassay. In contrast both patients with cancer showed an increased plasma concentration of vasopressin which remained elevated during the period of immersion. In spite of the persistently elevated concentration of vasopressin, one of the patients exhibited a marked increase in free water clearance during immersion. The complexity of the results of immersion experiments has been discussed in Chapter 9; added to that complexity in these observations are the destructive effects of the cancerous process. To allude that only the nerve fibres in the vagi attached to atrial receptors are destroyed in this process is bordering on fantasy. It does not appear that this sort of experiment, and particularly in only two patients, contributes anything at all towards explaining the mechanism involved during stimulation of atrial receptors. Such criticism, however, should not deter the search for, and investigation of, patients with purer autonomic nervous dysfunction, which could provide evidence for or against the involvement of these atrial reflexes in man.

The renin–angiotensin–aldosterone system has been

Atrial receptors in disease

implicated in the development of fluid retention which accompanies chronic heart failure in man (e.g. Nicholls, Espiner, Donald & Hughes, 1974) and in an animal model (e.g. Watkins, Burton, Haber, Cant, Smith & Barger, 1976). Brennan *et al.* (1971) using balloons in the right and left atria, suggested that right atrial receptors (and not left atrial receptors) affect the concentration of renin in plasma. They were attempting to involve atrial receptors in the renin–angiotensin–aldosterone theory but their evidence does not provide support; no reflex involvement at all was demonstrated. Zehr *et al.* (1976) distended a large balloon in the left atrium, obstructing the mitral orifice to raise the left atrial pressure about 0.5 kPa, and showed a reduction in plasma renin from an innervated kidney, but not denervated and with the vagi intact but not when sectioned. Atrial receptors obviously could be implicated but the possibility that other receptors were involved has not been eliminated; e.g. arterial baroreceptors will have changed their discharge and sectioning the vagi as a technique for demonstrating the previous involvement of afferent fibres from atrial receptors is not recommended (see Chapter 4). These two reports are examples of attempts to involve the atrial receptors and the renin–angiotensin–aldosterone system in an explanation of the retention of liquid in heart failure; their evidence is incomplete and they fail. However, it is an interesting idea in view of the evidence of changes in the transducer properties of the atrial receptors in heart failure (see earlier in this chapter). Though it is not possible to implicate atrial receptors in this way it should be valuable to continue to challenge this hypothesis. For example, an evaluation of the role of the left atrial receptors in the preparation of Gill *et al.* (1967) in which ascites is produced chronically by constriction of the thoracic inferior vena cava in conscious dogs in the manner described in Chapters 6 and 10, may unravel any chronic changes in their function. Better still would be the same proper evaluation in spontaneously occurring heart failure in animals, to continue the examination of the hypothesis that a lower discharge of left atrial receptors causes a retention of liquid.

In conclusion it is suggested that there is a considerable body of circumstantial evidence suggesting links between atrial receptors and various aspects of the syndrome of congestive

Atrial receptors and cardiac arrhythmias

An association between paroxysmal supraventricular tachycardia and urine flow has been observed clinically for many years (e.g. Wenkebach & Winterberg, 1927; Jones, 1954; Kilburn, 1963; Wood, 1963; Ghose, Jockes & Kyriacou, 1965; Luria, Adelson & Lockaya, 1966; Kinney, Stein & DiScala, 1974). One investigation was reported to the British Cardiac Society in 1961 by Paul Wood and later his observations were published posthumously (Wood, 1963). Wood (1963) related the diuresis to a rapid heart rate of long duration (> 10 min); diuresis was present in over 60% of patients with paroxysmal lone atrial fibrillation or flutter. Although Wood (1963) reported that in a typical attack the urine had a low specific gravity and electrolyte content, there was an increase in sodium excretion (Fig. 11.3). Wood (1963) was of the opinion that this diuresis was 'due to an increase in the volume of blood in the left atrium and resembles the diuresis produced experimentally by inflating a balloon in that chamber'. He was referring to the experiments of Henry *et al.* (1956). However, if reference is made to the evidence in Chapter 10 it will be seen that during distension of balloons in the left atrium the increased excretion of sodium does not parallel the increased excretion of water. If the atrial receptors are involved in this phenomenon there is also at least one other major component. That there is some other mechanism with which to explain this diuresis is suggested by work on animal models.

Tachycardia and diuresis in animal models

Goetz & Bond (1973) in conscious dogs examined the effect of atrial pacing on urine flow and the concentration of circulating antidiuretic hormone. In dogs with complete heart block rapid atrial pacing did not alter ventricular rate, mean arterial blood

Atrial receptors in disease

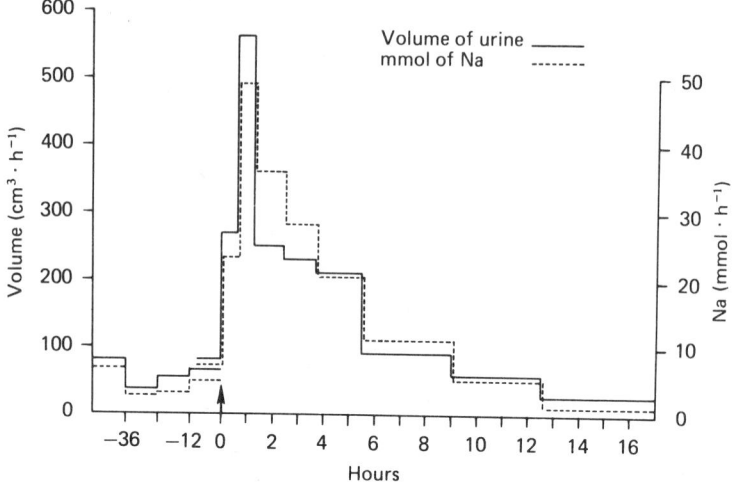

Fig. 11.3. Chart showing the increased volume of urine ($cm^3 \cdot h^{-1}$) and the increased output of sodium ($mmol \cdot h^{-1}$) during an attack of paroxysmal atrial fibrillation that lasted 18 h; the onset is indicated by an arrow. The increases started within 5–10 min, as was usual with this patient, and were considerable for $5\frac{1}{2}$ h, with a peak at about 1 h. The urine had been measured and analysed for 48 h, a week before this attack, and this is shown in the chart before the attack, as a control. From a woman, aged 60, with hypertension and a cardiomyopathy. (From Wood, 1963.)

pressure, atrial pulse pressure or central venous pressure and there were no significant changes in the urine flow or sodium excretion. In contrast in control dogs, atrial pacing resulted in a fall in pulse pressure but no significant changes in mean arterial pressure or central venous pressure (in superior vena cava) but there was a significant increase in urine flow and an increase in the excretion of sodium. There was no significant change in the concentration of antidiuretic hormone in either of the groups of animals. Although the changes in urine flow appeared to be similar to those described by Wood (1963), there were differences in that central venous pressure and arterial pressure did not change in the experiments of Goetz & Bond (1973). It is possible that a rise in atrial pressure (left and/or right), and not just a rise in heart rate, is necessary to produce the phenomenon. During an examination of the effect of ectopic tachycardia in dogs, Kahl, Flint, Szidon & Fishman (1972) showed that there was no change in the resistance in the renal

Atrial receptors and cardiac arrhythmias

vasculature in spite of generalised vasoconstriction attributed to the fall in blood pressure. They attributed this relative vasodilation in the kidney to the observed rise in left atrial pressure but no evidence was provided. The effects of stimulation of atrial receptors on the renal circulation in normal dogs has been discussed in Chapter 9 – a small vasodilatation was reflexly attributable to the stimulation of left atrial receptors.

Boykin, Cadnapaphornchai, McDonald & Schrier (1975), in anaesthetised dogs, by pacing the atria electrically increased the heart rate from approximately 140 beats·min^{-1} to approximately 240 beats·min^{-1}, which was accompanied by an increase in left atrial pressure from 0.8 to 2.0 kPa, and a decrease in mean arterial pressure from 18.1 to 16.4 kPa; the pressure in the renal artery was kept constant at 14.1 kPa by adjusting a Blalock clamp on the aorta. They observed an increase in urine volume, a fall in urine osmolarity with unchanged glomerular filtration rate and renal vascular resistance. The latter was calculated using values for renal blood flow measured by the clearance of para amino hippuric (PAH) acid. On the basis of these findings the authors claimed that the entire renal response was mediated by a fall in the concentration of antidiuretic hormone (which was not measured). However, the experimental protocol has several shortcomings which are outlined in Chapter 10. Another important feature relates to the claim that renal blood flow was kept constant by adjusting the clamp on the aorta. It is difficult to envisage how the authors managed to compensate for an average fall in mean arterial pressure of 1.7 kPa (with a much greater range) without a significant increase in renal blood flow. The fact that the PAH clearance technique failed to detect this change is an indictment of the latter.

Thus in conclusion animal models have so far failed to elucidate the mechanism of the increase in urine flow observed in some patients presenting with a supraventricular tachycardia.

Effect of arrhythmias on the discharge from atrial receptors

The effect of atrial pacing on the discharge from type B and type A atrial receptors was examined by Goetz & Bond (1973) in both intact dogs and in dogs with complete heart block. In the intact dogs they observed that the discharge from type B receptors expressed as impulses·s^{-1} was unchanged with increments in heart rate; thus as the diastolic interval was reduced the number of impulses per heart beat diminished progressively as the heart rate increased. In dogs with complete heart block, increasing the paced atrial rate resulted in a significant diminution of the number of impulses generated. They did not offer an explanation for this result but it is probable that there was reduction in the pressure in the atrium as more atrial contractions occurred during ventricular filling. The effect of pacing on type A receptors showed an increase in activity in both normal animals and in animals with complete heart block. Such results could be explained on the hypothesis suggested by Kappagoda, Linden & Mary (1976, 1977b; Chapter 3); a type A discharge occurred in receptors which were located in areas which were distorted by atrial contraction. Such distortions would occur more frequently as the rate of atrial pacing was increased. Hence the increase in the activity in type A receptors with pacing.

Zucker & Gilmore (1973) found that the activity, expressed as impulses·s^{-1}, in both type A and type B increased during atrial fibrillation as did the mean left atrial pressure. With the type A receptors, but not with type B receptors, the increase in activity was still evident even when the increase was expressed in terms of the impulses per heart beat; in the group in which the type A receptors were studied there was a greater increase in mean left atrial pressure.

In conclusion, there is circumstantial evidence linking atrial receptors to the diuresis observed in paroxysmal tachycardia, which in itself does not deny roles for other receptors in the cardiovascular system. It seems that the effect of these arrhythmias on the activity of the atrial receptors is governed mainly by the underlying events in the atrium, i.e. the intrinsic rhythms and the changes in pressure. It is known that stimulation of these receptors causes diuresis (Chapter 10).

Atrial receptors and renal circulation in 'shock'

Left atrial receptors have also been implicated in cardiogenic shock during several investigations in which the responses of the renal circulation in cardiogenic shock have been contrasted with, and shown to be different from, those in haemorrhagic shock

Atrial receptors and renal circulation in 'shock'

(e.g. Selkurt & Elpers, 1963; Lluch, Moguilevsky, Pietra, Shaffer, Hirsch & Fishman, 1969; Pelletier *et al.*, 1971; Gorfinkel, Szidon, Hirsch & Fishman, 1972; Hanley, Raizner, Inglesby & Skinner, 1972; Falicov, Mills & Gabe, 1973, 1975; Higgins, Vatner, Franklin & Braunwald, 1974; Kahl *et al.*, 1974; Peterson & Bishop, 1974). To take as an example the work of Lluch *et al.* (1969), they induced cardiogenic shock by the injection of mercury to cause emboli in the coronary vessels and haemorrhagic shock by gradual bleeding. Gorfinkel *et al.* (1972) obtained comparable decreases in cardiac output and blood pressure; however, renal blood flow fell by only 25% during cardiogenic shock but by 90% during haemorrhagic shock. Reduction in urine flow was also greatest in haemorrhagic shock (Gorfinkel *et al.*, 1972). Since they had consistently observed increases in left atrial pressure during cardiogenic shock and decreases during haemorrhagic shock they attributed the differences to increased and decreased stimulation of left atrial receptors respectively. From further experiments during which the pressure in the left atrium was raised by distending a balloon in the lumen and lowered by constricting the superior vena cava, Kahl *et al.* (1974) concluded that left atrial receptors were involved. They drew this conclusion because of the responses of renal vasodilatation and inhibition of activity in efferent renal nerves observed during stimulation of atrial receptors in normal animals (see Chapters 9 and 10) and the reduction of efferent nerve activity observed in experimental myocardial infarction (Kezdi, Kordenat & Misra, 1974).

However, they made no attempt by interruption of nervous pathways to investigate the particular reflex involved so that it must be concluded that the left atrial receptors are only one possible group of receptors which could be responsible for these results. As pointed out previously (Linden, 1973; Sleight, 1975; Donald & Shepherd, 1978; Thorén, 1979a) other reflexes are involved, particularly those which discharge into non-myelinated fibres in the vagi and 'sympathetic' afferent fibres mainly from the ventricle; for instance Donald & Shepherd (1978) refer to investigations showing that myocardial infarction, digitalis therapy and aortic stenosis have all been implicated in the stimulation of ventricular receptors causing responses of hypotension and bradycardia. In models of ischaemic heart disease

Atrial receptors in disease

an increased discharge in afferent vagal and 'sympathetic' fibres has been observed: in cardiac 'sympathetic' afferent fibres during myocardial ischaemia (Brown, 1967), in vagal fibres during myocardial infarction (Kolatat *et al.*, 1967; Recordati, Schwartz, Pagani, Malliani & Brown, 1971), in non-myelinated vagal afferent fibres (Thorén, 1976*b*) and in myelinated fibres from Paintal-type B atrial receptors (Zucker & Gilmore, 1974*a*), all these increases in discharge probably arising from the resulting distension of a chamber of the heart rather than a chemical or local mechanical disturbance in the infarct or in the ischaemic area.

Unfortunately, it is not immediately possible to extrapolate from this evidence to the probability that reflexes to, say the kidney, are involved – there being no complete analytical study – and it is pure speculation to extrapolate to man. But this investigation into models of disease is starting and promising and the special requirement is for good models of the chronic disease state of myocardial ischaemia on which to superimpose the acute intervention of infarction, with the subsequent careful analytical dissection of the mechanisms.

REFERENCES

Abrahám, A. (1955). Uber die Stelle und Struktur der Rezeptoren im Aorten-bogen des Rindes. *Acta Biol. Szeged.*, **1**, 125–59.
Abrahám, A. (1956). Uber die Struktur und die Endigungen der Aorticusfasernim Aortenbogen des Menschen mit Berücksichtigung der Cholinesterase-Aktivität der Pressorezeptorn. *Z. Mikrosk. Anat. Forsch.*, **62**, 194–228.
Abrahám, A. (1961). Struktur und Endigungsform der Fasern des Nervus aorticus im Aortenbogen des Schweines. *Z. Mikrosk. Anat. Forsch.*, **67**, 409–26.
Abrahám, A. (1964). *Die mikroskopische Innervation des Herzens und der Blutgetgefässe von Vertebraten*. Budapest: Akadēmiai Kiadō.
Abrahám, A. (1969). *Microscopic Innervation of the Heart and Blood Vessels in Vertebrates Including Man*. Oxford: Pergamon Press.
Abrahamsson, H. & Thorén, P. (1972). Reflex relaxation of the stomach elicited from receptors located in the heart. An analysis of the receptors and afferents involved. *Acta Physiol. Scand.*, **84**, 197–207.
Adair, J. R. & Manning, J. W. (1975). Hypothalamic modulation of baroreceptor afferent unit activity. *Am. J. Physiol.*, **229**, 1357–64.
Agostini, E., Chinnock, J. E., Daly, M. de Burgh & Murray, J. G. (1957). Functional and histological studies of the vagus nerve and its branches to the heart, lungs and abdominal viscera in the cat. *J. Physiol.*, **135**, 182–205.
Ahmad, G. & Nicoll, P. A. (1963). Chronotropic response to intravenous infusion in the anaesthetized dog. *Am. J. Physiol.*, **204**, 423–6.
Albrook, S. M., Bennion, G. R. & Ledsome, J. R. (1972). The effects of decerebration on the reflex response to pulmonary vein distension. *J. Physiol.*, **226**, 793–803.
Alexander, R. S. (1946). Tonic and reflex functions of medullary sympathetic cardiovascular centers. *J. Neurophysiol.*, **9**, 205–17.
Amman, A. & Schaefer, H. (1943). Uber sensible Impulse im Herznerven. *Pflügers Arch. ges. Physiol.*, **246**, 757–89.
Anderson, C. H., McCally, M. & Farrell, G. L. (1959). The effects of atrial stretch on aldosterone secretion. *Endocrinology*, **64**, 202–7.
Anderson, F. D. & Berry, C. M. (1956). An oscillographic study of the central pathways of the vagus nerve in the cat. *J. Comp. Neurol.*, **106**, 163–81.
Anrep, G. V., Pascual, W. & Rossler, R. (1936). Respiratory variations of

References

the heart rate. I. The reflex mechanism of the respiratory arrhythmia. *Proc. Roy. Soc. B*, **119**, 191–217.

Anrep, G. V. & Segall, H. N. (1926). The central and reflex regulation of the heart rate. *J. Physiol.*, **61**, 215–31.

Arborelius, M., Balldin, U. I., Lilja, B. & Lundgren, C. E. B. (1972). Hemodynamic changes in man during immersion with the head above water. *Aerospace Med.*, **43**, 592–8.

Ardill, B. L., Bannister, R. G., Fentem, P. H. & Greenfield, A. D. M. (1967). Circulatory responses of supine subjects to the exposure of parts of the body below the xiphisternum to subatmospheric pressure. *J. Physiol.*, **193**, 57–72.

Arndt, J. O., Brambring, P., Hindorf, K. & Röhnelt, M. (1971). The afferent impulse traffic from atrial A-type receptors in cats. Does the A-type receptor signal heart rate? *Pflügers Arch.*, **326**, 300–15.

Arndt, J. O., Brambring, P., Hindorf, K. & Röhnelt, M. (1974). The afferent discharge pattern of atrial mechano-receptors in the cat during sinusoidal stretch of atrial strip *in situ*. *J. Physiol.*, **240**, 33–52.

Arndt, J. O., Reineck, H. & Gauer, O. H. (1963). Ausscheidungsfunktion und Hämodynamik der Nieren bei Dehnung des linken Vorhofes am narkotisierten Hund. *Pflügers Arch.*, **277**, 1–15.

Aström, A. & Crafoord, J. (1968). Afferent and efferent activity in the renal nerves of cats. *Acta Physiol. Scand.*, **74**, 69–78.

Aviado, D. M. (1957). Hypotension and the autonomic nervous system. *Ann. N.Y. Acad. Sci.*, **66**, 998–1009.

Aviado, D. M., Li, T. H., Kalow, W., Schmidt, C. F., Turnbull, G. L., Peskin, G. W., Hess, M. E. & Weiss, A. J. (1951). Respiratory and circulatory reflexes from the perfused heart and pulmonary circulation of the dog. *Am. J. Physiol.*, **165**, 261–77.

Aviado, D. M. & Schmidt, C. F. (1955). Reflexes from stretch receptors in blood vessels, heart and lungs. *Physiol. Rev.*, **35**, 247–300.

Aviado, D. M. & Schmidt, C. F. (1959). Cardiovascular and respiratory reflexes from the left side of the heart. *Am. J. Physiol.*, **196**, 726–30.

Azer, M., Gannon, R. & Kaloyanides, G. J. (1972). Effect of renal denervation on the antinatriuresis of caval constriction. *Am. J. Physiol.*, **222**, 611–16.

Baertschi, A. J., Munzner, R. F., Ward, D. G., Johnson, R. N. & Gann, D. S. (1975). Right and left atrial B-fiber input to medulla of the cat. *Brain Res.*, **98**, 189–93.

Baertschi, A. J., Ward, D. G. & Gann, D. S. (1976). Role of atrial receptors in the control of ACTH. *Am. J. Physiol.*, **231**, 692–9.

Bainbridge, F. A. (1915). The influence of venous filling upon the rate of the heart. *J. Physiol.*, **50**, 65–84.

Baisset, A., Douste-Blazy, L. & Montastruc, P. (1959). Réduction de la sécrétion d'aldostérone sous l'effet d'une distension auriculaire. *J. Physiol. (Paris)*, **51**, 393–4.

Baisset, A. & Montastruc, P. (1957). Polyurie par distension auriculaire chez le chien; role de l'hormone antidiurétique. *J. Physiol. (Paris)*, **49**, 33–6.

References

Baker, D. G., Coleridge, H. M. & Coleridge, J. C. G. (1979). Vagal afferent C fibres from the ventricle. In *Cardiac Receptors*, ed. Hainsworth, R., Kidd, C. & Linden, R. J., pp. 117–37. Cambridge: Cambridge University Press.

Ballin, I. R. & Katz, L. N. (1941). Observations on the localization of the receptor area of the Bainbridge reflex. *Am. J. Physiol.*, **135**, 202–13.

Banzett, R. B., Coleridge, H. M., Coleridge, J. C. G. & Kidd, C. (1976). Multi-terminal afferent fibres from the thoracic viscera in sympathetic rami communicantes of cats and dogs. *J. Physiol.*, **254**, 57P–58P.

Baratz, R. A. & Ingraham, R. C. (1960). Renal hemodynamics and antidiuretic hormone release associated with volume regulation. *Am. J. Physiol.*, **198**, 565–70.

Baratz, R. A., Philbin, D. M. & Patterson, R. W. (1970). Urinary output and plasma levels of antidiuretic hormone during intermittent positive-pressure breathing in the dog. *Anesthesiology*, **32**, 17–22.

Barer, G. R. & Kottegoda, S. R. (1958). Changes in heart rate and blood pressure of the cat in response to increased pressure in the right side of the heart. *J. Physiol.*, **143**, 1–10.

Barger, A. C., Muldowney, F. P. & Liebowitz, M. R. (1959). Role of the kidney in the pathogenesis of congestive heart failure. *Circulation*, **20**, 273–85.

Baumgarten, R. von, Koepchen, P. & Aranda, L. (1959). Untersuchungen zur Lokalisation der bulbaren Kreislaufzentren. *Verh. Dtsch. ges. Kreisl. Forsch.*, **25**, 170–2.

Bazett, H. C. (1924). Studies on the effects of baths on man. I. Relationship between the effects produced and the temperature of the bath. *Am. J. Physiol.*, **70**, 412–29.

Bazett, H. C., Thurlow, S., Crowell, C. & Stewart, W. (1924). Studies on the effects of baths in man. II. The diuresis caused by warm baths, together with some observations on urinary tides. *Am. J. Physiol.*, **70**, 430–52.

Bergel, D. H. & Makin, G. S. (1967). Central and peripheral cardiovascular changes following chemical stimulation of the surface of the dog's heart. *Cardiovasc. Res.*, **1**, 80–90.

Berkley, H. J. (1895). The intrinsic nerve supply of the cardiac ventricles in certain vertebrates. *Johns Hopkins Hosp. Ref.*, **4**, 248–74.

Bernard, C. (1859). *Leçons sur les Propriétés Physiologiques et les Altérations Pathologiques des Liquides de l'Organisme*. Paris: Baillière.

Berne, R. M. (1952). Hemodynamics and sodium excretion of denervated kidney in anesthetized and unanesthetized dog. *Am. J. Physiol.*, **171**, 148–58.

Bevegard, S., Castenfors, J. & Lindblad, L. E. (1977). Effect of changes in blood volume distribution on circulatory variables and plasma renin activity in man. *Acta Physiol. Scand.*, **99**, 237–45.

Bezold, A. Von, & Hirt, L. (1867). Uber die physiologischen Wirkungen des essigsauren Veratrins. *Unter Physiol. Lab. Wurzburg*, **1**, 75–156.

Bianconi, R. & Green, J. H. (1959). Pulmonary baroreceptors in the cat. *Arch. Ital. Biol.*, **97**, 305–15.

References

Biscoe, T. J. & Millar, R. A. (1966). The effects of cyclopropane, halothane and ether on central baroreceptor pathways. *J. Physiol.*, **184**, 535–59.

Bishop, V. S., Lombardi, F., Malliani, A., Pagani, M. & Recordati, G. (1976). Reflex sympathetic tachycardia during intravenous infusions in chronic spinal cats. *Am. J. Physiol.*, **230**, 25–9.

Blatteis, C. M. & Horvath, S. M. (1964). Inexcitability of the Bainbridge, McDowall and Harrison reflexes. *Arch. Internat. Physiol.*, **72**, 535–52.

Blatteis, C. M. & Tucker, E. F. (1961). A prong-catheter for inducing vascular distension in the intact animal. *Am. Heart J.*, **61**, 236–7.

Blinks, J. R. (1956). Positive chronotropic effect of increasing right atrial pressure in the isolated mammalian heart. *Am. J. Physiol.*, **186**, 299–303.

Boasberg, P. D., Henry, J. P., Rosenbloom, A. A., Hall, T. C., Rose, M. & Fisher, D. A. (1977). Case reports and studies of paraneoplastic hypotension: abnormal low pressure baroreceptor responses. *Med. Pediat. Oncol.*, **3**, 59–66.

Bonjour, J. P., Churchill, P. C. & Malvin, R. L. (1969). Change of tubular reabsorption of sodium and water after renal denervation in the dog. *J. Physiol.*, **204**, 571–82.

Bonvallet, M. & Sigg, B. (1958). Etude électrophysiologique des afférences vagales au niveau de leur pénétration dans le bulbe. *J. Physiol. (Paris)*, **50**, 63–74.

Boura, A. L. A. & Green, A. F. (1959). The actions of bretylium: adrenergic neurone blocking and other effects. *Br. J. Pharmac. Chemother.*, **14**, 536–48.

Boykin, J., Cadnapaphornchai, P., McDonald, K. M. & Schrier, R. W. (1975). Mechanism of diuretic response associated with atrial tachycardia. *Am. J. Physiol.*, **229**, 1486–91.

Boylan, J. W. & Antkowiak, D. E. (1959). Mechanism of diuresis during negative pressure breathing. *J. Appl. Physiol.*, **14**, 116–20.

Brennan, L. A., Malvin, R. L., Jochim, K. E. & Roberts, D. E. (1971). The influence of right and left atrial receptors on plasma concentrations of ADH and renin. *Am. J. Physiol.*, **221**, 273–8.

Brod, J. (1972). Pathogenesis of cardiac oedema. *Br. Med. J.*, **1**, 222–8.

Brooks, C. McC., Hsin-Hsiang, L., Lange, G., Mangi, R., Shaw, R. B. & Geoly, K. (1966). Effects of localized stretch of the sinoatrial node region of the dog heart. *Am. J. Physiol.*, **211**, 1197–202.

Brooks, C. McC. & Koizumi, K. (1974). The hypothalamus and control of integrative processes. In *Medical Physiology*, 13th edn Mountcastle, V. B., pp. 813–36. St Louis: C. V. Mosley.

Brosnihan, K. B. & Bravo, E. L. (1978). Graded reductions of atrial pressure and renin release. *Am. J. Physiol.*, **235**, H175–H181.

Brown, A. M. (1964). A study of the afferent innervation of the coronary vessels and the cardiac chambers. Ph.D. Thesis, University of London.

Brown, A. M. (1965). Mechanoreceptors in or near the coronary arteries. *J. Physiol.*, **177**, 203–14.

Brown, A. M. (1966). The depressor reflex arising from the left coronary artery of the cat. *J. Physiol.*, **184**, 825–36.

References

Brown, A. M. (1967). Excitation of afferent cardiac sympathetic nerve fibres during myocardial ischaemia. *J. Physiol.*, **190**, 35–53.

Brown, E., Goei, J. S., Greenfield, A. D. M. & Plassaras, G. C. (1966). Circulatory responses to simulated gravitational shifts of blood in man induced by exposure of the body below the iliac crests to subatmospheric pressure. *J. Physiol.*, **183**, 607–27.

Brown, A. M. & Malliani, A. (1971). Spinal sympathetic reflexes initiated by coronary receptors. *J. Physiol.*, **212**, 685–705.

Browse, N. L., Shepherd, J. T. & Donald, D. E. (1966). Differences in response of veins and resistance vessels in limbs to same stimulus. *Am. J. Physiol.*, **211**, 1241–7.

Burkhart, S. M., Funnell, L. & Ledsome, J. R. (1977). Effects of medullary lesions on arterial baroreceptor reflexes and responses to distension of pulmonary vein–left atrial junctions in anaesthetized dogs. *J. Physiol.*, **273**, 69–81.

Burkhart, S. M. & Ledsome, J. R. (1974). The response to distension of the pulmonary vein–left atrial junctions in dogs with spinal section. *J. Physiol.*, **237**, 685–700.

Burkhart, S. M. & Ledsome, J. R. (1977). The response to distension of the pulmonary vein–left atrial junctions in anaesthetized dogs after section of the rostral medulla. *J. Physiol.*, **273**, 57–67.

Campbell, G. S. (1955). Cardiac arrest: further studies on the effect of pH changes on vagal inhibition of the heart. *Surgery*, **38**, 615–34.

Carswell, F., Hainsworth, R. & Ledsome, J. R. (1968). Elimination of agents possibly responsible for the diuretic response to left atrial distension. *J. Physiol.*, **198**, 23P–24P.

Carswell, F., Hainsworth, R. & Ledsome, J. R. (1970a). The effects of distension of the pulmonary vein–atrial junctions upon peripheral vascular resistance. *J. Physiol.*, **207**, 1–14.

Carswell, F., Hainsworth, R. & Ledsome, J. R. (1970b). The effects of left atrial distension upon urine flow from the isolated perfused kidney. *Q. J. Exp. Physiol.*, **55**, 173–82.

Casati, R., Lombardi, F. & Malliani, A. (1979). Afferent sympathetic unmyelinated fibres with left ventricular endings in cats. *J. Physiol.*, **292**, 135–48.

Cauna, N. (1959). The mode of termination of the sensory nerves and its significance. *J. Comp. Neurol.*, **113**, 169–209.

Chabarova, A. J. (1959). Die afferente Innervation des Herzens. *Z. Mikrosk. Anat. Forsch.*, **66**, 236–50.

Chapman, L. W. & Henry, J. P. (1973). The role of cardiac receptors in fluid balance. *Physiologist*, **16**, 194–201.

Chapman, L. W. & Mittman, U. (1975). An exchangeable intra-atrial balloon device. *J. Appl. Physiol.*, **38**, 558–9.

Chapman, L. W., Mittman, U., Prickett, C. & Richmond, W. (1978). Left atrial receptor inhibition of cardiac efferent vagal activity in the dog. *Clin. Exp. Pharmacol. Physiol.*, **5**, 471–6.

Chervova, I. A. (1965). Structural organization of intracardiac nerve apparatus. *Arkh. Anat.*, **48**, 60–6.

References

Christensen, K., Lewis, E. & Kuntz, A. (1951). Innervation of the renal blood vessels in the cat. *J. Comp. Neurol.*, **95**, 373–85.

Clement, D. L., Pelletier, C. L. & Shepherd, J. T. (1972). Role of vagal afferents in the control of renal sympathetic nerve activity in the rabbit. *Circ. Res.*, **31**, 824–30.

Coleridge, H. M. & Coleridge, J. C. G. (1972). Cardiovascular receptors. In *Modern Trends in Physiology*, ed. Downman, C. B. B., pp. 245–67. London: Butterworths.

Coleridge, H. M., Coleridge, J. C. G., Dangel, A., Kidd, C., Luck, J. C. & Sleight, P. (1973). Impulses in slowly conducting vagal fibers from afferent endings in the veins, atria and arteries of dogs and cats. *Circ. Res.*, **33**, 87–97.

Coleridge, H. M., Coleridge, J. C. G. & Kidd, C. (1964a). Role of the pulmonary arterial baroreceptors in the effects produced by capsaicin in the dog. *J. Physiol.*, **170**, 272–85.

Coleridge, H. M., Coleridge, J. C. G. & Kidd, C. (1964b). Cardiac receptors in the dog, with particular reference to two types of afferent ending in the ventricular wall. *J. Physiol.*, **174**, 323–39.

Coleridge, H. M., Coleridge, J. C. G. & Kidd, C. (1979). Afferent innervation of the heart and great vessels: a comparison of vagal and sympathetic components. *Acta Physiol. Polonica*, **29**, Suppl. 17, 55–79.

Coleridge, H. M., Coleridge, J. C. G., Rosenthal, F. & Dangel, A. (1973). Stimulation of C-fibers accompanying anodal polarization block of A-fibres in the vagus nerves of cats. *Fed. Proc.*, **32**, 355.

Coleridge, J. C. G., Hemingway, A., Holmes, R. L. & Linden, R. J. (1957). The location of atrial receptors in the dog: a physiological and histological study. *J. Physiol.*, **136**, 174–97.

Coleridge, J. C. G. & Kidd, C. (1960). Electrophysiological evidence of baroreceptors in the pulmonary artery of the dog. *J. Physiol.*, **150**, 319–31.

Coleridge, J. C. G. & Kidd, C. (1961). Relationship between pulmonary arterial pressure and impulse activity in pulmonary arterial baroreceptor fibres. *J. Physiol.*, **158**, 197–205.

Coleridge, J. C. G. & Kidd, C. (1963). Reflex effects of stimulating baroreceptors in the pulmonary artery. *J. Physiol.*, **166**, 197–210.

Coleridge, J. C. G., Kidd, C. & Sharp, J. A. (1961). The distribution, connexions and histology of baroreceptors in the pulmonary artery, with some observations on the sensory innervation of the ductus arteriosus. *J. Physiol.*, **156**, 591–602.

Coleridge, J. C. G. & Linden, R. J. (1955). The effect of intravenous infusions upon the heart rate of the anaesthetized dog. *J. Physiol.*, **128**, 310–19.

Comroe, J. H. & Mortimer, L. (1964). The respiratory and cardiovascular responses of temporarily separated aortic and carotid bodies to cyanide, nicotine, phenyldiguanide and serotonin. *J. Pharmacol. Exp. Ther.*, **146**, 33–41.

Coote, J. H. & McLeod, V. H. (1974). The influence of bulbospinal monoaminergic pathways on sympathetic nerve activity. *J. Physiol.*, **241**, 453–75.

References

Cottle, M. K. (1964). Degeneration studies of primary afferents of IXth and Xth cranial nerves in the cat. *J. Comp. Neurol.*, **122**, 329–45.

Cox, J. R., Davies-Jones, G. A. B., Leonard, P. J. & Singer, B. (1963). The effect of positive pressure respiration on urinary aldosterone excretion. *Clin. Sci.*, **24**, 1–5.

Cryer, G. L. & Gann, D. S. (1973). Location of vagal receptors controlling adrenal corticosteroid secretion. *Am. J. Physiol.*, **225**, 1346–50.

Cryer, G. L. & Gunn, D. S. (1974). Right atrial receptors mediate the adrenocortical response to small hemorrhage. *Am. J. Physiol.*, **227**, 325–8.

Cryer, G. L., Grayson, M. & Gann, D. S. (1974). Evidence that left atrial receptors are involved in the adrenocortical response to small hemorrhage. (Abstract.) *Physiologist*, **17**, 204.

Daly, I. de Burgh, Ludany, G., Todd, A. & Verney, E. B. (1937). Sensory receptors in the pulmonary vascular bed. *Q. J. Exp. Physiol.*, **27**, 123–46.

Daly, I. de Burgh & Verney, E. B. (1926). Cardiovascular reflexes. *J. Physiol.*, **61**, 268–74.

Daly, I. de Burgh & Verney, E. B. (1927). The localisation of receptors involved in the reflex regulation of the heart rate. *J. Physiol.*, **62**, 330–40.

Daly, M. de Burgh & Hazzledine, J. L. (1963). The effects of artificially induced hyperventilation on the primary reflex response to stimulation of the carotid bodies in the dog. *J. Physiol.*, **168**, 872–89.

Daly, M. de Burgh, Hazzledine, J. L. & Howe, A. (1965). Reflex respiratory and peripheral vascular responses to stimulation of the isolated perfused aortic arch chemoreceptors of the dog. *J. Physiol.*, **177**, 300–22.

Daly, M. de Burgh, Hazzledine, J. L. & Ungar, A. (1967). The reflex effects of alterations in lung volume on systemic vascular resistance in the dog. *J. Physiol.*, **188**, 331–51.

Daly, M. de Burgh & Robinson, B. H. (1968). An analysis of the reflex systemic vasodilator response elicited by lung inflation in the dog. *J. Physiol.*, **195**, 387–406.

Daly, M. de Burgh & Scott, M. J. (1958). The effects of stimulation of the carotid body chemoreceptors on heart rate in the dog. *J. Physiol.*, **144**, 148–66.

Daly, M. de Burgh & Scott, M. J. (1962). An analysis of the primary cardiovascular reflex effects of stimulation of the carotid body chemoreceptors in the dog. *J. Physiol.*, **162**, 555–73.

Davis, J. T. & DuBois, A. B. (1977). Immersion diuresis in dogs. *J. Appl. Physiol.*, **42**, 915–22.

Dawes, G. S. (1947). Studies on veratrum alkaloids. II. Receptor areas in the coronary arteries and elsewhere as revealed by the use of veratridine. *J. Pharmacol. Exp. Ther.*, **89**, 325–42.

Dawes, G. S. & Comroe, J. H. (1954). Chemoreflexes from the heart and lungs. *Physiol. Rev.*, **34**, 167–201.

Dawes, G. S. & Widdicombe, J. G. (1953). The afferent pathway of the Bezold reflex: the left vagal branches in dogs. *Br. J. Pharmacol.*, **8**, 395–8.

References

DeGraff, A. C. & Sands, J. (1925). Are reflexes from the large veins or auricle of importance in the regulation of the circulation? *Am. J. Physiol.*, **74**, 400–15.

Denn, M. J. & Stone, H. L. (1976). Autonomic innervation of dog coronary arteries. *J. Appl. Physiol.*, **41**, 30–5.

DiBona, G. F. (1977). Neurogenic regulation of renal tubular sodium reabsorption. *Am. J. Physiol.*, **233**, F73–F81.

Dickinson, C. J. (1950). Afferent nerves from the heart region. *J. Physiol.*, **111**, 399–407.

Dogiel, A. S. (1898). Die sensiblen Nervenendigungen im Herzen und im dem Blutgefässen der Säugetiere. *Arch. Mikrosk. Anat.*, **52**, 44–70.

Donald, D. E., Ferguson, D. A. & Milburn, S. E. (1968). Effects of beta-adrenergic receptor blockade on racing performance of greyhounds with normal and with denervated hearts. *Circ. Res.*, **22**, 127–34.

Donald, D. E. & Shepherd, J. T. (1963). Changes in heart rate on intravenous infusion in dogs with chronic cardiac denervation. *Proc. Soc. Exp. Biol. Med.*, **113**, 315–19.

Donald, D. E. & Shepherd, J. T. (1978). Reflexes from the heart and lungs: physiological curiosities or important regulatory mechanisms. *Cardiovasc. Res.*, **12**, 449–69.

Donoghue, S., Fox, R. E., Kidd, C. & Koley, B. N. (1977). The projection of vagal, cardiac C-fibres to the brain stem of the cat. *J. Physiol.*, **270**, 44P–45P.

Donoghue, S., Fox, R. E., Kidd, C. & Koley, B. N. (1981). The distribution in the cat brainstem of neurones activated by vagal nonmyelinated afferent fibres from the heart and lungs. *Q. J. Physiol.* (In press.)

Drury, D. R., Henry, J. P. & Goodman, J. (1947). The effects of continuous pressure breathing on kidney function. *J. Clin. Invest.*, **26**, 945–51.

Echtenkamp, S. F. & Gilmore, J. P. (1980). Intravascular mechanoreceptor modulation of renal sympathetic nerve activity in the cat. *Am. J. Physiol.*, **238**, H801–H808.

Edgeworth, F. H. (1892). On a large-fibred sensory supply of the thoracic and abdominal viscera. *J. Physiol.*, **13**, 260–71.

Edis, A. J., Donald, D. E. & Shepherd, J. T. (1970). Cardiovascular reflexes from stretch of pulmonary vein–atrial junctions in the dog. *Circ. Res.*, **27**, 1091–100.

Edis, A. J. & Shepherd, J. T. (1969). Circulatory reflexes from stretch of pulmonary vein–atrial junctions. *Physiologist*, **12**, No. 3, 213.

Ellison, J. P. & Hibbs, R. G. (1974). Catecholamine-containing cells of the guinea pig heart: an ultrastructural study. *J. Mol. Cardiol.*, **6**, 17–26.

Epstein, A. N., Kissileff, H. R. & Stellar, E. (1973). *The Neurophysiology of Thirst: New Findings and Advances in Concepts.* Washington: Winston.

Epstein, M. (1976). Cardiovascular and renal effects of head-out water immersion in man. Application of the model in the assessment of volume homeostasis. *Circ. Res.*, **39**, 619–28.

Epstein, M. (1978). Renal effects of head-out water immersion in man:

implications for an understanding of volume homeostasis. *Physiol. Rev.*, **58**, 529–81.

Epstein, M., Pins, D. S. & Miller, M. (1975). Suppression of ADH during water immersion in normal man. *J. Appl. Physiol.*, **38**, 1038–44.

Eyster, J. A. E. & Middleton, W. S. (1924). Cardio-vascular reactions to hemorrhage and transfusion in man. *Am. J. Physiol.*, **68**, 581–4.

Falicov, R. E., Mills, C. J. & Gabe, I. T. (1973). Response of renal and femoral vascular beds to experimental myocardial infarction. *Br. Heart J.*, **35**, 550.

Falicov, R. E., Mills, C. J. & Gabe, I. T. (1975). The response of the renal and femoral vascular beds to coronary embolization in the dog. *Cardiovasc. Res.*, **9**, 151–60.

Feigl, E. O. (1975). Reflex parasympathetic coronary vasodilation elicited from cardiac receptors in the dog. *Circ. Res.*, **37**, 175–82.

Fenn, W. O., Otis, A. B., Rahn, H., Chadwick, L. E. & Hegnauer, A. H. (1947). Displacement of blood from the lungs by pressure breathing. *Am. J. Physiol.*, **151**, 258–69.

Fillenz, M. (1969). Innervation of pulmonary capillaries. *Experientia*, **25**, 842.

Fisher, S. J. & Malvin, R. L. (1980). Role of neural pathways in renin response to intravascular volume expansion. *Am. J. Physiol.*, **238**, H611–H617.

Fitzsimons, J. T. (1972). Thirst. *Physiol. Rev.*, **52**, 468–561.

Fitzsimons, J. T. (1979). *The Physiology of Thirst and Sodium Appetite*, p. 221. Cambridge: Cambridge University Press.

Fitzsimons, J. T. & Moore-Gillon, M. J. (1980). Pulmo–atrial junctional receptors and the inhibition of drinking. *J. Physiol.*, **307**, 74P–75P.

Floyd, K. (1979). Light microscopy of nerve endings in the atrial endocardium. In *Cardiac Receptors*, ed. Hainsworth, R., Kidd, C. & Linden, R. J., pp. 3–26. Cambridge: Cambridge University Press.

Floyd, K., Linden, R. J. & Saunders, D. A. (1972). Presumed receptors in the left atrial appendage of the dog. *J. Physiol.*, **227**, 27P–28P.

Floyd, K., Linden, R. J. & Saunders, D. A. (1974). The morphological variation of nervous structures in the atrial endocardium of the dog. *J. Physiol.*, **238**, 19P.

Ford, L. E. (1976). Heart size. *Circ. Res.*, **39**, 297–303.

Forsling, M.L. (1974). Extraction of neurohypophyseal hormones for bioassay. *J. Physiol.*, **241**, 3P–5P.

Franz, D. N. & Iggo, A. (1968). Conduction failure in myelinated and non-myelinated axons at low temperatures. *J. Physiol.*, **199**, 319–45.

Furnival, C. M., Linden, R. J. & Snow, H. M. (1970). Inotropic changes in the left ventricle: the effect of changes in heart rate, aortic pressure and end-diastolic pressure. *J. Physiol.*, **211**, 359–87.

Furnival, C. M., Linden, R. J. & Snow, H. M. (1971). Reflex effects on the heart of stimulating left atrial receptors. *J. Physiol.*, **218**, 447–63.

Fussey, I. F., Kidd, C. & Whitwam, J. G. (1967). Single unit activity associated with cardiovascular events in the brain stem of the dog. *J. Physiol.*, **191**, 57P–58P.

References

Fussey, I. F., Kidd, C. & Whitwam, J. G. (1973). Activity evoked in the brain stem by stimulation of C fibres in cervical vagus nerve of the dog. *Brain Res.*, **49**, 436–40.

Gabriel, M. & Seller, H. (1970). Interaction of baroreceptor afferents from carotid sinus and aorta at the nucleus tractus solitarii. *Pflügers Arch.*, **318**, 7–20.

Gann, D. S. (1966). Carotid vascular receptors and control of adrenal corticosteroid secretion. *Am. J. Physiol.*, **211**, 193–7.

Ganong, W. F. (1977). The renin–angiotensin system and the central nervous system. *Fed. Proc.*, **36**, 1771–5.

Gauer, O. H. (1955). Volume changes of the left ventricle during blood pooling and exercise in the intact animal. Their effects on left ventricular performance. *Physiol. Rev.*, **35**, 143–55.

Gauer, O. H. & Henry, J. P. (1963). Circulatory basis of fluid volume control. *Physiol. Rev.*, **43**, 423–81.

Gauer, O. H. & Henry, J. P. (1976). Neurohormonal control of plasma volume. In Internat. Rev. Physiol., *Cardiovascular Physiol.* II, Vol. 9, ed. Guyton, A. C. & Cowley, A. W., pp. 145–90. Baltimore: University Park Press.

Gauer, O. H., Henry, J. P. & Behn, C. (1970). The regulation of extracellular fluid volume. *Ann. Rev. Physiol.*, **32**, 547–95.

Gauer, O. H., Henry, J. P., Sieker, H. O. & Wendt, W. E. (1954). The effect of negative pressure breathing on urine flow. *J. Clin. Invest.*, **33**, 287–96.

Ghose, R. R., Joekes, A. M. & Kyriacou, E. H. (1965). Renal response to paroxysmal tachycardia. *Br. Heart J.*, **27**, 684–7.

Gill, J. R., Carr, A. A., Fleischmann, L. E., Casper, A. G. T. & Bartter, F. C. (1967). Effects of pentolinium on sodium excretion in dogs with constriction of the vena cava. *Am. J. Physiol.*, **212**, 191–6.

Gillespie, D. J., Sandberg, R. L. & Koike, T. I. (1973). Dual effect of left atrial receptors on excretion of sodium and water in the dog. *Am. J. Physiol.*, **225**, 706–10.

Gilmore, J. P. (1968). Contribution of cardiac nerves to the control of the body salt and water. *Fed. Proc.*, **27**, 1156–9.

Gilmore, J. P. & Daggett, W. M. (1966). Response of the chronic cardiac denervated dog to acute volume expansion. *Am. J. Physiol.*, **210**, 509–12.

Gilmore, J. P., Peterson, T. V. & Zucker, I. H. (1979). Neither dorsal root nor baroreceptor afferents are necessary for eliciting the renal responses to acute intravascular volume expansion in the primate *Macaca fascicularis*. *Circ. Res.*, **45**, 95–9.

Gilmore, J. P. & Weisfeldt, M. L. (1965). Contribution of intravascular receptors to the renal responses following intravascular volume expansion. *Circ. Res.*, **17**, 144–54.

Gilmore, J. P. & Zucker, I. H. (1974a). Failure of the type B atrial receptors to respond to increase in osmolality in the dog. *Am. J. Physiol.*, **227**, 1005–7.

Gilmore, J. P. & Zucker, I. H. (1974b). Discharge of the type B atrial receptors during changes in vascular volume and depression of atrial contractility. *J. Physiol.*, **239**, 207–23.

Gilmore, J. P. & Zucker, I. H. (1978a). Contribution of vagal pathways to the renal responses to head-out immersion in the nonhuman primate. *Circ. Res.*, **42**, 263–7.

Gilmore, J. P. & Zucker, I. H. (1978b). Failure of left atrial distension to alter renal function in the nonhuman primate. *Circ. Res.*, **42**, 267–70.

Glick, G., Wechsler, A. S. & Epstein, S. E. (1969). Reflex cardiovascular depression produced by stimulation of pulmonary stretch receptors in the dog. *J. Clin. Invest.*, **48**, 467–75.

Godley, J. A., Myers, J. W. & Rosenbaum, D. A. (1967). Cardiovascular and renal function during continuous negative pressure breathing in dogs. *J. Appl. Physiol.*, **22**, 568–72.

Goetz, K. L. (1965). Effect of increased pressure within a right heart cul-de-sac on heart rate in dogs. *Am. J. Physiol.*, **209**, 507–12.

Goetz, K. L., Bloxham, D. D., Bond, G. C. & Sharma, J. N. (1976). Persistence of the renal response to atrial tamponade after cardiac denervation. *Proc. Soc. Exp. Biol. Med.*, **152**, 423–7.

Goetz, K. L. & Bond, G. C. (1973). Reflex diuresis during tachycardia in the dog. Evaluation of the role of atrial and sinoaortic receptors. *Circ. Res.*, **32**, 434–41.

Goetz, K. L., Bond, G. C. & Bloxham, D. D. (1975). Atrial receptors and renal function. *Physiol. Rev.*, **55**, 157–205.

Goetz, K. L., Bond, G. C., Hermreck, A. S. & Trank, J. W. (1970). Plasma ADH levels following a decrease in mean atrial transmural pressure in dogs. *Am. J. Physiol.*, **219**, 1424–8.

Goetz, K. L., Hermreck, A. S., Slick, G. L. & Starke, H. S. (1970). Atrial receptors and renal function in conscious dogs. *Am. J. Physiol.*, **219**, 1417–23.

Goldreyer, B. N. & Damato, A. N. (1971). The essential role of atrioventricular conduction delay in the initiation of paroxysmal supraventricular tachycardia. *Circulation*, **43**, 679–87.

Goodman, L. S. & Gilman, A. (1970). *The Pharmacological Basis of Therapeutics*. London: Collier-Macmillan.

Gorfinkel, H. J., Szidon, J. P., Hirsch, L. J. & Fishman, A. P. (1972). Renal performance in experimental cardiogenic shock. *Am. J. Physiol.*, **222**, 1260–8.

Graveline, D. E. & Jackson, M. M. (1962). Diuresis associated with prolonged water immersion. *J. Appl. Physiol.*, **17**, 519–24.

Greenberg, T. T., Richmond, W. H., Stocking, R. A., Gupta, P. D., Meehan, J. P. & Henry, J. P. (1973). Impaired atrial receptor responses in dogs with heart failure due to tricuspid insufficiency and pulmonary artery stenosis. *Circ. Res.*, **32**, 424–33.

Greenwood, P. V., Hainsworth, R., Karim, F., Morrison, G. W. & Sofola, O. A. (1980). Reflex inotropic responses of the heart from lung inflation in anaesthetized dogs. *Pflügers Arch.*, **386**, 199–205.

Greenwood, P. V. & Kappagoda, C. T. (1979). Summation of reflex increases in heart rate from stimulation of left and right atrial receptors in the dog. *J. Physiol.*, **296**, 24P–25P.

References

Greenwood, P. V. & Kappagoda, C. T. (1980). 'Summation' of the increase in heart rate from stimulation of atrial receptors. *Can. J. Physiol. Pharmacol.*, **58**, 666–72.

Gribbe, P., Lind, J., Linko, E. & Wegelius, C. (1958). The events of the left side of the normal heart as studied by cineradiography. *Cardiologia*, **33**, 293–304.

Grizzle, W. E., Dallman, M. F., Schramm, L. P. & Gann, D. S. (1974). Inhibitory and facilitatory hypothalamic areas mediating ACTH release in the cat. *Endocrinology*, **95**, 1450–61.

Grizzle, W. E., Johnson, R. N., Schramm, L. P. & Gann, D. S. (1975). Hypothalamic cells in an area mediating ACTH release respond to right atrial stretch. *Am. J. Physiol.*, **228**, 1039–45.

Gross, R. & Kirchheim, H. (1978). Effects of bilateral common carotid occlusion on sympathetic activity and renal function in conscious dogs. *J. Physiol.*, **284**, 64P–65P.

Guazzi, M., Libretti, A. & Zanchetti, A. (1962). Tonic reflex regulation of the cat's blood pressure through vagal afferents from the cardiopulmonary region. *Circ. Res.*, **11**, 7–16.

Gupta, B. N. (1977a). The location and distribution of type A and type B atrial endings in cats. *Pflügers Arch.*, **367**, 271–5.

Gupta, B. N. (1977b). Studies on the adaptation rate and frequency distribution of type A and type B atrial endings in cats. *Pflügers Arch.*, **367**, 277–81.

Gupta, P. D. (1975). Spinal autonomic afferents in elicitation of tachycardia in volume infusion in the dog. *Am. J. Physiol.*, **229**, 303–8.

Gupta, P. D., Henry, J. P., Sinclair, R. & Baumgarten, R. von (1966). Responses of atrial and aortic baroreceptors to nonhypotensive hemorrhage and to transfusion. *Am. J. Physiol.*, **211**, 1429–37.

Gupta, P. D. & Singh, M. (1977). Autonomic afferents at T_1 in elicitation of volume-induced tachycardia in the dog. *Am. J. Physiol.*, **232**, H464–H469.

Guyton, A. C., Coleman, T. C. & Granger, H. J. (1972). Circulation: overall regulation. *Ann. Rev. Physiol.*, **34**, 13–46.

Hainsworth, R. (1974). Circulatory responses from lung inflation in anaesthetized dogs. *Am. J. Physiol.*, **226**, 247–55.

Hainsworth, R. & Karim, F. (1973). Left ventricular inotropic and peripheral vasomotor responses from independent changes in pressure in the carotid sinuses and cerebral arteries in anaesthetized dogs. *J. Physiol.*, **228**, 139–55.

Hainsworth, R., Karim, F. & Sofola, O. A. (1979). Left ventricular inotropic responses to stimulation of carotid body chemoreceptors in anaesthetized dogs. *J. Physiol.*, **287**, 455–66.

Hainsworth, R., Kidd, C. & Linden, R. J. (1979). *Cardiac Receptors.* Cambridge: Cambridge University Press.

Hainsworth, R., Ledsome, J. R. & Carswell, F. (1971). Reflex responses from aortic baroreceptors. *Am. J. Physiol.*, **218**, 423–9.

Hakumäki, M. O. K. (1970). Function of the left atrial receptors. *Acta Physiol. Scand.*, Suppl. 344, 1–54.

Hakumäki, M. O. K. (1972). Vagal and sympathetic efferent discharge in the Bainbridge reflex of dogs. *Acta Physiol. Scand.*, **85**, 414–17.

References

Hakumäki, M. O. K. (1979). Influence of intravenous infusion on heart rate, sympathetic and vagal efferentation and left atrial and aortic baroreceptor activity in dogs. *Acta Physiol. Scand.*, **107**, 127–33.

Hanker, J. S., Dixon, A. D. & Moore, H. G. (1973). Cytochrome oxidase activity of mitochondria in sensory nerve endings of mouse palatal rugae. *J. Anat.*, **116**, 93–102.

Hanley, H. G., Raizner, A. E., Inglesby, T. V. & Skinner, N. S. (1972). Response of the renal vascular bed to acute experimental coronary arterial occlusion. *Am. J. Cardiol.*, **29**, 803–8.

Harrison, F. & Bruesch, S. A. (1954). Intermedullary potentials following stimulation of the cervical vagus. *Anat. Res.*, **91**, 280.

Harry, J. D., Kappagoda, C. T., Linden, R. J. & Snow, H. M. (1971). Depression of the reflex tachycardia from the left atrial receptors by acidaemia. *J. Physiol.*, **218**, 465–75.

Harry, J. D., Kappagoda, C. T., Linden, R. J. & Snow, H. M. (1973). Action of propranolol on the dog heart. *Cardiovasc. Res.*, **7**, 729–39.

Hartshorne H. (1847). *Water Versus Hydrotherapathy or An Essay on Water and its True Relations to Medicine*, p. 28. Philadelphia: Lloyd P. Smith Press.

Hayashi, K. D. (1969). Responses of systemic arterial pressure and the heart rate to increased intrapulmonary pressure in anaesthetized dogs. *Proc. Soc. Exp. Biol. Med.*, **131**, 426–9.

Hayward, J. N. (1977). Functional and morphological aspects of hypothalamic neurons. *Physiol. Rev.*, **57**, 574–658.

Hellner, K. & Baumgarten, R. von (1961). Uber ein Endigungsgebiet afferenter, Kardiovasculärer Fasern des Nervus vagus im Rautenhirn der Katze. *Pflügers Arch.*, **273**, 223–34.

Henry, J. P., Gauer, O. H. & Reeves, J. L. (1956). Evidence of the atrial location of receptors influencing urine flow. *Circ. Res.*, **4**, 85–90.

Henry, J. P. & Pearce, J. W. (1956). The possible role of cardiac atrial stretch receptors in the induction of changes in urine flow. *J. Physiol.*, **131**, 572–85.

Hess, G. L., Zuperku, E. J., Coon, R. L. & Kampine, J. P. (1974). Sympathetic afferent nerve activity of left ventricular origin. *Am. J. Physiol.*, **227**, 543–6.

Heymans, C. & Neil, E. (1958). *Reflexogenic Areas of the Cardiovascular System*. London: Churchill.

Higgins, C. B., Vatner, S. F., Franklin, D. & Braunwald, E. (1974). Pattern of differential vasoconstriction in response to acute and chronic low-output states in the conscious dog. *Cardiovasc. Res.*, **8**, 92–8.

Hirsch, L. J., Boyd, E. & Katz, L. N. (1964). Effect of intravenous volume infusion on heart rate in unanaesthetized dogs. *Am. J. Physiol.*, **206**, 992–6.

Hirsch, E. F., Nigh, C. A., Kaye, M. P. & Cooper, T. (1964). Terminal innervation of the heart. II. Studies of the perimysial innervation apparatus and of the sensory receptors in the rabbit and in the dog with techniques of total extrinsic denervation, bilateral, cervical vagotomy and bilateral thoracic sympathectomy. *Arch. Path.*, **77**, 172–87.

References

Hirsch, E. F. & Orme, J. F. (1947). Sensory nerves of the human heart. *Arch. Path.*, **44**, 325–35.

Hodge, R. L., Lowe, R. D., Ng, K. K. F. & Vane, J. R. (1969). Role of the vagus nerve in the control of the concentration of angiotensin II in the circulation. *Nature*, **221**, 177–9.

Hodge, R. L., Lowe, R. D. & Vane, J. R. (1966). Increased angiotensin formation in response to carotid occlusion in the dog. *Nature*, **211**, 491–3.

Holmes, R. L. (1956). Further observations on the nerve endings in the adult dog heart. *J. Anat.*, **90**, 600.

Holmes, R. L. (1957a). Structures in the atrial endocardium of the dog which stain with methylene blue, and the effects of unilateral vagotomy. *J. Anat.*, **91**, 259–66.

Holmes, R. L. (1957b). Cholinesterase activity in the atrial wall of the dog and cat heart. *J. Physiol.*, **137**, 421–6.

Holmes, R. L. (1958). Nervous structures in the mammalian atrial wall. *J. Physiol.*, **142**, 46P–47P.

Holmes, R. L. & Torrance, R. W. (1959). Afferent fibres of the stellate ganglion. *Q. J. Exp. Physiol.*, **44**, 271–81.

Holton, A. (1977). Characteristics of cardiac receptors with fibres in the rami communicantes. Ph.D. thesis, University of Leeds.

Homma, S. & Suzuki, S. (1966). Phasic properties of aortic and atrial receptors observed from their afferent discharge. *Jpn. J. Physiol.*, **16**, 31–41.

Hopp, F. A., Zuperku, E. J., Coon, R. L. & Kampine, J. P. (1980). Effect of anodal blockade of myelinated fibers on vagal C-fiber afferents. *Am. J. Physiol.*, **239**, R454–R462.

Horvath, R. S. (1969). Variability of cortical auditory evoked response. *J. Neurophysiol.*, **32**, 1056–63.

Horwitz, L. D. & Bishop, V. S. (1972). Effect of acute volume loading on heart rate in the conscious dog. *Circ. Res.*, **30**, 316–21.

Howard, P. (1965). The physiology of positive acceleration. In *A Textbook of Aviation Physiology*, ed. Gillies, J. A., pp. 551–687. Oxford: Pergamon Press.

Hubay, C. A., Waltz, R. C., Brecher, G. A., Praglin, J. & Hingson, R. A. (1954). Circulatory dynamics of venous return during positive–negative pressure respiration. *Anesthesiology*, **15**, 445–61.

Humphrey, D. R. (1967). Neuronal activity in the medulla oblongata of cat evoked by stimulation of the carotid sinus nerve. In *Baroreceptors and Hypertension*, ed. Kezdi, P., pp. 131–68. Oxford: Pergamon Press.

Hyman, A. L. (1968). Pulmonary vasoconstriction due to nonocclusive distension of large pulmonary arteries in the dog. *Circ. Res.*, **23**, 401–13.

Hyman, A. L. & Sanchez, G. (1969). Active response of pulmonary veins to distension of a single pulmonary vein in intact dogs. *J. Lab. Clin. Med.*, **73**, 476–85.

Ito, C. S. & Scher, A. M. (1973). Arterial baroreceptor fibers from the aortic region of the dog in the cervical vagus nerve. *Circ. Res.*, **32**, 442–6.

Ito, C. S. & Scher, A. M. (1974). Reflexes from the aortic baroreceptor fibers in the cervical vagus of the cat and the dog. *Circ. Res.*, **34**, 51–60.

References

Jarecki, M., Thorén, P. N. & Donald, D. E. (1978). Release of renin by the carotid baroreflex in anesthetized dogs. Role of cardiopulmonary vagal afferents and renal arterial pressure. *Circ. Res.*, **42**, 614–19.

Jarisch, A. & Henze, C. (1937). Uber Blutdrucksenkung durch chemische Erregun depressorischer Nerven. *Arch. Exp. Path. Pharmak.*, **187**, 706–30.

Jarisch, A. & Richter, H. (1939). Die Kreislaufwirkung des Veratrins. *Arch. Exp. Path. Pharmak.*, **193**, 347–54.

Jarisch, A. & Zotterman, Y. (1948). Depressor reflexes from the heart. *Acta Physiol. Scand.*, **16**, 31–51.

Johns, E. J., Lewis, B. A. & Singer, B. (1976). Angiotensin release and the sodium-retaining effect of renal nerve activity in the cat. *J. Physiol.*, **257**, 49P–50P.

Johnson, J. A., Davis, J. O. & Witty, R. T. (1971). Effects of catecholamines and renal nerve stimulation on renin release in the nonfiltering kidney. *Circ. Res.*, **29**, 646–53.

Johnson, J. A., Moore, W. W. & Segar, W. E. (1969). Small changes in left atrial pressure and plasma antidiuretic hormone titers in dogs. *Am. J. Physiol.*, **217**, 210–14.

Johnson, J. M., Rowell, L. B., Niederburger, M. & Eisman, M. M. (1974). Human splanchnic and forearm vasoconstrictor responses to reductions of right atrial and aortic pressures. *Circ. Res.*, **34**, 515–24.

Johnson, J. A., Zehr, J. E. & Moore, W. W. (1970). Effects of separate and concurrent osmotic and volume stimuli on plasma ADH in sheep. *Am. J. Physiol.*, **218**, 1273–80.

Johnston, B. D. (1968). Nerve endings in the human endocardium. *Am. J. Anat.*, **122**, 621–9.

Jones, G. M. (1954). Paroxysmal auricular tachycardia: observations in 47 cases. *Ann. Intern. Med.*, **40**, 581–7.

Jones, J. J. (1962). The Bainbridge reflex. *J. Physiol.*, **160**, 298–305.

Kaczmarczyk, G., Eigenheer, F., Gatzka, M., Kuhl, U. & Reinhardt, H. W. (1978). No relation between atrial natriuresis and renal blood flow in conscious dogs. *Pflügers Arch.*, **373**, 49–58.

Kaczmarczyk, G., Kuhl, U., Riedel, J., Arnold, B., Gatzka, M., Eigenheer, F. & Reinhardt, H. W. (1976). Modification of postprandial (PP) water and sodium excretion by exogeneous ADH – studies in conscious dogs on different levels of sodium intake. *Pflügers Arch.*, **362**, Suppl., Abstract 50.

Kaczmarczyk, G., Reinhardt, H. W., Riedel, J., Eisele, R., Gatzka, M. & Kuhl, U. (1977). Left atrial pressure and postprandial diuresis in conscious dogs on a high sodium intake. *Pflügers Arch.*, **368**, 181–4.

Kahl, F. R., Flint, J. F. & Szidon, J. P. (1974). Influence of left atrial distension on renal vasomotor tone. *Am. J. Physiol.*, **226**, 240–6.

Kahl, F. R., Flint, J. F., Szidon, J. P. & Fishman, A. P. (1972). Effects of ectopic tachycardias on the renal circulation. *Circulation*, **45**, Suppl. II, 172.

Kaiser, D., Eckert, P., Gauer, O. H. & Linkenbach, H. J. (1969). Die diurese bei immersion in ein thermoindefferentes Vollbad. *Pflügers Arch.*, **306**, 247–61.

References

Kappagoda, C. T., Knapp, M. F., Linden, R. J., Pearson, M. J. & Whitaker, E. M. (1979). Diuresis from left atrial receptors: effect of plasma on the secretion of the Malpighian tubules of *Rhodnius prolixus*. *J. Physiol.*, **291**, 381–91.

Kappagoda, C. T., Knapp, M. F., Linden, R. J. & Whitaker, E. M. (1976). A possible bioassay for the humoral agent responsible for the diuresis from atrial receptors. *J. Physiol.*, **254**, 59P–60P.

Kappagoda, C. T., Linden, R. J. & Mary, D. A. S. G. (1975). Gradation of the reflex response from atrial receptors. *J. Physiol.*, **251**, 561–7.

Kappagoda, C. T., Linden, R. J. & Mary, D. A. S. G. (1976). Atrial receptors in the cat. *J. Physiol.*, **262**, 431–6.

Kappagoda, C. T., Linden, R. J. & Mary, D. A. S. G. (1977a). Patterns of discharge from atrial receptors in the dog. *J. Physiol.*, **270**, 65P–66P.

Kappagoda, C. T., Linden, R. J. & Mary, D. A. S. G. (1977b). Atrial receptors in the dog and rabbit. *J. Physiol.*, **272**, 799–815.

Kappagoda, C. T., Linden, R. J. & Mary, D. A. S. G. (1979). Chloralose anaesthesia using a continuous infusion system in dogs. *J. Physiol.*, **290**, 10P.

Kappagoda, C. T., Linden, R. J., Mary, D. A. S. G. & Weatherill, D. (1978). Atrial receptors which effect a reflex decrease in renal sympathetic activity. *J. Physiol.*, **280**, 61P–62P.

Kappagoda, C. T., Linden, R. J. & Pashley, M. (1980). Increased sensitivity of ADH bio-assay in rats by change of diet. *J. Physiol.*, **299**, 425–35.

Kappagoda, C. T., Linden, R. J. & Saunders, D. (1972a). The effect of distending the right and left atrial appendages in the dog. *J. Physiol.*, **222**, 35P–36P.

Kappagoda, C. T., Linden, R. J. & Saunders, D. A. (1972b). The effect on heart rate of distending the atrial appendages in the dog. *J. Physiol.*, **225**, 705–19.

Kappagoda, C. T., Linden, R. J., Scott, E. M. & Snow, H. M. (1975). Atrial receptors and heart rate: the efferent pathway. *J. Physiol.*, **249**, 581–90.

Kappagoda, C. T., Linden, R. J. & Sivananthan, N. (1977). The receptors which mediate a reflex increase in heart rate. *J. Physiol.*, **266**, 89P–90P.

Kappagoda, C. T., Linden, R. J. & Sivananthan, N. (1978). Atrial receptors and the urine response. *J. Physiol.*, **282**, 49P.

Kappagoda, C. T., Linden, R. J. & Sivananthan, N. (1979). The nature of the atrial receptors responsible for a reflex increase in heart rate in the dog. *J. Physiol.*, **291**, 393–412.

Kappagoda, C. T., Linden, R. J. & Snow, H. M. (1970). An approach to the problems of acid–base balance. *Clin. Sci.*, **39**, 169–82.

Kappagoda, C. T., Linden, R. J. & Snow, H. M. (1972a). A reflex increase in heart rate from distension of the junction between the superior vena cava and the right atrium. *J. Physiol.*, **220**, 177–97.

Kappagoda, C. T., Linden, R. J. & Snow, H. M. (1972b). The effect of stretching the superior vena caval–right atrial junction on right atrial receptors in the dog. *J. Physiol.*, **227**, 875–87.

References

Kappagoda, C. T., Linden, R. J. & Snow, H. M. (1972c). The effect of distending the atrial appendages on urine flow in the dog. *J. Physiol.*, **227**, 233–42.

Kappagoda, C. T., Linden, R. J. & Snow, H. M. (1973). Effect of stimulating right atrial receptors on urine flow in the dog. *J. Physiol.*, **234**, 493–502.

Kappagoda, C. T., Linden, R. J., Snow, H. M. & Whitaker, E. M. (1974). Left atrial receptors and the antidiuretic hormone. *J. Physiol.*, **237**, 663–83.

Kappagoda, C. T., Linden, R. J., Snow, H. M. & Whitaker, E. M. (1975). Effect of destruction of the posterior pituitary on the diuresis from left atrial receptors. *J. Physiol.*, **244**, 757–70.

Kappagoda, C. T., Linden, R. J. & Sreeharan, N. (1979). The role of renal nerves in the diuresis and natriuresis caused by stimulation of atrial receptors. *J. Physiol.*, **287**, 17P–18P.

Kappagoda, C. T., Stoker, J. B., Snow, H. M. & Linden, R. J. (1972). The CO_2 titration curve of mixed venous blood. *Clin. Sci.*, **43**, 553–9.

Karim, F., Hainsworth, R., Sofola, O. A. & Wood, L. M. (1980). Responses of the heart to stimulation of aortic body chemoreceptors in dogs. *Circ. Res.*, **46**, 77–83.

Karim, F., Kidd, C., Malpus, C. M. & Penna, P. E. (1972). The effects of stimulation of the left atrial receptors on sympathetic efferent nerve activity. *J. Physiol.*, **227**, 243–60.

Keatinge, W. R. (1959). The effect of increased filling pressure on rhythmicity and atrioventricular conduction in isolated mammalian hearts. *J. Physiol.*, **149**, 193–208.

Keith, I. C., Kidd, C., Linden, R. J. & Snow, H. M. (1975). Modification of neuronal activity in the dog medulla oblongata by stimulation of left atrial receptors. *J. Physiol.*, **245**, 80P–81P.

Kent, B. J., Drane, J. W. & Manning, J. W. (1971). Suprapontine contributions to the carotid sinus reflex in the cat. *Circ. Res.*, **29**, 534–41.

Kezdi, P., Kordenat, R. K. & Misra, S. N. (1974). Reflex inhibitory effects of vagal afferents in experimental myocardial infarction. *Am. J. Cardiol.*, **33**, 853–60.

Khabarova, A. I. (1963). *The Afferent Innervation of the Heart.* Tr. Haigh, B. New York: Consultants Bureau.

Kidd, C. (1979). Central neurons activated by cardiac receptors. In *Cardiac Receptors*, ed. Hainsworth, R., Kidd, C. & Linden, R. J., pp. 377–403. Cambridge: Cambridge University Press.

Kidd, C. (1980). Central connections of vagal cardiac receptors. In *Central Interaction between Respiratory and Cardiovascular Control Systems*, ed. Koepchen, P., Hilton, S. M. & Trzebski, A., pp. 104–15. Heidelberg: Springer-Verlag.

Kidd, C., Ledsome, J. R. & Linden, R. J. (1966). Left atrial receptors and heart rate. *J. Physiol.*, **185**, 78P–79P.

Kidd, C., Ledsome, J. R. & Linden, R. J. (1978). The effect of distension of the pulmonary vein–atrial junction on activity of left atrial receptors. *J. Physiol.*, **285**, 445–53.

References

Kilburn, K. H. (1963). Diuresis with paroxysmal tachycardia. *Circulation*, **28**, 749.

Kilburn, K. H. & Sieker, H. O. (1960). Hemodynamic effects of continuous positive and negative pressure breathing in normal man. *Circ. Res.*, **8**, 660–9.

King, A. B. (1939). Nerve endings in the cardiac muscle of the rat. *Bull. Johns Hopkins Hosp.*, **65**, 489–99.

Kinney, M. J. & DiScala, V. A. (1972). Renal clearance studies of effect of atrial distension in the dog. *Am. J. Physiol.* **222**, 1000–3.

Kinney, M. J., Stein, R. M. & DiScala, V. A. (1974). The polyuria of paroxysmal atrial tachycardia. *Circulation*, **50**, 429–35.

Kirchheim, H. R. (1976). Systemic arterial baroreceptor reflexes. *Physiol. Rev.*, **56**, 100–76.

Kjellberg, S. R. & Olsson, S-E. (1954). Roentgenologic studies of the sphincter mechanism of the caval and pulmonary veins. *Acta Radiol.*, **41**, 481–97.

Knapp, M. F., Linden, R. J. & Pearson, M. J. (1981). Diuresis from stimulation of left atrial receptors: ADH on the Malpighian tubules of *Rhodnius prolixus*. *Q. J. Exp. Physiol.* **66**, 333–8.

Knutsson, E. & Sjöstrand, T. (1974). Impulse discharges from the low pressure side varying with the central blood volume. *Pflügers Arch.*, **352**, 105–14.

Koepchen, H. P., Langhorst, P., Seller, H., Polster, J. & Wagner, P. H. (1967). Neuronale Activität im unterem Hirnstamm mit Beziehung zum Kreislauf. *Pflügers Arch.*, **294**, 40–64.

Koizumi, K., Ishikawa, T., Nishino, H. & Brooks, C. McC. (1975). Cardiac and autonomic system reactions to stretch of the atria. *Brain Res.*, **87**, 247–61.

Koizumi, K., Nishino, H. & Brooks, C. McC. (1977). Centers involved in the autonomic reflex reactions originating from stretching of the atria. *Proc. Nat. Acad. Sci. U.S.A.*, **74**, 2177–81.

Koizumi, K. & Yamashita, H. (1977). Effects of stretch of the cardiac atrial on neurosecretory cells in the hypothalamus. *Physiologist*, **20**, 52.

Koizumi, K. & Yamashita, H. (1978). Influence of atrial stretch receptors on hypothalamic neurosecretory neurones. *J. Physiol.*, **285**, 341–58.

Kolatat, T., Ascanio, G., Tallarida, R. J. & Oppenheimer, M. J. (1967). Action potentials in the sensory vagus at the time of coronary infarction. *Am. J. Physiol.*, **213**, 71–8.

Kollai, M., Koizumi, K., Yamashita, H. & Brooks, C. McC. (1978). Study of cardiac sympathetic and vagal efferent activity during reflex responses produced by stretch of the atria. *Brain Res.*, **150**, 519–32.

Korner, P. I. (1971). Integrative neural cardiovascular control. *Physiol. Rev.*, **51**, 312–67.

Korner, P. I. (1979). Central nervous control of autonomic cardiovascular function. In *Handbook of Physiology, The Cardiovascular System, I. The Heart*, ed. Berne, R. M., Sporelakis, N. & Geiger, S. R., pp. 691–739. Bethesda, Maryland: American Physiological Society.

Korner, P. I., Shaw, J., West, M. J. & Oliver, J. R. (1972). Central

References

nervous control of baroreceptor reflexes in the rabbit. *Circ. Res.*, **31**, 637–52.

Kostreva, D. R., Zuperku, E. J., Purtock, R. V., Coon, R. L. & Kampine, J. P. (1975). Sympathetic afferent nerve activity of right heart origin. *Am. J. Physiol.*, **229**, 911–15.

Kumar, S. (1971). Nerve endings in the heart of amphibia. *Mikroskopie*, **27**, 235–41.

LaGrange, R. G., Sloop, C. H. & Schmid, H. E. (1973). Selective stimulation of renal nerves in the anesthetized dog: effect on renin release during control changes in renal haemodynamics. *Circ. Res.*, **33**, 704–12.

Lam, R. L. & Tyler, H. R. (1952). Electrical responses evoked in the visceral afferent nucleus of the rabbit by vagal stimulation. *J. Comp. Neurol.*, **97**, 21–36.

Lange, G., Hsin-Hsiang, L., Chang, A. & Brooks, C. McC. (1966). Effect of stretch in the isolated cat sinoatrial node. *Am. J. Physiol.*, **211**, 1192–6.

Lange, L., Lange, S., Echt, M. & Gauer, O. H. (1974). Heart volume in relation to body posture and immersion in a thermo-neutral bath. *Pflügers Arch.*, **352**, 219–26.

Langrehr, D. (1960). Entladungsmuster und Allgemeine Reizbedingungen von Vorhofsreceptoren bei Hund und Katze. *Pflügers Arch.*, **271**, 257–69.

Larsell, O. (1921). Nerve terminations in the lung of the rabbit. *J. Comp. Neurol.*, **33**, 105–32.

Laubie, M. & Schmitt, H. (1979). Destruction of the nucleus tractus solitarii in the dog: comparison with sinoaortic denervation. *Am. J. Physiol.*, **236**, H736–H743.

Lauson, H. D. & Bocanegra, M. (1961). Clearance of exogenous vasopressin from plasma of dogs. *Am. J. Physiol.*, **200**, 493–7.

Lavrenter, B. I. (1946). Innervation of heart. *Am. Rev. Soc. Med.*, **3**, 229–35.

Lawrence, M., Ledsome, J. R. & Mason, J. M. (1973). The time course of the diuretic response to left atrial distension. *Q. J. Exp. Physiol.*, **58**, 219–27.

Lawrentjew, B. J. (1929). Experimentell-morphologische Studien über den feineren Bau des autonomen Nervensystems. I. Die Beteiligung des Vagus und der Herzinnervation. *Z. Mikrosk. Anat. Forsch.*, **16**, 383–411.

Ledsome, J. R. (1979). The effects of medullary lesions on the reflex response to distension of the pulmonary vein–left atrial junctions. In *Cardiac Receptors*, ed. Hainsworth, R., Kidd, C. & Linden, R. J., pp. 405–17. Cambridge: Cambridge University Press.

Ledsome, J. R. & Hainsworth, R. (1970). The effects upon respiration of distension of the pulmonary vein–atrial junctions. *Resp. Physiol.*, **9**, 86–94.

Ledsome, J. R. & Kan, W-O. (1977). Reflex changes in hindlimb and renal vascular resistance in response to distension of the isolated pulmonary arteries of the dog. *Circ. Res.*, **40**, 64–72.

References

Ledsome, J. R. & Linden, R. J. (1962). The effects of distension of the junctional regions of the pulmonary veins and left atrium. *J. Physiol.*, **165**, 44P–45P.

Ledsome, J. R. & Linden, R. J. (1964a). The effect of bretylium tosylate on some cardiovascular reflexes. *J. Physiol.*, **170**, 442–55.

Ledsome, J. R. & Linden, R. J. (1964b). A reflex increase in heart rate from distension of the pulmonary vein–atrial junctions. *J. Physiol.*, **170**, 456–73.

Ledsome, J. R. & Linden, R. J. (1967). The effect of distending a pouch of the left atrium on the heart rate. *J. Physiol.*, **193**, 121–9.

Ledsome, J. R. & Linden, R. J. (1968). The role of the left atrial receptors in the diuretic response to left atrial distension. *J. Physiol.*, **198**, 487–503.

Ledsome, J. R., Linden, R. J. & Norman, J. (1965). The use of sympathetic B-receptor blocking agents in the investigation of reflex changes in heart rate. *Br. J. Pharmac. Chemother.*, **24**, 781–8.

Ledsome, J. R., Linden, R. J. & Norman, J. (1971). The effect of light chloralose and pentobarbitone anaesthesia on the acid–base state and oxygenation of arterial blood in dogs. *J. Physiol.*, **212**, 611–27.

Ledsome, J. R., Linden, R. J. & O'Connor, W. J. (1961). The mechanisms by which distension of the left atrium produces diuresis in anaesthetized dogs. *J. Physiol.*, **159**, 87–100.

Ledsome, J. R. & Mason, J. M. (1972). The effects of vasopressin on the diuretic response to left atrial distension. *J. Physiol.*, **211**, 427–40.

Lenfant, C. & Howell, B. J. (1960). Cardiovascular adjustments in dogs during continuous pressure breathing. *J. Appl. Physiol.*, **15**, 425–8.

Levinson, R., Epstein, M., Sackner, M. A. & Begin, R. (1977). Comparison of the effects of water immersion and saline infusion on central hemodynamics in man. *Clin. Sci. Mol. Med.*, **52**, 343–50.

Levy, M. N. & Zieske, H. (1969). Effect of enhanced contractility on the left ventricular response to vagus nerve stimulation in dogs. *Circ. Res.*, **24**, 303–11.

Lifschitz, M. D. (1978). Lack of a role for the renal nerves in renal sodium reabsorption in conscious dogs. *Clin. Sci. Mol. Med.*, **54**, 567–72.

Lind, J. & Wegelius, C. (1956). The relationship between electrical and mechanical events in the heart as demonstrated by angiocardiography. (Frank Norman Wilson lecture.) *Univ. Michigan Med. Bull.*, **22**, 447–63.

Linden, R. J. (1973). Function of cardiac receptors. *Circulation*, **48**, 463–80.

Linden, R. J. (1975). Reflexes from the heart. *Prog. Cardiovasc. Dis.*, **18**, 201–21.

Linden, R. J. (1976). Reflexes from receptors in the heart. *Cardiology*, **61**, (Suppl. 1): 7–30.

Linden, R. J. (1979a). Atrial receptors and heart rate. In *Cardiac Receptors*, ed. Hainsworth, R., Kidd, C. & Linden, R. J., pp. 165–91. Cambridge: Cambridge University Press.

Linden, R. J. (1979b). Atrial receptors and renal function. *Am. J. Cardiol.*, **44**, 879–83.

References

Linden, R. J., Malpus, C. M., Saunders, D. A. & Snow, H. M. (1974). Correlation of a cardiovascular reflex response with the auditory evoked potential in the dog during changes of depths of anaesthesia. *J. Physiol.*, **238**, 9P–10P.

Linden, R. J., Mary, D. A. S. G. & Weatherill, D. (1979a). Atrial receptors which effect reflex inhibition in renal nerves in dogs. *J. Physiol.*, **290**, 11P.

Linden, R. J., Mary, D. A. S. G. & Weatherill, D. (1979b). The response of renal nerve inhibition to stimulation of atrial receptors during changes in carotid sinus pressure in the dog. *J. Physiol.*, **290**, 32P–33P.

Linden, R. J., Mary, D. A. S. G. & Weatherill, D. (1980a). The nature of the atrial receptors responsible for a reflex decrease in activity in renal nerves in the dog. *J. Physiol.*, **300**, 31–40.

Linden, R. J., Mary, D. A. S. G. & Weatherill, D. (1980b). The effects of changes in carotid sinus pressure on activity in efferent cardiac sympathetic nerves which respond to stimulation of atrial receptors. *J. Physiol.*, **308**, 106P–107P.

Linden, R. J., Mary, D. A. S. G. & Weatherill, D. (1981a). The effect of cooling on transmission of impulses in vagal nerve fibres attached to atrial receptors in the dog. *Q. J. Exp. Physiol.* **66**, 321–2.

Linden, R. J., Mary, D. A. S. G. & Weatherill, D. (1981b). The responses in renal nerves to stimulation of atrial receptors, carotid sinus baroreceptors and carotid chemoreceptors. *Q. J. Exp. Physiol.*, **66**, 179–91.

Linden, R. J. & Norman, J. (1969). The effect of acidaemia on the response to stimulation of the autonomic nerves to the heart. *J. Physiol.*, **200**, 51–71.

Linden, R. J. & Sreeharan, N. (1979). Does the renal humoral response to stimulation of atrial receptors include a natriuresis? *J. Physiol.*, **291**, 43P–44P.

Linden, R. J. & Sreeharan, N. (1981). Humoral nature of the urine response to stimulation of atrial receptors. *Q. J. Exp. Physiol.*, **66**, 431–8.

Linkenbach, H. J., Eckert, P. & Gauer, O. H. (1967). Nachweis eins diuretischen Faktors im menschlichen Serum während der durch Expansion des intrathorakalen Blutvolumens ausgelösten Diurese. *Pflügers Arch.*, **293**, 107–14.

Lioy, F., Malliani, A., Pagani, M., Recordati, G. & Schwartz, P. J. (1974). Reflex hemodynamic responses initiated from the thoracic aorta. *Circ. Res.*, **34**, 78–84.

Little, R., Wennergren, G. & Oberg, B. (1975). Aspects of the central integration of arterial baroreceptor and cardiac ventricular receptor reflexes in the cat. *Acta Physiol. Scand.*, **93**, 85–96.

Lloyd, T. C. (1972). Control of systemic vascular resistance by pulmonary and left heart baroreflexes. *Am. J. Physiol.*, **222**, 1151–517.

Lloyd, T. C. (1975). Cardiopulmonary baroreflexes: effects of staircase, ramp and square-wave stimulation. *Am. J. Physiol.*, **228**, 470–6.

Lloyd, T. C. & Freidman, J. J. (1977). Effect of a left atrium–pulmonary

vein baroreflex on peripheral vascular beds. *Am. J. Physiol.*, **233**, H587–H591.
Lloyd, T. C. & Schneider, A. J. L. (1969). Relation of pulmonary arterial pressure to pressure in the pulmonary venous system. *J. Appl. Physiol.*, **27**, 489–97.
Lloyd, T. C. & Schneider, A. J. L. (1970). Reflex pulmonary vascular response to distension of lung vessels and left heart. *J. Appl. Physiol.*, **29**, 318–22.
Lluch, S., Moguilevsky, H. C., Pietra, G., Shaffer, A. B., Hirsch, L. J. & Fishman, A. P. (1969). A reproducible model of cardiogenic shock in the dog. *Circulation*, **39**, 205–18.
Lowenstein, W. R. & Altamirano-Orrego, R. (1956). Enhancement of activity in a Pacinian corpuscle by sympathomimetic agents. *Nature*, **178**, 1292–3.
Luria, M. H., Adelson, E. I. & Lochaya, S. (1966). Paroxysmal tachycardia with polyuria. *Ann. Intern. Med.*, **65**, 461–70.
Lydtin, H. & Hamilton, W. F. (1964). Effect of acute changes in left atrial pressure on urine flow in unanaesthetized dogs. *Am. J. Physiol.*, **207**, 530–6.
McCall, R. B., Gebber, G. L. & Barman, S. M. (1977). Spinal interneurones in the baroreceptor reflex arc. *Am. J. Physiol.*, **232**, H657–H665.
MacMillan, J. B. & Lev, M. (1959). The ageing heart. I. Endocardium. *J. Gerontol.*, **14**, 268–83.
Malliani, A. (1979). Afferent cardiovascular sympathetic nerve fibres and their function in the neural regulation of the circulation. In *Cardiac Receptors*, ed. Hainsworth, R., Kidd, C. & Linden, R. J., pp. 319–38. Cambridge: Cambridge University Press.
Malliani, A., Pagani, M., Recordati, G. & Schwartz, P. J. (1971). Spinal sympathetic reflexes elicited by increases in arterial blood pressure. *Am. J. Physiol.*, **220**, 128–34.
Malliani, A., Parks, M., Tuckett, R. P. & Brown, A. M. (1973). Reflex increases in heart rate elicited by stimulation of afferent cardiac sympathetic nerve fibers in the cat. *Circ. Res.*, **32**, 9–14.
Malliani, A., Peterson, D. F., Bishop, V. S. & Brown, A. M. (1972). Spinal sympathetic cardiocardiac reflexes. *Circ. Res.*, **30**, 158–66.
Malliani, A., Recordati, G. & Schwartz, P. J. (1973). Nervous activity of efferent cardiac sympathetic fibres with atrial and ventricular endings. *J. Physiol.*, **229**, 457–69.
Malliani, A., Schwartz, P. J. & Zanchetti, A. (1969). A sympathetic reflex elicited by experimental coronary occlusion. *Am. J. Physiol.*, **217**, 703–9.
Mancia, G. & Donald, D. E. (1975). Demonstration that the atria, ventricles and lungs each are responsible for a tonic inhibition of the vasomotor center in the dog. *Circ. Res.*, **36**, 310–18.
Mancia, G., Donald, D. E. & Shepherd, J. T. (1973). Inhibition of adrenergic outflow to peripheral blood vessels by vagal afferents from the cardiopulmonary region in the dog. *Circ. Res.*, **33**, 713–21.

References

Mancia, G., Romero, J. C. & Shepherd, J. T. (1975). Continuous inhibition of renin release in dogs by vagally innervated receptors in the cardiopulmonary region. *Circ. Res.*, **36**, 529–35.

Mancia, G., Romero, J. C. & Strong, C. G. (1974). Neural influence on canine renal prostaglandin secretion. *Acta Physiol. Lat.*, **24**, 555–60.

Mancia, G., Shepherd, J. T. & Donald, D. E. (1975). Role of cardiac, pulmonary and carotid mechanoreceptors in the control of hind-limb and renal circulation in dogs. *Circ. Res.*, **37**, 200–8.

Mancia, G., Shepherd, J. T. & Donald, D. E. (1976). Interplay among carotid sinus, cardiopulmonary and carotid body reflexes in dogs. *Am. J. Physiol.*, **230**, 19–24.

Mason, J. M. & Ledsome, J. R. (1974). Effects of obstruction of the mitral orifice or distension of the pulmonary vein–atrial junctions on renal hind-limb vascular resistance in the dog. *Circ. Res.*, **35**, 24–32.

Meek, W. J. & Eyster, J. A. E. (1922). The effect of plethora and variations in venous pressure on diastolic size and output of the heart. *Am. J. Physiol.*, **61**, 186–202.

Mendell, L. M. & Wall, P. D. (1964). Presynaptic hyperpolarization: a role for fine afferent fibres. *J. Physiol.*, **172**, 274–94.

Menninger, R. P. (1979). Response of supraoptic neurosecretory cells to changes in left atrial distension. *Am. J. Physiol.*, **236**, R261–R267.

Menninger, R. P. & Frazier, D. T. (1972). Effects of blood volume and atrial stretch on hypothalamic single-unit activity. *Am. J. Physiol.*, **223**, 288–93.

Meyling, H. A. (1953). Structure and significance of the peripheral extensions of the autonomic nervous system. *J. Comp. Neurol.*, **99**, 495–543.

Michailow, S. (1908). Die Nerven des Endocardiums. *Anat. Anz.*, **32**, 87–101.

Middleton, S., Woolsey, C. N., Burton, H. & Rose, J. E. (1973). Neural activity with cardiac periodicity in medulla oblongata of the cat. *Brain Res.*, **50**, 297–314.

Milhorn, H. T. (1966). *The Application of Control Theory to Physiological Systems.* London: W. B. Saunders.

Miller, M. R. & Kasahara, M. (1964). Studies on the nerve endings in the heart. *Am. J. Anat.*, **115**, 217–34.

Miller, R. A. & Morris, M. E. (1961). Sympatho-adrenal responses during general anaesthesia in the dog and man. *Can. Anaesth. Soc. J.*, **8**, 356–86.

Mills, I. H. & Osbaldiston, G. W. (1968). The effect of stretch of the right atrium on arterial pressure and renal function in the dog. *J. Physiol.*, **197**, 40P–41P.

Mitchell, G. A. G. (1950). The renal nerves. *Br. J. Urol.*, **22**, 269–80.

Mitchell, G. A. G. (1956). *Cardiovascular Innervation.* Edinburgh: E. & S. Livingstone.

Miura, M. & Reis, D. J. (1972). The role of the solitary and paramedian reticular nuclei in mediating cardiovascular reflex responses from carotid baro- and chemoreceptors. *J. Physiol.*, **223**, 525–48.

References

Moe, G. K., Cohen, W. & Vick, R. L. (1963). Experimentally induced paroxysmal A-V nodal tachycardia in the dog. *Am. Heart J.*, **65**, 87–92.

Moran, W. H. Jr, Miltenberger, F. W., Shu'ayb, W. A. & Zimmermann, B. (1964). The relationship of antidiuretic hormone secretion to surgical stress. *Surgery*, **56**, 99–108.

Moravec-Mochet, M., Moravec, J. & Hatt, P. Y. (1977). Presence of synaptic and muscle spindle-like structures in the atrioventricular junction of the rat heart: an electron microscopic study. *J. Ultrastruct. Res.*, **58**, 196–209.

Muers, M. F. & Sleight, P. (1972a). The reflex cardiovascular depression caused by occlusion of the coronary sinus in the dog. *J. Physiol.*, **221**, 259–82.

Muers, M. F. & Sleight, P. (1972b). Action potentials from ventricular mechanoreceptors stimulated by occlusion of the coronary sinus in the dog. *J. Physiol.*, **221**, 283–309.

Murdaugh, H. V., Sieker, H. O. & Manfredi, F. (1959). Effect of altered intrathoracic pressure on renal haemodynamics, electrolyte excretion and water clearance. *J. Clin. Invest.*, **38**, 834–42.

Nashat, F. S. (1974). Topics in renal physiology. In *Recent Advances in Physiology*, ed. Linden, R. J., pp. 191–238. London: Churchill.

Nashat, F. S., Scholefield, F. R., Tappin, J. W. & Wilcox, C. S. (1969). The effect of acute changes in haematocrit in the anaesthetized dog on the volume and character of the urine. *J. Physiol.*, **205**, 305–16.

Neil, E. & Joels, N. (1961). The impulse activity in cardiac afferent vagal fibres. *Naunyn Schmiedebergs Arch. Pharmacol.*, **240**, 453–60.

Neil, E. & Zotterman, Y. (1950). Cardiac vagal afferent fibres in the cat and the frog. *Acta, Physiol. Scand.*, **20**, 160–5.

Nettleship, W. A. (1936). Experimental studies on the afferent innervation of the cat's heart. *J. Comp. Neurol.*, **64**, 115–33.

Nevalainen, T. O., Hakumaki, M. O. K., Hyodynmaa, S. J., Narhi, M. V. O. & Sarajas, H. S. S. (1980). Distension of pulmonary vein–left atrial junction: heart rate responses in conscious and anaesthetized dogs. *Acta Physiol. Scand.*, **110**, 47–52.

Nicholls, M. G., Espiner, E. A., Donald, R. A. & Hughes, H. (1974). Aldosterone and its regulation during diuresis in patients with gross congestive heart failure. *Clin. Sci. Mol. Med.*, **47**, 301–15.

Nonidez, J. F. (1937). Identification of the receptor areas in the venae cavae and the pulmonary veins which initiate reflex cardiac acceleration (Bainbridge's reflex). *Am. J. Anat.*, **61**, 203–31.

Nonidez, J. F. (1939). Studies on the innervation of the heart. I. Distribution of the cardiac nerves, with special reference to the identification of sympathetic and parasympathetic post-ganglionics. *Am. J. Anat.*, **65**, 361–413.

Nonidez, J. F. (1941). Studies on innervation of the heart. II. Afferent nerve endings in the large arteries and veins. *Am. J. Anat.*, **68**, 151–89.

Nonidez, J. F. (1943). The structure and innervation of the conductive system of the heart of the dog and rhesus monkey, as seen with a silver impregnation technique. *Am. Heart J.*, **26**, 577–97.

References

Oberg, B. & Thorén, P. (1972a). Studies on left ventricular receptors, signalling in non-medullated vagal afferents. *Acta Physiol. Scand.*, **85**, 145–63.

Oberg, B. & Thorén, P. (1972b). Increased activity in left ventricular receptors during hemorrhage or occlusion of caval veins in the cat. A possible cause of the vaso-vagal reaction. *Acta Physiol. Scand.*, **85**, 164–73.

Oberg, B. & Thorén P. (1973). Circulatory responses to stimulation of medullated and non-medullated afferents in the cardiac nerve in the cat. *Acta Physiol. Scand.*, **87**, 121–32.

Oberg, B. & White, S. (1970a). Circulatory effects of interruption and stimulation of cardiac vagal afferents. *Acta Physiol. Scand.*, **80**, 383–94.

Oberg, B. & White, S. (1970b). The role of vagal cardiac nerves and arterial baroreceptors in the circulatory adjustments to hemorrhage in the cat. *Acta Physiol. Scand.*, **80**, 395–403.

O'Connor, W. J. & Summerill, R. A. (1979). Sodium excretion in normal conscious dogs. *Cardiovasc. Res.*, **13**, 22–30.

Orloff, J., Wagner, H. N. & Davidson, D. G. (1958). The effect of variations in solute excretion and vasopressin dosage on the excretion of water in the dog. *J. Clin. Invest.*, **37**, 458–64.

Pagani, M., Schwartz, P. J., Bishop, V. S. & Malliani, A. (1975). Reflex sympathetic changes in aortic diastolic pressure–diameter relationship. *Am. J. Physiol.*, **229**, 286–90.

Paintal, A. S. (1953a). A study of right and left atrial receptors. *J. Physiol.*, **120**, 596–610.

Paintal, A. S. (1953b). The response of pulmonary and cardiovascular vagal receptors to certain drugs. *J. Physiol.*, **121**, 182–90.

Paintal, A. S. (1953c). The conduction velocities and respiratory and cardiovascular afferent fibres in the vagus nerve. *J. Physiol.*, **121**, 341–59.

Paintal, A. S. (1955). A study of ventricular pressure receptors and their role in the Bezold reflex. *Q. J. Exp. Physiol.*, **40**, 348–63.

Paintal, A. S. (1957). The influence of certain chemical substances on the initiation of sensory discharges in pulmonary and gastric stretch receptors and atrial receptors. *J. Physiol.*, **135**, 486–510.

Paintal, A. S. (1962). Determination of intrathoracic conduction time in cardiovascular afferent fibres of the vagus nerve. *J. Physiol.*, **163**, 222–38.

Paintal, A. S. (1963a). Vagal afferent fibres. *Ergeb. Physiol.*, **52**, 74–156.

Paintal, A. S. (1963b). Natural stimulation of type B atrial receptors. *J. Physiol.*, **169**, 116–36.

Paintal, A. S. (1964). Effects of drugs on vertebrate mechanoreceptors. *Pharmacol. Rev.*, **16**, 341–80.

Paintal, A. S. (1965a). Block of conduction in mammalian myelinated nerve fibres by low temperatures. *J. Physiol.*, **180**, 1–19.

Paintal, A. S. (1965b). Effects of temperature on conduction in single vagal and saphenous myelinated nerve fibres of the cat. *J. Physiol.*, **180**, 20–49.

References

Paintal, A. S. (1966). Re-evaluation of respiratory reflexes. *Q. J. Exp. Physiol.*, **51**, 151–63.
Paintal, A. S. (1972). Cardiovascular receptors. In *Handbook of sensory physiology*, Vol. III/I. *Enteroreceptors*, ed. Neil, E., pp. 1–45. Berlin: Springer-Verlag.
Paintal, A. S. (1973a). Vagal sensory receptors and their reflex effects. *Physiol. Rev.*, **53**, 159–227.
Paintal, A. S. (1973b). Sensory mechanisms involved in the Bezold–Jarisch effect. *Aust. J. Exp. Biol. Sci.*, **51** (1), 3–15.
Paley, H. W., Leonard, J. J., Eggers, G. W. N. Jr, deGroot, W. J. & Warren, J. V. (1960). Hemodynamic effects of full phase negative pressure breathing. *Circulation*, **22**, 794.
Pannese, E. (1969). Unusual membrane-particle complexes within nerve cells of the spinal ganglia. *J. Ultrastruct. Res.*, **29**, 334–42.
Pannier, R. (1940). Contribution a l'étude de l'innervation pressor-et chemo-sensible des oreillettes et des vaisseaux de la base du coeur. *Archs Int. Pharmacodyn. Ther.*, **64**, 476–84.
Pathak, C. L. (1958). Effects of changes in intraluminal pressure on inotropic and chronotropic responses of isolated mammalian hearts. *Am. J. Physiol.*, **194**, 197–9.
Pathak, C. L. (1959). Alternative mechanism of cardiac acceleration in Bainbridge's infusion experiments. *Am. J. Physiol.*, **197**, 441–4.
Pathak, C. L. (1966). The fallacy of the Bainbridge reflex. *Am. Heart J.*, **72**, 577–81.
Payne, R. M., Stone, H. L. & Engelken, E. J. (1971). Atrial function during volume loading. *J. Appl. Physiol.*, **31**, 326–31.
Pearce, J. W. (1959). The effect of vagotomy and denervation of the carotid sinus on diuresis following plasma volume expansion. *Can. J. Biochem. Physiol.*, **37**, 81–90.
Pelletier, C. L., Clement, D. L. & Shepherd, J. T. (1972). Comparison of afferent activity of canine aortic and sinus nerves. *Circ. Res.*, **31**, 557–68.
Pelletier, C. L., Edis, A. J. & Shepherd, J. T. (1971). Circulatory reflex from vagal afferents in response to hemorrhage in the dog. *Circ. Res.*, **29**, 626–34.
Pelletier, C. L. & Shepherd, J. T. (1973). Circulatory reflexes from mechanoreceptors in the cardio-aortic area. *Circ. Res.*, **33**, 131–8.
Perlmutt, J. H. (1961). Renal activity of vasopressin in anesthetized dogs. *Am. J. Physiol.*, **200**, 400–4.
Peterson, D. F. & Bishop, V. S. (1974). Reflex blood pressure control during acute myocardial ischaemia in the conscious dog. *Circ. Res.*, **34**, 226–32.
Peterson, D. F. & Brown, A. M. (1971). Pressor reflexes produced by stimulation of afferent fibres in the cardiac sympathetic nerves of the cat. *Circ. Res.*, **28**, 605–10.
Pillsbury, H. R. C., Guazzi, M. & Freis, E. D. (1969). Vagal afferent depressor nerves in the rabbit. *Am. J. Physiol.*, **217**, 768–70.
Plechkova, E. K. (1936). On the morphology of the antagonistic innervation of the heart. *Bull. Biol. Med. Exp. U.R.S.S.*, **1**, 402.

References

Pomeranz, B. H., Birtch, A. G. & Barger, A. C. (1968). Neural control of intrarenal blood flow. *Am. J. Physiol.*, **215**, 1067–81.

Porter, R. (1963). Unit responses evoked in the medulla oblongata by vagus nerve stimulation. *J. Physiol.*, **168**, 717–35.

Potkay, S., Daggett, W. M. & Gilmore, J. P. (1970). Role of the vagus in body water regulation. *Am. J. Physiol.*, **218**, 1333–6.

Price, H. L. & Cohen, P. J. (1964). *The Effects of Anesthetics on the Circulation.* Springfield, Ill.: Thomas.

Prosnitz, E. H. & DiBona, G. F. (1978). Effect of decreased renal-sympathetic nerve activity on renal tubular sodium reabsorption. *Am. J. Physiol.*, **235**, F557–F563.

Purtock, R. V., von Colditz, J. H., Seagard, J. L., Igler, F. O., Zuperku, E. J. & Kampine, J. P. (1977). Reflex effects of thoracic sympathetic afferent nerve stimulation on the kidney. *Am. J. Physiol.*, **233**, H580–H586.

Randall, W. C., Pace, J. P., Wecshsler, J. S. & Kim, K. S. K. (1969). Cardiac responses to separate stimulation of sympathetic and parasympathetic components of the vagosympathetic trunk in the dog. *Cardiologia*, **54**, 104–18.

Rao, P. S., Fahim, M. & Gupta, B. N. (1975). Relative distribution of types A and B atrial receptors in dogs, cats, monkeys and rabbits. *Experientia*, **31**, 1174–5.

Recordati, G. M. (1978). Type A atrial receptors in the cat: effects of changes in atrial volume and contractility. *J. Physiol.*, **280**, 303–17.

Recordati, G., Lombardi, F., Bishop, V. S. & Malliani, A. (1975). Response of type B atrial vagal receptors to changes in wall tension during atrial filling. *Circ. Res.*, **36**, 682–91.

Recordati, G., Lombardi, F., Bishop, V. S. & Malliani, A. (1976). Mechanical stimuli exciting type A atrial vagal receptors in the cat. *Circ. Res.*, **38**, 397–403.

Recordati, G., Lombardi, F., Malliani, A. & Brown, A. M. (1974). Instantaneous dimensional changes of the right atrium in the cat. *J. Appl. Physiol.*, **36**, 686–92.

Recordati, G., Schwartz, P. J., Pagani, M., Malliani, A. & Brown, A. M. (1971). Activation of cardiac vagal receptors during myocardial ischaemia. *Experientia*, **27**, 1423–4.

Reeves, J. L., Henry, J. P. & Gauer, O. H. (1956). Three methods of inducing graded obstruction of the pulmonary circulation. *Am. J. Vet. Res.*, **17**, 98–102.

Reimann, K. A. & Weaver, L. C. (1980). Contrasting reflexes evoked by chemical activation of cardiac afferent nerves. *Am. J. Physiol.*, **239**, H316–H325.

Reinhardt, H. W., Kaczmarczyk, G., Eisele, R., Arnold, B., Eigenheer, F. & Kuhl, U. (1977). Left atrial pressure and sodium balance in conscious dogs on a low sodium intake. *Pflügers Arch.*, **370**, 59–66.

Reinhardt, H. W., Kaczmarczyk, G., Eisele, R., Reidel, J., Kuhl, U. & Gatzka, M. (1975). Water and electrolyte excretion during acute reversible mitral stenosis in conscious dogs on a low and a high sodium intake. *Pflügers Arch.*, Suppl. **355**, abst. 103.

References

Reinhardt, H. W., Kaczmarczyk, G., Mohnhaupt, R. & Simgen, B. (1980a). Atrial natriuresis under the condition of a constant renal perfusion pressure. *Pflügers Arch.*, **389**, 9–15.

Reinhardt, H. W., Kaczmarczyk, G., Mohnhaupt, R. & Simgen, B. (1980b). The possible mechanism of atrial natriuresis – experiments on chronically instrumented dogs. In *Hormonal Regulation of Sodium Excretion*, ed. Lichardus, B., Schrier, R. W. & Ponec, J., pp. 63–72. Proceedings of an International Symposium, Bratislava. Elsevier/North Holland Biomedical Press.

Reitz, B. A., Dong, E. & Stinson, E. B. (1971). The Bainbridge reflex in canine cardiac autotransplants. *Circulation* (Suppl. 1) **43**, 136–40.

Ricksten, S.-E., Noresson, E. & Thorén, P. (1979). Inhibition of renal sympathetic nerve traffic from cardiac receptors in normotensive and spontaneously hypertensive rats. *Acta Physiol. Scand.*, **106**, 17–22.

Risch, W. D., Koubenec, H-J., Beckmann, U., Lange, S. & Gauer, O. H. (1978). The effect of graded immersion on heart volume, central venous pressure, pulmonary blood distribution and heart rate in man. *Pflügers Arch.*, **374**, 115–18.

Risch, W. D., Koubenec, H-J., Gauer, O. H. & Lange, S. (1978). Time course of cardiac distension with rapid immersion in a thermo-neutral bath. *Pflügers Arch.*, **374**, 119–20.

Robertson, J. D., Swan, A. A. B. & Whitteridge, D. (1956). Effect of anaesthetics on systemic baroreceptors. *J. Physiol.*, **131**, 463–72.

Roddie, I. C., Shepherd, J. T. & Whelan, R. F. (1957). Reflex changes in vasoconstrictor tone in human skeletal muscle in response to stimulation of receptors in a low-pressure area of the intra thoracic vascular bed. *J. Physiol.*, **139**, 369–76.

Rogge, J. D., Moore, W. W., Segar, W. E. & Fasola, A. F. (1967). Effect of $+G_z$ and $+G_x$ acceleration on peripheral venous ADH levels in humans. *J. Appl. Physiol.*, **23**, 870–3.

Romero, J. C., Dunlop, C. L. & Strong, C. G. (1976). The effect of indomethacin and other anti-inflammatory drugs on the renin-angiotensin system. *J. Clin. Invest.*, **58**, 282–8.

Ross, J., Frahm, C. J. & Braunwald, E. (1961). The influence of intracardiac baroreceptors on venous return, systemic vascular volume and peripheral resistance. *J. Clin. Invest.*, **40**, 563–72.

Salmoiraghi, G. C. (1962). 'Cardiovascular' neurones in brainstem of cat. *J. Neurophysiol.*, **25**, 182–97.

Santini, M. (1969). New fibers of sympathetic nature in the inner core region of Pacinian corpuscles. *Brain Res.*, **16**, 535–8.

Saunders, D. A. (1979). Evaluation of a new cardiovascular reflex. Ph.D. Thesis, University of Leeds.

Sassa, K. & Miyazaki, H. (1920). The influence of venous pressure upon the heart-rate. *J. Physiol.*, **54**, 203–12.

Schoultz, T. W. & Swett, J. E. (1972). The fine structure of the Golgi tendon organ. *J. Neurocytol.*, **1**, 1–26.

Schrier, R. W., Berl, T. & Anderson, R. J. (1979). Osmotic and nonosmotic control of vasopressin release. *Am. J. Physiol.*, **236**, F321–F332.

References

Schwartz, P. J., Pagani, M., Lombardi, F., Malliani, A. & Brown, A. M. (1973). A cardiocardiac sympathovagal reflex in the cat. *Circ. Res.*, **32**, 215–20.

Schwartz, P. J., Stone, H. L. & Brown, A. M. (1976). Effects of unilateral stellate ganglion blockade on the arrhythmias associated with coronary occlusion. *Am. Heart J.*, **92**, 589–99.

Scott, E. M. (1975). The efferent pathway of the reflex responses to stimulation of left atrial receptors in the dog. Ph.D. Thesis, University of Leeds.

Seal, J. B. & Zbrozyna, A. W. (1978). Renal vasoconstriction and its habituation in the course of repeated auditory stimulation and naturally elicited defence reactions in dogs. *J. Physiol.*, **280**, 56P–57P.

Selkurt, E. E. & Elpers, M. J. (1963). Influence of hemorrhagic shock on renal hemodynamics and osmolar clearance in the dog. *Am. J. Physiol.*, **205**, 147–52.

Selkurt, E. E., Womark, I. & Dailey, W. N. (1965). Mechanism of natriuresis and diuresis during elevated renal arterial pressure. *Am. J. Physiol.*, **209**, 95–9.

Seller, H. & Illert, M. (1969). The localization of the first synapse in the carotid sinus baroreceptor reflex pathway and its alteration of the afferent input. *Pflügers Arch.*, **306**, 1–19.

Semenov, S. P. (1963). Experimental-morphological study of afferent endings of different cardiac nerves. *Arkh. Anat.*, **45**, 72–83.

Share, L. (1961). Acute reduction in extracellular fluid volume and the concentration of antidiuretic hormone in blood. *Endocrinology*, **69**, 925–33.

Share, L. (1965). Effects of carotid occlusion and left atrial distension on plasma vasopressin titer. *Am. J. Physiol.*, **208**, 219–23.

Shepherd, J. T. (1973). Intrathoracic baroreceptors. In *Mayo Clinic Proceedings*, **48**, 426–37.

Shu'ayb, W. A., Moran, W. H. & Zimmerman, B. (1965). Studies of the mechanism of antidiuretic hormone secretion and post-commissurotomy dilutional syndrome. *Ann. Surg.*, **162**, 690–701.

Sieker, H. O., Gauer, O. H. & Henry, J. P. (1954). The effect of continuous negative pressure breathing on water and electrolyte excretion by the human kidney. *J. Clin. Invest.*, **33**, 572–7.

Siggaard-Andersen, O. (1963). Blood acid–base alignment nomogram. *Scand. J. Clin. Lab. Invest.*, **15**, 211–17.

Siggaard-Andersen, O. (1971). An acid–base chart for arterial blood with normal and pathophysiological reference areas. *Scand. J. Clin. Lab. Invest.*, **27**, 239–45.

Sivananthan, N., Kappagoda, C. T. & Linden, R. J. (1981). The nature of atrial receptors responsible for the increase in urine flow caused by distension of the left atrium. *Q. J. Exp. Physiol.*, **66**, 51–9.

Sleight, P. (1964). A cardiovascular depressor reflex from the epicardium of the left ventricle of the dog. *J. Physiol.*, **173**, 321–43.

Sleight, P. (1975). Neural control of the cardiovascular system. In *Modern Trends in Cardiology*, ed. Oliver, M. F., pp. 1–43. London: Butterworth.

References

Sleight, P. (1979). Possible physiological stimuli for ventricular receptors and their significance in man. In *Cardiac Receptors*, ed. Hainsworth, R., Kidd, C. & Linden, R. J., pp. 241–58. Cambridge: Cambridge University Press.

Sleight, P., Lall, A. & Muers, M. (1969). Reflex cardiovascular effects of epicardial stimulation by acetylstrophanthidin in dogs. *Circ. Res.*, **25**, 705–11.

Sleight, P. & Widdicombe, J. G. (1965). Action potentials in fibres from receptors in the epicardium and myocardium of the dog's left ventricle. *J. Physiol.*, **181**, 235–58.

Slick, G. L., DiBona, G. F. & Kaloyanides, G. J. (1974). Renal sympathetic nerve activity in sodium retention of acute caval constriction. *Am. J. Physiol.*, **226**, 925–30.

Smirnow, A. (1895). Uber die sensiblen Nervenendigungen im Herzen bei Amphibien und Säugertieren. *Anat. Anz.*, **10**, 737–49.

Smith, R. S. & Pearce, J. W. (1961). Microelectrode recordings from the region of the nucleus tractus solitarius in the cat. *Can. J. Biochem. Physiol.*, **39**, 933–9.

Snow, H. M. (1973). The effects of hypoxia on the resistance to blood flow in the pulmonary veins. Ph.D. Thesis, University of Leeds.

Snyder, D. W. & Gebber, G. L. (1973). Relationship between medullary depressor region and central vasopressor pathways. *Am. J. Physiol.*, **225**, 1129–37.

Sonnenberg, H. & Pearce, J. W. (1962). Renal response to measured blood volume expansion in differently hydrated dogs. *Am. J. Physiol.*, **203**, 344–52.

Steiner, S. M., Frayser, R. & Ross, J. C. (1965). Alterations in pulmonary diffusing capacity and pulmonary capillary blood volume with negative pressure breathing. *J. Clin. Invest.*, **44**, 1623–30.

Stitzer, S. O. & Malvin, R. L. (1975). Right atrium and renal sodium excretion. *Am. J. Physiol.*, **228**, 184–90.

Stoker, J. B., Kappagoda, C. T., Grimshaw, V. A. & Linden, R. J. (1972). A new method for assessing states of acute acidaemia in man. *Clin. Sci.*, **42**, 455–63.

Stricker, E. M., Vagnucci, A. H. McDonald, R. H. & Leenen, F. H. (1979). Renin and aldosterone secretions during hypovolemia in rats: relation to NaCl intake. *Am. J. Physiol.*, **237**, R45–R51.

Stroh-Werz, M., Langhorst, P. & Camerer, H. (1977a). Neuronal activity with cardiac rhythm in the nucleus of the solitary tract in cats and dogs. I. Different discharge patterns related to the cardiac cycle. *Brain Res.*, **133**, 65–80.

Stroh-Werz, M., Langhorst, P. & Camerer, H. (1977b). Neuronal activity with cardiac rhythm in the nucleus of the solitary tract in cats and dogs. II. Activity modulation in relation to the respiratory cycle. *Brain Res.*, **133**, 81–93.

Surtshin, A., Hoeltzenbein, J. & White, H. L. (1955). Some effects of negative pressure breathing on urine excretion. *Am. J. Physiol.*, **180**, 612–16.

References

Swan, A. A. & Whitteridge, D. (1956). Baroreceptor fibres from the pulmonary artery. *Abstr. XX Int. Physiol. Congr.* 867–8.

Takeshita, A., Mark, A. L., Eckberg, D. L. & Abboud, F. M. (1979). Effect of central venous pressure on arterial baroreceptor control of heart rate. *Am. J. Physiol.*, **236**, H42–H47.

Takino, M. (1951). Reflex cardiac acceleration by the stimulating of the receptor area of the pulmonary veins and their vicinity in the left atrium. *Nippon J. Angio-Cardiol.*, **15**, 1–4.

Tanigawa, H., Dua, S. L. & Assaykeen, T. A. (1974). Effect of renal and adrenal denervation on the renin response to slow haemorrhage in dogs. *Clin. Exp. Pharmacol. Physiol.*, **1**, 325–32.

Thames, M. D. (1977). Reflex suppression of renin release by ventricular receptors with vagal afferents. *Am. J. Physiol.*, **233**, H181–H184.

Thames, M. D. (1979). Behaviour of left atrial receptors with non-medullated vagal afferents in spontaneously breathing cats. In *Cardiac Receptors*, ed. Hainsworth, R., Kidd, C. & Linden, R. J., p. 161. Cambridge: Cambridge University Press.

Thames, M. D., Donald, D. E. & Shepherd, J. T. (1977). Behavior of cardiac receptors with non-myelinated vagal afferents during spontaneous respiration in cats. *Circ. Res.*, **41**, 694–701.

Thames, M. D. & Schmid, P. G. (1979). Cardiopulmonary receptors with vagal afferents tonically inhibit ADH release in the dogs. *Am. J. Physiol.*, **237**, H299–H304.

Thames, M. D., Zubair-Ul-Hassan, Brackett, N. C., Lower, R. R. & Krontos, H. A. (1971). Plasma renin responses to hemorrhage after cardiac autotransplantation. *Am. J. Physiol.*, **221**, 1115–19.

Thomas, S. (1967). Reflex increase in urine flow by veratridine. *Q. J. Exp. Physiol.*, **52**, 313–18.

Thorén, P. (1972). Left ventricular receptors activated by severe asphyxia and by coronary artery occlusion. *Acta Physiol. Scand.*, **85**, 455–63.

Thorén, P. (1973). Reflex bradycardia elicited from left ventricular receptors during acute severe hypoxia in cats. *Acta Physiol. Scand.*, **87**, 103–12.

Thorén, P. N. (1976a). Atrial receptors with nonmedullated vagal afferents in the cat. Discharge frequency and pattern in relation to atrial pressure. *Circ. Res.*, **38**, 357–62.

Thorén, P. (1976b). Activation of left ventricular receptors with non-medullated vagal afferent fibres during occlusion of a coronary artery in the cat. *Am. J. Cardiol.*, **37**, 1046–51.

Thorén, P. (1979a). Role of cardiac vagal C-fibers in cardiovascular control. *Rev. Physiol. Biochem. Pharmacol.*, **86**, 1–94.

Thorén, P. (1979b). Reflex effects of left ventricular receptors and their significance in man. In *Cardiac Receptors*, ed. Hainsworth, R., Kidd, C. & Linden, R. J., pp. 259–77. Cambridge: Cambridge University Press.

Thorén, P., Donald, D. E. & Shepherd, J. T. (1976). Role of heart and lung receptors with nonmedullated vagal afferents in circulatory control. *Circ. Res.*, **38**, Suppl. II, 2–9.

References

Thorén, P. N., Mancia, G. & Shepherd, J. T. (1975). Vasomotor inhibition in rabbits by vagal nonmedullated fibers from cardiopulmonary area. *Am. J. Physiol.*, **229**, 1410–13.

Thorén, P., Noresson, E. & Ricksten, S.-E. (1979). Cardiac receptors with non-medullated vagal afferents in the rat. *Acta Physiol. Scand.*, **105**, 295–303.

Thorén, P., Ricksten, S.-E. & Noresson, E. (1978). Characteristics of cardiac vagal afferents in normotensive and hypertensive rat. *Acta Physiol. Scand.*, **102**, 53A–54A.

Thorén, P., Shepherd, J. T. & Donald, D. E. (1977). Anodal block of medullated cardiopulmonary vagal afferents in cats. *J. Appl. Physiol.*, **42**, 461–5.

Tiitso, M. von (1939). Uber die Bedingungen des Zustandekommens des chronotropen Effektes der Dehnung des rechten Vorhofes Beim Hunde. *Pflügers Arch.*, **242**, 685–90.

Torii, H. (1962). Electron microscope observations of the S-A and A-V nodes and Purkinje fibers of the rabbit. *Jpn Circ. J.*, **26**, 39–50.

Torrente, A. de, Robertson, G. L., McDonald, K. M. & Schrier, R. W. (1975). Mechanism of diuretic response to increased left atrial pressure in the anaesthetized dog. *Kidney Int.*, **8**, 355–61.

Tranum-Jensen, J. (1975). The ultrastructure of the sensory end-organs (baroreceptors) in the atrial wall of young mini-pigs. *J. Anat.*, **119**, 255–75.

Tranum-Jensen, J. (1979). Ultrastructural studies on atrial nerve-end formations in mini-pigs. In *Cardiac Receptors*, ed. Hainsworth, R., Kidd, C. & Linden, R. J., pp. 27–50. Cambridge: Cambridge University Press.

Tsakiris, A. G., Padiyar, R., Gordon, D. A. & Lipton, I. (1977). Left atrial size and geometry in the intact dog. *Am. J. Physiol.*, **232**, H167–H172.

Uchida, Y. (1975). Afferent sympathetic nerve fibers with mechanoreceptors in the right heart. *Am. J. Physiol.*, **228**, 223–30.

Uchida, Y. (1979). Mechanisms of excitation of cardiac 'sympathetic' afferents. In *Cardiac Receptors*, ed. Hainsworth, R., Kidd, C. & Linden, R. J., pp. 301–17. Cambridge: Cambridge University Press.

Uchida, Y. & Murao, S. (1974a). Potassium-induced excitation of afferent cardiac sympathetic nerve fibers. *Am. J. Physiol.*, **226**, 603–7.

Uchida, Y. & Murao, S. (1974b). Excitation of afferent cardiac sympathetic nerve fibers during coronary occlusion. *Am. J. Physiol.*, **226**, 1094–9.

Uchida, Y. & Murao, S. (1974c). Afferent sympathetic nerve fibers originating in the left atrial wall. *Am. J. Physiol.*, **227**, 753–8.

Uchida, Y. & Murao, S. (1975). Acid-induced excitation of afferent cardiac sympathetic nerve fibers. *Am. J. Physiol.*, **228**, 27–33.

Uther, J. B., Hunyor, S. N., Shaw, J. & Korner, P. I. (1970). Bulbar and suprabulbar control of the cardiovascular autonomic effects during arterial hypoxia in the rabbit. *Circ. Res.*, **26**, 491–506.

Van Citters, R. L., Franklin, D. L. & Rushmer, R. F. (1964). Left ventricular dynamics in dogs during anesthesia with alpha-chloralose and sodium pentobarbital. *Am. J. Cardiol.*, **13**, 349–54.

References

Vatner, S. F., Beottcher, D. H., Heyndrickx, G. R. & McRitchie, R. J. (1975). Reduced baroreflex sensitivity with volume loading in conscious dogs. *Circ. Res.*, **37**, 236–42.

Vick, R. L. (1963). Effects of increased transmural pressures upon atrial and ventricular rhythms in the dog heart–lung preparation. *Circ. Res.*, **13**, 39–47.

Volostchenko, A. A. (1964). On afferent innervation of atrioventricular valves. *Arkh. Anat.*, **47**, 81–6.

Wahab, N. S., Zucker, I. H. & Gilmore, J. P. (1975). Lack of a direct effect of efferent cardiac vagal nerve activity on atrial receptor activity. *Am. J. Physiol.*, **229**, 314–17.

Walsh, E. G. & Whitteridge, D. (1944). Vagal activity and the tachypnoea produced by multiple pulmonary emboli. *J. Physiol.*, **103**, 37P–38P.

Ward, D. G., Baertschi, A. J. & Gann, D. S. (1977). Neurons in medullary areas controlling ACTH: atrial input and rostral projections. *Am. J. Physiol.*, **233**, R116–R126.

Wardener, H. E. de (1973). The control of sodium excretion. In *Handbook of Physiology, Section 8, Renal Physiology*, ed. Orloff, J. & Berliner, R. W., pp. 677–720. Washington, D.C.: American Physiological Society.

Warner, H. B. & Cox, A. (1962). A mathematical model of heart rate control by sympathetic and vagus efferent information. *J. Appl. Physiol.*, **17**, 349–55.

Warren, D. J. & Ledingham, J. G. G. (1975). Renal circulatory responses to general anaesthesia in the rabbit: studies using radioactive microspheres. *Clin. Sci. Mol. Med.*, **48**, 61–6.

Warren, D. J. & Ledingham, J. G. G. (1978). Renal vascular response to haemorrhage in the rabbit after pentobarbitone, chloralose–urethane and ether anaesthesia. *Clin. Sci. Mol. Med.*, **54**, 489–94.

Watkins, L., Burton, J. A., Haber, E., Cant, J. R., Smith, F. W. & Barger, C. (1976). The renin–angiotensin–adolesterone system in congestive failure in conscious dogs. *J. Clin. Invest.*, **57**, 1606–17.

Watson, J. F. & Rapp, R. M. (1962). Effect of forward acceleration on renal function. *J. Appl. Physiol.*, **17**, 413–16.

Weaver, L. C. (1977). Cardiopulmonary sympathetic afferent influences on renal activity. *Am. J. Physiol.*, **233**, H592–H599.

Weaver, L. C., Macklem, L. J., Reimann, K. A., Meckler, R. L. & Oehl, R. S. (1979). Organization of thoracic sympathetic afferent influences on renal nerve activity. *Am. J. Physiol.*, **237**, H44–H50.

Webb-Peploe, M. W. (1969). The isovolumetric spleen: index of reflex changes in splanchnic vascular capacity. *Am. J. Physiol.*, **216**, 407–13.

Webb-Peploe, M. W. & Shepherd, J. T. (1968). Response of large hindlimb veins of the dog to sympathetic nerve stimulation. *Am. J. Physiol.*, **215**, 299–307.

Wenckebach, K. F. & Winterberg, H. (1927). *Die Unregelmassige Hertztatigkeit*, p. 252. Leipzig: Verlag von Wilhelm Engelmann.

Wennergren, G., Little, R. & Oberg, B. (1976). Studies on the central integration of excitatory chemoreceptor influences and inhibitory

References

baroreceptor and cardiac receptor influences. *Acta Physiol. Scand.*, **96**, P1–P18.

Westenfelder, C., Arruda, J. A. L., Lockwood, R., Boonjarern, S., Nascimento, L. & Kurtzman, N. A. (1976). Distribution of renal blood flow in dogs with congestive heart failure. *Am. J. Physiol.*, **230**, 537–42.

Whitaker, E. M. (1977). Blood borne agents involved in the diuretic response to stimulation of atrial receptors. Ph.D. Thesis, University of Leeds.

Whitteridge, D. (1948). Afferent nerve fibres from the heart and lungs in the cervical vagus. *J. Physiol.*, **107**, 496–512.

Wiberg, T., Vaage, J. & Scott, E. (1979). Release of prostaglandin-like substances during elevations of left atrial pressure in the cat. *Acta Physiol. Scand.*, **107**, 97–103.

Widdicombe, J. G. (1954). Respiratory reflexes elicited by inflation of the lungs. *J. Physiol.*, **123**, 105–15.

Widdicombe, J. G. (1973). Reflex control of breathing. In International Review of Science, Physiology Series 1, Vol. 2. *Respiratory Physiology*, ed. Widdicombe, J. G., pp. 273–301. Baltimore: University Park Press.

Wiggers, C. J. (1949). *Physiology in Health and Disease*, 5th edn. London: Kimpron.

Wilcox, C. S., Aminoff, M. J. & Slater, J. D. H. (1977). Sodium homeostasis in patients with autonomic failure. *Clin. Sci. Mol. Med.*, **53**, 321–28.

Williams, T. H. (1964). Mitral and tricuspid valve innervation. *Br. Heart J.*, **26**, 105–15.

Wood, P. (1963). Polyuria in paroxysmal tachycardia and paroxysmal atrial flutter and fibrillation. *Br. Heart J.*, **25**, 273–82.

Wood, E. H., Sutterer, W. F. & Marshall, H. W. (1961). Effect of headward and forward accelerations on the cardiovascular system. *Wright-Patterson Air Force Base, Wright Air Develop. Div. Tech. Rept.* 60–634.

Woollard, H. H. (1926). The innervation of the heart. *J. Anat.*, **60**, 345–73.

Yamauchi, A. (1979). Comparisons of the fine structure of receptor end-organs in the heart and aorta. In *Cardiac Receptors*, ed. Hainsworth, R., Kidd, C. & Linden, R. J., pp. 51–70. Cambridge: Cambridge University Press.

Yaron, M. & Bennett, C. M. (1978). Mechanism of impaired water excretion in acute right ventricular failure in conscious dogs. *Circ. Res.*, **42**, 801–5.

Yoon, M. S., Han, J., Tse, W. W. & Rogers, R. (1977). Effects of vagal stimulation, atropine and propranolol on fibrillation threshold of normal and ischemic ventricles. *Am. Heart J.*, **93**, 60–5.

Yun, J. C. G., Delea, C. S., Bartter, F. C. & Kelly, G. (1976). Increase in renin release after sinoaortic denervation and cervical vagotomy. *Am. J. Physiol.*, **230**, 777–83.

Zanchetti, A., Stella, A., Leonetti, G., Morganti, A. & Terzoli, L. (1976). Control of renin release: a review of experimental evidence and clinical implications. *Am. J. Cardiol.*, **37**, 675–91.

References

Zapata, P. (1975). Effects of dopamine on carotid chemo- and baroreceptors in vitro. *J. Physiol.*, **244**, 235–51.

Zehr, J. E., Hasbargen, J. A. & Kurz, K. D. (1976). Reflex suppression of renin secretion during distension of cardiopulmonary receptors in dogs. *Circ. Res.*, **38**, 232–9.

Zehr, J. E., Hawe, A., Tsakiris, A. G., Rastelli, G., McGoon, D. C. & Seger, W. E. (1971). ADH levels following nonhypotensive hemorrhage in dogs with chronic mitral stenosis. *Am. J. Physiol.*, **221**, 312–17. *J. Clin. Invest.*, **60**, 323–31.

Zehr, J. E., Johnson, J. A. & Moore, W. W. (1969). Left atrial pressure, plasma osmolality and ADH levels in the unanesthetized ewe. *Am. J. Physiol.*, **217**, 1672–80.

Zoller, R. P., Mark, A. L., Abboud, F. M., Schmid, P. G. & Heistad, D. D. (1972). The role of low pressure baroreceptors in reflex vasoconstrictor responses in man. *J. Clin. Invest.*, **51**, 2967–72.

Zucker, I. H., Earle, A. M. & Gilmore, J. P. (1977). The mechanism of adaptation of left atrial stretch receptors in dogs with chronic congestive heart failure. *J. Clin Invest.*, **60**, 323–31.

Zucker, I. H. & Gilmore, J. P. (1973). Left atrial receptor discharge during atrial arrhythmias in the dog. *Circ. Res.*, **33**, 672–7.

Zucker, I. H. & Gilmore, J. P. (1974a). Atrial receptor discharge during acute coronary occlusion in the dog. *Am. J. Physiol.*, **227**, 360–3.

Zucker, I. H. & Gilmore, J. P. (1974b). Evidence for an indirect sympathetic control of atrial stretch receptor discharge in the dog. *Circ. Res.*, **34**, 441–6.

Zucker, I. H. & Gilmore, J. P. (1975). Responsiveness of type B atrial receptors in the monkey. *Brain Res.*, **95**, 159–65.

Zucker, I. H. & Gilmore, J. P. (1976). The response of atrial stretch receptors to increases in heart rate in dogs. *Circ. Res.*, **38**, 15–19.

Zucker, I. H. & Gilmore, J. P. (1977). Cardiopulmonary vagal afferents in the monkey: A survey of receptor activity. *Basic Res. Cardiol.*, **72**, 392–401.

Zucker, I. H., Share, L. & Gilmore, J. P. (1979). Renal effects of left atrial distension in dogs with chronic congestive heart failure. *Am. J. Physiol.*, **236**, H554–H560.

INDEX

ACTH, 247–8
acceleration, 225–6
acid–base balance, 94–100
  nomogram, 98
acidosis, 95–100
ADH, 221–30, 260, 262, 274–87, 317–19
  bioassay, 285
  immunoassay, 282, 314–15
adaptation, 83–5
adrenaline
  in conversion of pattern of discharge, 42, 44
afferent pathways (nerve fibres) 2, 31, 102, 113, 116, 137, 268–73
  differential cooling, 144, 268
  'sympathetic', 2, 31, 65–73, 155, 180, 195, 322
    multiterminal, 66, 68, 71–2
    non-myelinated, 57–73
    rami communicantes, 66, 68, 195
    receptor fields, 71
    termination of, 203–5
  vagal, 31, 137, 247, 268
    myelinated, 2, 31–2, 83, 180–8, 204–5, 269–70; conduction velocity, 37; histological studies, 36; intermediate type discharge, 33, 40–57, 141; relation to atrial pressure pulse, 32; trains of impulses, 32, 83; type A discharge, 32, 40–57, 319–20; type B discharge, 32–4, 40–57, 139, 319–20
    non-myelinated (C-fibres), 2, 31, 57, 59, 63–5, 124, 127, 144–5, 151–5, 180, 187–95, 204–5, 230, 301
aldosterone, 244–6, 315–16
amphibia, 12

anaesthesia, 94–7
  oxygen, partial pressure of, 97–100
angiotensin, 240–5, 304, 315–16
anodal block (*see* blockade)
ansae subclaviae, 126, 129, 156, 158
area postrema, 204
arrhythmia, 317–20
atenolol, 158, 163
atrial appendage, 19, 121, 129–34, 268
  distension of balloon (*see also* balloons), 69, 79, 117–18, 129, 265–6
atrial distension (*see also* balloons), 48, 291, 322
atrial fibrillation (*see* fibrillation)
atrial muscle, isolated, 37, 38
atrial pressure (*see also* blood pressure), 45, 52, 105, 115, 117, 220, 222–3, 233, 251–2, 260
  and pattern of discharge, 44
  changes in, 52, 59, 113, 135
  monitoring, 80
  threshold pressure, 51
  volume, 47
atrial tachycardia (*see* tachycardia)
atrial tamponade, 260, 276
atrium (*see also* balloons)
  distortion of, 51–53
  left, 120–3, 243
    atrial pouch, 79–80, 87, 129, 131, 134–5
  right, 67, 113, 117–19, 135, 143, 262
  size, 52, 56
atropine, 94, 108, 113, 202, 214

Bainbridge reflex, 75, 101–6, 161
balloons, 148–56, 162, 167–71, 181, 186, 188–92, 235, 249, 251–5, 263–8
  distension in appendage, 69, 79, 117–18, 128, 265–6

Index

balloons (*cont.*)
  large, 170, 219, 235, 251–2
  pulmonary vein–atrial junction, 69, 129
  superior vena caval–right atrial junction, 77, 117, 135
baroreceptors, arterial, 122–3, 178–9, 205–18, 236, 246–7
  aortic, 178
  carotid sinus, 181, 211–12, 215–16, 231, 239, 275, 288, 291, 292
B-receptor antagonists, 3, 163–7
Bezold–Jarisch reflex, 126–7, 174–5, 191
bioassay (*see* ADH)
blockade, nerves, 156–8, 176
  anodal, 92, 126
  cold, 92, 134, 241, 295
  of tonic activity, 126
  pharmacological, 93, 108–9, 111
blood borne agent, 285–7, 308
blood gases, 97–100
blood pressure (*see also* hypotension), 96, 188, 192, 228–9, 260, 302–5, 318–21
blood volume, 220–3, 225, 227, 231, 244, 246, 291, 295, 299, 307–9
bradycardia, 106, 109–127, 135–6, 175, 178–80, 198, 321
  initial heart rate (*see* heart rate)
bretylium tosylate, 143, 156–8, 163–7, 214, 295
butanol, 286

calf, 12
capacitance vessels
  tone, 186
capsaicin, 59
cardiac nerves (*see* efferent pathways)
  inferior, 196–9
cardiac output, 121, 162, 223, 251, 260–2
cardiac receptors (*see also* receptors), 174–6
'cardiopulmonary' receptors (*see also* receptors), 176–7, 217–18, 236, 283, 291
carotid body, chemoreceptors (*see* receptors)
carotid sinus baroreceptors (*see* baroreceptors)
cat, 12, 20, 39, 42, 56–7, 59, 63–4, 71, 174, 188, 196

central nervous connections, 3, 203–18
  input, 89
  physiological range, 89
  second order neurone, 34–5, 87
    effective signal from atrial receptors, 35
centrifugation, 225–7
C-fibres (*see* afferent pathway)
chemoreceptors (*see* receptors)
choralose (*see also* anaesthesia), 96–7, 136
cholinesterase, 24
CO_2
  partial pressure of, 97–100
  titration curve, 99
compliance, atrial wall, 47
conduction velocity of nerve fibres, 2, 37, 57, 59, 66, 124, 145
contractility, 171, 196, 199
convergence, 213–6
cooling vagi, 59, 126, 129, 134–6, 138, 144–56, 189, 208–9, 238–9, 261, 263, 266, 268–73, 286, 296
coronary arteries, 175, 196
coronary receptors, 58
corticosteroids, 246

decerebration, 121, 162, 207, 211
degeneration studies, 17, 20–3
denervation
  heart, 110
  kidney, 274, 284, 287–8, 298–302, 304
  sino-aortic, 242, 284, 299
deoxycortisone acetate, 259
dextran, 291
diabetes insipidus, 281
dialysis, 231, 234
diffuse stimulation (*see also* receptors), 101–17, 219–49
discrete stimulation (*see also* receptors), 117, 263
diuresis (*see also* urine flow), 128, 219–20, 224–5, 230, 263, 274, 317–20
dog, 12, 39, 42–3, 52, 56–8, 63, 71, 174, 181–3, 191, 259, 319
  decerebrate, 121, 207, 211
  denervated heart, 110
  denervated kidney, 242, 302, 304
  peripheral veins, 182
  spleen preparation, 182
  unanaesthetised, 136
  venous tone, 183

359

Index

efferent pathways, 102, 113, 156–72, 274–97
  sympathetic nerve fibres, 6, 30
electron microscopy, 23–9
electrophysiology, 31–73, 139–41, 158–61
end-net, 10, 13, 21–3
end-organ (*see* receptors and unencapsulated endings)
endocardium
  atrial, 13, 17, 24, 50
  ventricular, 21
extracellular recording, 204–5

fibrillation, 317, 320
fluid retention, 316
fluid volume, 230, 241
free water clearance, 224, 227–30, 232, 255–7

germitridine, 45
glomerular filtration rate, 223, 226, 228–9, 232, 262, 287–8, 319
gravitational force, 219, 225–7
guinea-pig, 20

haemorrhage, 46, 59, 73, 109–10, 175, 233, 244, 246, 290–1, 321
  in converting pattern of discharge, 42, 44
heart block, 320
heart failure, 282–3, 290, 312–7
heart rate (*see also* bradycardia and tachycardia), 96, 111, 117, 303–5
  control, 34, 49
  increase, in 34, 47, 97, 111, 117–36, 164–77, 186, 192, 216, 263, 273, 295, 304
  initial, 106–7, 121, 167, 170
heart rhythm, 57–9, 320
heart volumes, 47, 65, 228, 308
histochemical methods, 24
histology, 6–30, 268, 314
homeostasis
  sodium, 290
horse, 12
humoral agents (*see also* ADH), 274
hydrocortisone, 245
hypophysectomy, 246, 276–7, 281
hypotension (*see also* haemorrhage), 113, 116–17, 170, 174–5, 177, 192, 198, 321

hypothalamus, 122, 245, 248, 284
hypovolaemia (*see also* haemorrhage), 244, 246
hysteresis, 47

immersion, 75, 219, 227–30, 315
indomethacin, 249
infarction, 175, 322
infusion, 46, 59, 75, 102–9, 231–4, 300
  vagal pathways, 105, 299
  sectioning of vagus, 105
inotropic response, 121, 128, 171, 179, 308
interaction, central nervous, 214–7
inter-atrial septum (*see* location of receptors)
ischaemia, 66, 196, 322

kidney (*see also* diuresis), 128, 182, 188–9, 219–33
  isolated, 274
  nerves, 196, 217–18, 287, 301–2
  vascular resistance in, 236

latency responses, CNS, 204
light microscopy, 7, 25
location of receptors
  endocardium, 9, 13, 17
    atrial appendage, 19
    inferior vena cava, 13, 24
    inter-atrial septum, 24
    position, 24
    pulmonary veins, 10
    superior vena cava, 9, 13, 24
    pulmonary vein/left atrial junction, 13, 24, 50, 53–4, 61, 76, 80
    vena cavae/right atrium, 13, 24
  epicardium, 10
  myocardium, 12
  punctate location, 39
lung, 71, 125, 173–4
  congestion, 179
  inflation, 179
  irritants, 179
  J-receptors, 179
  oedema, 179
  receptors in, 179–80

Malpighian tubule, 285–6
man, 17, 21, 217
mechanoreceptors (*see* receptors)

Index

medulla (*see also* nucleus and tractus solitarius), 203–12
methylene blue, 7, 10
microscopy
 electron, 23–9
 light, 7, 25
 histochemical technique, 24
  fluorescent, 30
  phase contrast, 25, 30
monkey, 41, 52, 56
multifocal origin, 200
myelinated nerves (*see* afferent pathways and receptors), 2
 in the vagi, 6
myocardial infarction, 175, 322

neck suction, 217
negative pressure, 183–5
 breathing, 220–4, 244
Nembutal (*see* pentobarbitone)
nerve ending
 end-net, 10, 13, 21–3, 29–30
  efferent adrenergic fibres, 23
 free fibre, 10
 species: amphibia, 12; calf, 12; cat, 12, 20; dog, 12; man, 17, 21; pig, 12; rabbit, 20; rat, 12; sheep, 12
 unencapsulated, 4, 10, 13, 15, 20, 29–30, 31, 74
  collagenous fibrils, 24, 27
  complex, 13–7
  discharging into myelinated fibres (Paintal type), 31, 73, 137, 141, 150, 214, 269, 273, 295–6
  distribution ratio, 17, 19
  glycogen granules, 28
  mitochondria, 27–8
  nerve fibre size, numbers, 17
  Schwann cell, 25
  smooth muscle cells, 24
  thin fibres, fluorescent, 25
nerve fibres (*see also* afferent and efferent pathways, and receptors)
 connection between unencapsulated endings and end-net, 23
 sensory 7, 20
neurone
 medullary, 122, 209
 second order, 87
non-myelinated nerves (*see* afferent and efferent pathways, and receptors)

non-respiratory pH, 98
nucleus (*see also* medulla and tractus solitarius)
 ambiguus, 204
 dorsal motor, 203–4
 intercalatus, 203
 of hypoglossal nerve, 208
 of tractus solitarius, 203–12
 supraoptic, 284

oxygen
 partial pressure of, 97–100

Paintal-type receptors (*see* nerve ending)
para-aminohippuric acid, 262
parahypoglossal area (*see also* nucleus), 204, 208
pentobarbitone, 136, 282
perfusion, 112–17, 177, 181
 pressure, 303–4
pericardium, 68, 71
 pouch, 284
pericoronary nerves, 196–9
peripheral resistance, 181–2, 189, 192, 315
 skeletal muscle, 188–9
 skin, 189
pH of blood, 97–100
pharmacological denervation (*see* denervation)
phenoxybenzamine, 196, 198
phenyldiguanide, 59, 179
phenylephrine, 217
pig, 12
 mini, 24
pituitrin, 45
plasma
 concentration of ADH, 226, 276, 280, 282
 concentration of renin, 244–5
 hypotonicity, 233
 osmolarity, 45, 232–3
 renal flow, 226, 262
 volume, 279–80, 298
plastic beads
 injection of, 251
pleura, 68, 71
positive pressure breathing, 220, 224
posture, 183
potassium excretion, 257, 262
propranolol, 156–8, 164, 288
prostaglandin, 219, 249

361

Index

pulmonary artery, 21, 71
　receptors, 177
pulmonary circulation, 200–2
　termination of afferent fibres from 203–5
pulmonary veins, 71, 120, 129
pulmonary vein–atrial junction (*see also* location of receptors), 50, 53–4, 61, 76, 80, 82, 121–2, 128, 180, 189, 192, 201, 235–7, 240, 263–6, 285, 295, 300

rabbit, 20, 39, 42–3, 56, 189, 299
rat, 64
　spontaneously hypertensive, 292
receptors (*see also* unencapsulated endings), 1
　anatomical position of, 54
　chemoreceptor, 45, 108, 178–9, 215–16
　control theory, 2
　malfunction of atrial, 314
　generator membrane, 27
　mechanoreceptors, 27, 29, 58, 63, 125
　multi-terminal, 66
　pattern of discharge, 38, 40, 41, 68
　　atrial, 38, 42, 200–2: attached to myelinated nerves (Paintal type), 74; attached to non-myelinated nerves, 74, 283; intermediate (*see* afferent pathways); 'sympathetic', 74; type A (*see* afferent pathways); type B (*see* afferent pathways)
　　change of pattern, 40, 41, 42, 43, 203–5
　　incidence of type, 39, 40
　　outside atrial endocardium 39–40, 42, 57, 244; type A, 39; type B, 39
　　stimulus, 1, 2, 102
　　chemical, 44–5, 63
　　cul-de-sac preparation, 115
　　distension of small balloons, 34, 61, duration of, 83
　　gradation of, 82, 141–3
　　mechanical, 44–57, 63–5, 68, 73, 123
　　natural, 33, 44–57, 63–5, 73, wall tension, 53, 64–5
　　obstruction to blood flow, 118–19, 235–6, 240, 260–3, 315

　　physiological, 81–2
　　specificity, 90
　　ventricular, 57–8, 62–5, 67–8, 175
　　　pattern of discharge, 68
reflex arc, 1, 3, 74–100
　afferent pathway, 2, 92
　efferent pathway, 3, 93–4
　pharmacological blockade, 3
reflex response, 75, 93, 97, 101, 169, 180, 209–11, 268–73, 296, 308
renal blood flow, 228, 235–41, 262, 288
　vascular resistance, 236, 240
renal denervation (*see also* denervation), 241–3, 287–8
renal nerves (*see also* kidney), 161, 196, 274, 287–307
renin, 219, 240–5, 249, 288–9, 304, 315–16
renin–angiotensin system (*see* renin and angiotensin)
respiration (*see also* negative pressure and positive pressure breathing), 200, 220–3
Rhodnius prolixus, 285–6
Ringer lactate infusion, 315

sheep, 12, 25, 232
shock, 320–1
silver impregnation, 7, 9, 12
sinu-atrial node, 110–11, 115, 123, 128
sodium bicarbonate
　infusion of, 99
sodium excretion, 219–20, 224, 227–30, 246, 257–60, 262, 267, 307–9, 317–19
sodium thioglycolate, 287
solute excretion (*see also* sodium and potassium excretion), 255–60
spinal section, 162
splanchnic nerves, 287, 292
spontaneous discharge (*see* receptor, pattern of discharge)
stellate ganglion, 22, 197
　removal, 22
steroids, 219, 245–9
stimulation, (*see* receptors, diffuse stimultion and discrete stimulation)
subclavian artery, 71
summation, interaction 214
sympathetic nerve (*see* unencapsulated endings, afferent and efferent pathways, and receptors)

Index

sympathetic nerve (*cont.*)
   afferent fibres, 2
   efferent to the nerve ending, 6, 25, 30
synapse, 204–5

tachycardia (*see also* heart rate), 109–126, 164–71, 177–80, 186, 188, 216, 317–20
   paroxysmal supraventricular, 317, 320
tachypnoea, 125, 201
temperature (*see also* blockade and cooling vagi), 94, 144–56, 177
thirst, 309
thorax
   sympathetic trunk, 196–7
   intrathoracic blood volume, 225–7
   intrathoracic circulation, 220
   intrathoracic pressures, 222
   intrathoracic receptors, 302
trachea, 71
tractus solitarius (*see also* nucleus), 122, 203–12
transplants
   in dog, 110
tubules
   Malpighian, 285–6
   reabsorption by, 290–1

unencapsulated endings (*see also* receptors), 4, 10, 13, 15, 20, 74, 244, 294
   complex, 13–17, 186–7
   distribution ratio, 17, 19
   efferent adrenergic fibres, 23

mitochondria, 27, 28
nerve fibres from, 17
photographic evidence, 15
Schwann cell, 25
urine flow, 219, 225–7, 231–4, 251–309, 314, 317–19

vagotomy (see vagal nerves, section of)
vagal nerves (*see also* afferent pathways), 203, 205, 211–12, 268
   cooling of (*see* blockade and cooling)
   myelinated afferent, 2, 141
   non-myelinated afferent fibres, 2
   section of, 21, 23, 105–8, 111, 113, 115–18, 123, 129, 138–9, 176, 231, 236–7, 242–5, 273, 282, 284, 291, 297, 299, 301
   tone, 108, 235–6, 239, 242
vasoconstriction, 173–4, 180, 183, 188, 287–8, 319
vasomotor centre, 188, 191, 207
vasopressin (*see also* ADH), 226, 230, 257, 277, 279, 281, 315
vena cavae/right atrial junction (*see also* location of receptors), 13, 19, 79, 87, 129, 268
venous inflow, 101
venous pressure, 102, 104, 105
veratridine, 45, 58–9, 127, 174–5, 234–5, 299
volume receptors, 307–9

water excretion (*see also* ADH and vasopressin), 246, 305–9, 314
wire cage (expanding), 119, 143

363

RAYMOND H. FOGLER LIBRARY
DATE DUE

BOOKS ARE SUBJECT TO
RECALL AFTER TWO